FIRST AID FOR THE®

Surgery Clerkship

Second Edition

SERIES EDITORS:

MATTHEW S. KAUFMAN, MD
Attending Physician and Co-investigator
Chronic Lymphocytic Leukemia Research and Treatment Program
Department of Hematology-Oncology
North Shore–Long Island Jewish Health System
Manhasset and New Hyde Park, New York

S. MATTHEW STEAD, MD, PhD
Epilepsy Research Fellow
Department of Neurology
Mayo Clinic and Mayo School of Graduate Medical
   Education
Rochester, Minnesota

LATHA G. STEAD, MD, FACEP
Professor and Chair, Department of Emergency Medicine
University of Rochester
Rochester, New York

VOLUME EDITOR:

NITIN MISHRA, MBBS, MS, MRCS (UK)
Resident in General Surgery
North Shore–Long Island Jewish Health System
Manhasset and New Hyde Park, New York

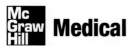 **Medical**

New York / Chicago / San Francisco / Lisbon / London / Madrid / Mexico City
Milan / New Delhi / San Juan / Seoul / Singapore / Sydney / Toronto

First Aid for the® Surgery Clerkship, Second Edition

Copyright © 2009 by The McGraw-Hill Companies, Inc. All rights reserved. Printed in the United States of America. Except as permitted under the United States Copyright Act of 1976, no part of this publication may be reproduced or distributed in any form or by any means, or stored in a data base or retrieval system, without the prior written permission of the publisher.

Previous edition copyright © 2003 by The McGraw-Hill Companies, Inc.

First Aid for the® is a registered trademark of The McGraw-Hill Companies, Inc.

3 4 5 6 7 8 9 0   QDB/QDB   14 13 12

ISBN   978-0-07-144871-0
MHID 0-07-144871-3

Notice

Medicine is an ever-changing science. As new research and clinical experience broaden our knowledge, changes in treatment and drug therapy are required. The authors and the publisher of this work have checked with sources believed to be reliable in their efforts to provide information that is complete and generally in accord with the standards accepted at the time of publication. However, in view of the possibility of human error or changes in medical sciences, neither the authors nor the publisher nor any other party who has been involved in the preparation or publication of this work warrants that the information contained herein is in every respect accurate or complete, and they disclaim all responsibility for any errors or omissions or for the results obtained from use of the information contained in this work. Readers are encouraged to confirm the information contained herein with other sources. For example and in particular, readers are advised to check the product information sheet included in the package of each drug they plan to administer to be certain that the information contained in this work is accurate and that changes have not been made in the recommended dose or in the contraindications for administration. This recommendation is of particular importance in connection with new or infrequently used drugs.

This book was set in Electra LH by Rainbow Graphics.
The editors were Catherine A. Johnson and Robert Pancotti.
The production supervisor was Catherine Saggese.
The illustration manager was Armen Ovsepyan.
Project management was provided by Rainbow Graphics.
The index was prepared by Rainbow Graphics.
Quad/Graphics Dubuque was printer and binder.

This book is printed on acid-free paper.

Library of Congress Cataloging-in-Publication Data
Kaufman, Matthew S.
   First aid for the surgery clerkship / Matthew S. Kaufman, Latha G.
Stead, S. Matthew Stead. – 2nd ed.
      p. ; cm.
   Includes index.
   ISBN-13: 978-0-07-144871-0 (pbk. : alk. paper)
   ISBN-10: 0-07-144871-3 (pbk. : alk. paper)
 1. Surgery–Outlines, syllabi, etc. 2. Clinical clerkship–Outlines,
syllabi, etc. I. Stead, Latha G. II. Stead, S. Matthew. III. Title.
   [DNLM: 1. Clinical Clerkship–Examination Questions. 2. Surgical
Procedures, Operative–Examination Questions. WO 18.2 K21f 2009]
   RD37.3.K38 2009
   617.0076–dc22
                                              2008054761

My work in the book is dedicated to my grandmother, Frances Jacobson.

—Matthew S. Kaufman, MD

My work in this book is dedicated to my parents, Mr. Rajeshwar Mishra and Mrs. Indu Mishra.

—Nitin Mishra, MBBS, MS, MRCS (UK)

CONTENTS

CONTRIBUTORS

MUHAMMAD AFTAB, MB, BS, MD

Resident in General Surgery
North Shore–Long Island Jewish Health System
Manhasset and New Hyde Park, New York
Cardiothoracic Surgery

MALATHY APPASAMY, MD

Resident in General Surgery
North Shore–Long Island Jewish Health System
Manhasset and New Hyde Park, New York
Orthopedics

MICHAEL P. AST, MD

Resident in Orthopedic Surgery
North Shore–Long Island Jewish Health System
Manhasset and New Hyde Park, New York
The Hand

LUKAS R. AUSTIN-PAGE

Medical Student
Class of 2010
Albert Einstein College of Medicine
Bronx, New York
The Pancreas

NETANEL BERKO, MD

Intern
Department of Medicine
New York Medical College
Sound Shore Medical Center of Westchester
New Rochelle, New York
The Surgical Patient

RONEN ELEFANT, MS, MD

Resident in General Surgery
Montefiore Medical Center
Albert Einstein College of Medicine Program
Bronx, New York
Fluids, Electrolytes, and Nutrition

TOVA C. FISCHER

Medical Student
Class of 2009
Albert Einstein College of Medicine
Bronx, New York
The Esophagus; Ear, Nose, and Throat Surgery

REBECCA PARVER GAMSS

Medical Student
Class of 2009
Albert Einstein College of Medicine
Bronx, New York
The Spleen

ARIELLE GLUECK, MD

Resident in Pediatrics
Children's Hospital at Montefiore
Albert Einstein College of Medicine
Bronx, New York
Acute Abdomen

EDWIN GULKO

Medical Student
Class of 2009
Albert Einstein College of Medicine
Bronx, New York
Neurosurgery

ANUNAYA R. JAIN, MBBS, MCEM (UK)

Research Fellow
Instructor of Emergency Medicine
Department of Emergency Medicine
Mayo Clinic College of Medicine
Rochester, Minnesota
Section IV: Classified

VIJAY KAMATH, MBBS

Resident in General Surgery
North Shore–Long Island Jewish Health System
Manhasset and New Hyde Park, New York
The Breast

JONATHAN D. KAYE, MD

Fellow in Pediatric Urologic Surgery
Emory University School of Medicine
Children's Healthcare of Atlanta
Atlanta, Georgia
The Genitourinary System

ASHLEY KEILER-GREEN, MD

Resident in Emergency Medicine
University of New Mexico
Albuquerque, New Mexico
The Hepatobiliary System

SILVIA KURTOVIC, MD

Resident in General Surgery
Cedars-Sinai Medical Center
Los Angeles, California
Critical Care

CHARLES F. LANZILLO III, MD

Resident in Ophthalmology
University of Colorado
Denver, Colorado
Wounds

JONATHAN MAZUREK, MD

Resident in Internal Medicine
Beth Israel Medical Center
New York, New York
Small Bowel

NITIN MISHRA, MBBS, MS, MRCS (UK)

Resident in General Surgery
North Shore–Long Island Jewish Health System
Manhasset and New Hyde Park, New York
Trauma; Transplant

SNEHA MISHRA, MBBS

Resident in Internal Medicine
Wyckoff Heights Medical Center
Brooklyn, New York
Burns; Anesthesia

SAMUEL T. OSTROWER, MD

Fellow in Pediatric Otolaryngology
Children's Hospital Boston
Boston, Massachusetts
Ear, Nose, and Throat Surgery

TAMAR RUBINSTEIN

Medical Student
Class of 2009
Albert Einstein College of Medicine
Bronx, New York
Pediatric Surgery

DAVUT SAVASER, MD

Resident in Emergency Medicine
University of California–San Diego
San Diego, California
Hernia and Abdominal Wall Problems

CASEY SEIDEMAN

Medical Student
Class of 2009
Albert Einstein College of Medicine
Bronx, New York
The Genitourinary System; Colon, Rectum, and Anal Canal

ANAND SHAH, MD, MPH

Resident in Radiology
Hospital of the University of Pennsylvania
Philadelphia, Pennsylvania
Vascular Surgery

EDAN SHAPIRO

Medical Student
Class of 2009
Albert Einstein College of Medicine
Bronx, New York
The Endocrine System

GRACE L. YU, MD

Resident in Plastic and Reconstructive Surgery
University of Southern California
Los Angeles, California
The Stomach

LISA ZUCKERWISE

Medical Student
Class of 2009
Albert Einstein College of Medicine
Bronx, New York
The Appendix

INTRODUCTION

This book is designed in the tradition of the *First Aid* series of books. It is formatted in the same way as the other books in the series. You will find that, apart from preparing you for success on the clerkship exam, this resource will also help guide you in the clinical diagnosis and treatment of common surgical conditions.

The content of the book is based on the objectives for medical students as determined by the Association for Surgical Education (ASE). Each chapter contains the major topics central to the practice of general surgery and has been specifically designed for the medical student. The book is divided into general surgery, which contains topics that comprise the core of the surgery rotation, and subspecialty surgery, which may be of interest but is generally considered less high yield for the clerkship. Knowledge of a subspecialty topic may be useful if observing a related surgery or if requesting a letter from a surgeon in that field.

The content of the text is organized in the format similar to other texts in the *First Aid* series. Topics are listed with bold headings, and the "body" of the topic provides essential information. The outside margins contain mnemonics, diagrams, summary or warning statements, and tips. Tips are categorized into Exam Tip ⬛ , Ward Tip ✎ , and OR tip ✎ .

HOW TO CONTRIBUTE

To continue to produce a high-yield review source for the surgery clerkship, you are invited to submit any suggestions or correction. Please send us your suggestions for:

- New facts, mnemonics, diagrams, and illustrations
- Low-yield facts to remove

For each entry incorporated into the next edition, you will receive personal acknowledgment. Diagrams, tables, partial entries, updates, corrections, and study hints are also appreciated, and significant contributions will be compensated at the discretion of the authors. Also let us know about material in this edition that you feel is low yield and should be deleted. You are also welcome to send general comments and feedback, although due to the volume of e-mails, we may not be able to respond to each of these.

The **preferred way** to submit entries, suggestions, or corrections is via **electronic mail**. Please include name, address, school affiliation, phone number, and e-mail address (if different from the address of origin). If there are multiple entries, please consolidate into a single e-mail or file attachment. Please send submissions to:

firstaidclerkships@gmail.com

Otherwise, please send entries, neatly written or typed or on disk (Microsoft Word), to:

Latha G. Stead, MD
C/o Catherine A. Johnson
Senior Editor
McGraw-Hill Medical
Two Penn Plaza, 23rd Floor
New York, NY 10121

All entries become property of the authors and are subject to editing and reviewing. Please verify all data and spellings carefully. In the event that similar or duplicate entries are received, only the first entry received will be used. Include a reference to a standard textbook to facilitate verification of the fact. Please follow the style, punctuation, and format of this edition if possible.

INTERNSHIP OPPORTUNITIES

The author team is pleased to offer part-time and full-time internships in medical education and publishing to motivated physicians. Internships may range from three months (e.g., a summer) up to a full year. Participants will have an opportunity to author, edit, and earn academic credit on a wide variety of projects, including the popular *First Aid* series. Writing/editing experience, familiarity with Microsoft Word, and Internet access are desired. For more information, e-mail a résumé or a short description of your experience along with a cover letter to **latha.stead@gmail.com.**

NOTE TO CONTRIBUTORS

All entries become properties of the authors and are subject to review and edits. Please verify all data and spelling carefully. In the event that similar or duplicate entries are received, only the first entry received will be used. Include a reference to a standard textbook to facilitate verification of the fact. Please follow the style, punctuation, and format of this edition if possible.

CONTRIBUTION FORM

Contributor Name: _____

School/Affiliation: _____

Address: _____

Telephone: _____

E-mail: _____

Topic:

Location:

Cause:

Image findings:

Notes, Diagrams, Tables, and Mnemonics:

Reference:

You will receive personal acknowledgment for each entry that is used in future editions.

How to Succeed in the Surgery Clerkship

The surgery clerkship is unique among all the medical school rotations. Even if you are dead sure you do not want to be a surgeon, it can be a very fun and rewarding experience if you approach it prepared. There are three key components to the rotation: (1) what to do in the OR, (2) what to do on the wards, and (3) how to study for the exam.

▶ IN THE OPERATING ROOM . . .

One of the most fun things on the surgery rotation is the opportunity to scrub in on surgical cases. The number and types of cases you will scrub in on depends on the number of residents and students on that service and how busy the service is that month. At some places, being able to go to the OR is considered a privilege rather than a routine part of the rotation. A few tips:

- **Eat before you begin the case.** Some cases can go on for longer than planned and it isn't cool to leave early because you are hungry (read unprepared!) or, worse, to pass out from exhaustion. As a student, your function in the OR will most likely be to hold retraction. This can be tedious, but it is important to pay attention and do a good job. Not pulling in the right direction obscures the view for your attending, and pulling too hard can destroy tissue. Many students get light-headed standing in one position for an extended period of time, especially when they are not used to it. Make sure you shift your weight and bend your knees once in a while so you don't faint. If you feel you are going to faint, then say something—ask one of the surgical techs to take over or state discreetly that you need relief. Do not hold on to the bitter end, pass out, and take the surgical field with you (believe it or not, this has actually happened; we print this advice from real experience).
- **Find out about the case as much as possible beforehand.** Usually, the OR schedule is posted the night before, so you should be able to tell. Read up on the procedure as well as the pathophysiology of the underlying condition. Know the important anatomic landmarks.
- **Find out who you are working with.** If you can, do a quick bibliography search on the surgeon you will be working with. It can never hurt to know which papers (s)he has written, and this may help to spark conversation and distinguish you among the many other students they will have met.
- **Assess the mood in the OR.** The amount of conversation in the OR directed to you varies by attending. Some are very into teaching and will engage you during most of the surgery. Many others act as if you aren't even there. Some will interact if you make the first move; others nuke all efforts at interaction. You'll have to figure it out based on the situation. Generally, if your questions and comments reflect that you have read about the procedure and disease, things will go well.
- **Keep a log of all surgeries** you have attended, scrubbed on, or assisted with (see Figure I-1). If you are planning to go into general surgery or a surgical subspecialty, it can be useful during residency interviews for conveying how much exposure/experience you have had. This is particularly true if your school's strength is clinical experience. The log can also be useful if you are requesting a letter from the chairman of surgery whom you have never worked with. It gives her/him an idea of what you have been doing with your rotation. Many rotations will set a minimum number of surgeries you are to attend. Try to attend as many as possible, and document them. This serves both to increase your exposure, and confirm your interest.

Operation	S/O	Attending	Date	MR #	Comments
1 Cholecystectomy	S	Dr. Wolfe	5/28/2003	123456	Got to close, placed 28 nonabsorbable sutures
2 Appendectomy	S	Dr. Tau	5/30/2003	246800	Used laparoscope
3 Cataract surgery	O	Dr. Mia	6/1/2003	135791	

S, scrubbed in; O, observed; MR, patient's medical record number.

FIGURE 1-1.   Example of an operative case log.

▶ ON THE WARDS . . .

Be on Time

Most surgical ward teams begin rounding between 6 and 7 A.M. If you are expected to "pre-round," you should give yourself at least 10 minutes per patient that you are following to see the patient and learn about the events that occurred overnight. Like all working professionals, you will face occasional obstacles to punctuality, but make sure this is occasional. When you first start a rotation, try to show up at least 15 minutes early until you get the routine figured out.

Dress in a Professional Manner

Even if the resident wears scrubs and the attending wears stiletto heels, you must dress in a professional, conservative manner. Wear a *short* white coat over your clothes unless discouraged.

> **Men** should wear long pants, with cuffs covering the ankle, a long collared shirt, and a tie. No jeans, no sneakers, no short-sleeved shirts.
> **Women** should wear long pants or knee-length skirt, blouse or dressy sweater. No jeans, no sneakers, no heels greater than 1½ inches, no open-toed shoes.
> **Both men and women** may wear scrubs occasionally, especially during overnight call or in the operating room. Do not make this your uniform.

Be Pleasant

The surgical rotation is often difficult, stressful, and tiring. Smooth out your experience by being nice to be around. Smile a lot and learn everyone's name. If you do not understand or disagree with a treatment plan or diagnosis, do not "challenge." Instead, say "I'm sorry, I don't quite understand, could you please explain . . ." Be empathetic toward patients.

Be Aware of the Hierarchy

The way in which this will affect you will vary from hospital to hospital and team to team, but it is always present to some degree. In general, address your questions regarding ward functioning to interns or residents. Address your medical questions to attendings; make an effort to be somewhat informed on your subject prior to asking attendings medical questions.

Address Patients and Staff in a Respectful Way

Address patients as Sir, Ma'am, or Mr., Mrs., or Miss. Do not address patients as "honey," "sweetie," and the like. Although you may feel that these names are friendly, patients will think you have forgotten their name, that you are being inappropriately familiar, or both. Address attending physicians as "doctor" unless told otherwise.

Take Responsibility for Your Patients

Know everything there is to know about your patients, their history, test results, details about their medical problem, and prognosis. Keep your intern or resident informed of new developments that he or she might not be aware of, and ask for any updates you might not be aware of. Assist the team in developing a plan and speaking to radiology, consultants, and family. Never give bad news to patients or family members without the assistance of your supervising resident or attending.

Respect Patients' Rights

1. All patients have the right to have their personal medical information kept private. This means do not discuss the patient's information with family members without that patient's consent, and do not discuss any patient in hallways, elevators, or cafeterias.
2. All patients have the right to refuse treatment. This means they can refuse treatment by a specific individual (you, the medical student) or of a specific type (no nasogastric tube). Patients can even refuse life-saving treatment. The only exceptions to this rule are if the patient is deemed to not have the capacity to make decisions or understand situations (in which case a health care proxy should be sought) or if the patient is suicidal or homicidal.
3. All patients should be informed of the right to seek advanced directives on admission. Often, this is done by the admissions staff, in a booklet. If your patient is chronically ill or has a life-threatening illness, address the subject of advanced directives with the assistance of your attending.

Volunteer

Be self-propelled, self-motivated. Volunteer to help with a procedure or a difficult task. Volunteer to give a 20-minute talk on a topic of your choice. Volunteer to take additional patients. Volunteer to stay late.

Be a Team Player

Help other medical students with their tasks; teach them information you have learned. Support your supervising intern or resident whenever possible. Never steal the spotlight, steal a procedure, or make a fellow medical student look bad.

Be Honest

If you don't understand, don't know, or didn't do it, make sure you always say that. Never say or document information that is false (a common example: "bowel sounds normal" when you did not listen).

Keep Patient Information Handy

Use a clipboard, notebook, or index cards to keep patient information, including a miniature history and physical, lab, and test results at hand.

Present Patient Information in an Organized Manner

Here is a template for the "bullet" presentation:

> This is a [age] year old [gender] with a history of [major history such as HTN, DM, coronary artery disease, CA, etc.] who presented on [date] with [major symptoms, such as cough, fever and chills], and was found to have [working diagnosis]. [Tests done] showed [results]. Yesterday the patient [state important changes, new plan, new tests, new medications]. This morning the patient feels [state the patient's words], and the physical exam is significant for [state major findings]. Plan is [state plan].

The newly admitted patient generally deserves a longer presentation following the complete history and physical format.

Some patients have extensive histories. The whole history can and probably should be present in the admission note, but in ward presentation it is often too much to absorb. In these cases it will be very much appreciated by your team if you can generate a **good summary** that maintains an accurate picture of the patient. This usually takes some thought, but it's worth it.

Presenting the Chest Radiograph (CXR)

A sample CXR presentation may sound like:

> This is the CXR of Mr. Jones. The film is an AP view with good inspiratory effort. There is an isolated fracture of the 8th rib on the right. There is no tracheal deviation or mediastinal shift. There is no pneumo- or hemothorax. The cardiac silhouette appears to be of normal size. The diaphragm and heart borders on both sides are clear; no infiltrates are noted. There is a central venous catheter present, the tip of which is in the superior vena cava.

The key elements of presenting a CXR are summarized in Figure I-2.

- First, confirm that the CXR belongs to your patient
- If possible, compare to a previous film

Then, present in a systematic manner:

1. *Technique*
   Rotation, anteroposterior (AP) or posteroanterior (PA), penetration, inspiratory effort.

2. *Bony structures*
   Look for rib, clavicle, scapula, and sternum fractures.

3. *Airway*
   Look for tracheal deviation, pneumothorax, pneumomediastinum.

FIGURE I-2. **How to present a chest radiograph (CXR).**

4. *Pleural space*

Look for fluid collections, which can represent hemothorax, chylothorax, pleural effusion.

5. *Lung parenchyma*

Look for infiltrates and consolidations: These can represent pneumonia, pulmonary contusions, hematoma, or aspiration. The location of an infiltrate can provide a clue to the location of a pneumonia:

- Obscured right (R) costophrenic angle = right lower lobe
- Obscured left (L) costophrenic angle = left lower lobe
- Obscured R heart border = right middle lobe
- Obscured L heart border = left upper lobe

6. *Mediastinum*

- Look at size of mediastinum—a widened one (> 8 cm) goes with aortic rupture.
- Look for enlarged cardiac silhouette (> ½ thoracic width at base of heart), which may represent congestive heart failure (CHF), cardiomyopathy, hemopericardium, or pneumopericardium.

7. *Diaphragm*

- Look for free air under the diaphragm (suggests perforation).
- Look for stomach, bowel, or NGT tube above diaphragm (suggests diaphragmatic rupture).

8. *Tubes and lines*

- Identify all tubes and lines.
- An endotracheal tube should be 2 cm above the carina. A common mistake is right mainstem bronchus intubation.
- A chest tube (including the most proximal hole) should be in the pleural space (not in the lung parenchyma).
- An NGT tube should be in the stomach, and uncoiled.
- The tip of a central venous catheter (central line) should be in the superior vena cava (not in the right atrium).
- The tip of a Swan–Ganz catheter should be in the pulmonary artery.
- The tip of a transvenous pacemaker should be in the right atrium.

FIGURE I-2. **(Continued)**

Types of Notes

In addition to the admission H&P and the daily progress note, there are a few other types of notes you will write on the surgery clerkship. These include the preoperative, operative, postoperative, and procedure notes. Samples of these are depicted in Figures I-3 through I-6.

Under sterile conditions following anesthesia with 5 cc of 2% lidocaine with epinephrine and negative wound exploration for foreign body, the laceration was closed with 3-0 Ethilon sutures. Wound edges were well approximated and no complications occurred. Wound was dressed with sterile gauze and triple antibiotic ointment.

FIGURE I-3. **Sample procedure note (for wound repair).**

Pre-op diagnosis:	Abdominal pain
Procedure:	Exploratory laparotomy
Pre-op tests:	List results of labs (CBC, electrolytes, PT, aPTT, urinalysis), ECG, CXR
	(Most adult patients require coagulation studies; patients over 40 usually need ECG and CXR—these are institution specific.)
Blood:	How many units of what type were crossmatched and available; or, "none" if no blood needed
Orders:	For example, colon prep, NPO after midnight, preoperative antibiotics

FIGURE I-4. **Sample preoperative note.**

Pre-op diagnosis:	Abdominal pain
Post-op Dx:	Small bowel obstruction
Procedure:	Segmental small bowel resection with end-to-end anastomosis
Surgeon:	Dr. Attending
Assistant:	Your Name Here
Anesthesia:	GETA (general endotracheal anesthesia)
	EBL (estimated blood loss): 100 cc
	Fluid replacement: 2000 cc crystalloid, 2 units FFP
	UO = 250 cc
Findings:	10 cm of infarcted small bowel
	Dermoid tumor, left ovary
Complications:	None

Wound was clean/clean contaminated/contaminated/dirty. (pick one)

Closure: 0-0 prolene for fascia, 3-0 vicryl SQ staples for skin.

Procedure tolerated well, patient remained hemodynamically stable throughout. Instrument, sponge, and needle counts were correct. Patient was extubated in the OR and transferred to the recovery room in stable condition.

FIGURE I-5. **Sample operative note.**

Postoperative day:	1
Procedure:	Colon resection with diverting colostomy
Vitals:	
Intake and output:	For intake include all oral and parenteral fluids and TPN
	For output include everything from all drains, tubes, and Foley
Physical examination:	Note particularly lung and abdominal exam, and comment on wound site.
Labs:	
Assessment:	
Plan:	

FIGURE I-6. **Sample postoperative note.**

7

Many students worry about their grade in this rotation. There is the perception that not getting honors in surgery pretty much closes the door to obtaining a residency spot in general or subspecialty surgery (ophthalmology, otorhinolaryngology, neurosurgery, plastic surgery, urology). While this is not necessarily true, the medicine and surgery clerkships are considered to be among the most important in medical school, so doing well in these is handy for all students. Usually, the clerkship grade is broken down into three or four components.

- *Inpatient evaluation.* This includes evaluation of your ward time by residents and attendings and is based on your performance on the ward. Usually, this makes up about half your grade and can be largely subjective.
- *Ambulatory evaluation.* This includes your performance in clinic, including clinic notes and any procedures performed in the outpatient setting.
- *Written examination.* Most schools use the NBME or "Shelf" examination. Some schools have their own homemade version, very similar to the NBME's. The test is multiple choice. This portion of the grade is anywhere from 20% to 40%, so performance on this multiple-choice test is vital to achieving honors in the clerkship. More on this below.
- *Objective Structured Clinical Examination (OSCE).* Some schools now include an OSCE as part of their clerkship evaluation. This is basically an exam that involves a standardized patient and allows assessment of a student's bedside manner and physical examination skills. This may comprise up to one fourth of a student's grade. It is a tool that will probably become more and more popular over the next few years.

▶ HOW TO STUDY

Make a List of Core Material to Learn

This list should reflect common symptoms, illnesses, and areas in which you have particular interest, or in which you feel particularly weak. Do not try to learn every possible topic. The Association for Surgical Education (*www.surgicaleducation.com*) has put forth a manual of surgical objectives for the medical student surgery clerkship, on which this book is based. The ASE emphasizes:

Symptoms and Lab Tests
- Abdominal masses
- Abdominal pain
- Altered mental status
- Breast mass
- Jaundice
- Lung nodule
- Scrotal pain and swelling
- Thyroid mass
- Fluid, electrolyte, and acid–base disorders
- Multi-injured trauma patient

Common Surgeries
- Appendectomy
- Coronary artery bypass grafting (CABG)
- Cholecystectomy
- Exploratory laparotomy
- Breast surgery
- Herniorraphy
- Peptic ulcer disease (PUD) surgery
- Bariatric surgery

We also recommend:

- Preoperative care
- Postoperative care
- Wound infection
- Shock

The core of the general surgery rotation consists of the following chapters:
1. The Surgical Patient
2. Wounds
3. Acute Abdomen
4. Trauma
5. Critical Care
6. Fluids, Electrolytes, and Nutrition
7. The Esophagus
8. The Stomach
9. Small Bowel
10. Colon, Rectum, and Anal Canal
11. The Appendix
12. Hernia and Abdominal Wall Problems
13. The Hepatobiliary System
14. The Pancreas
15. Endocrine System
16. The Spleen
17. The Breast
18. Burns
20. Vascular Surgery
24. Cardiothoracic Surgery

The other chapters are somewhat less important, as they focus on subspecialty surgery. The subspecialty chapters are comprehensive and less "high yield" than the abdominal chapters, but they are an excellent primer for anyone considering going into subspecialty surgery. We kept the detail in these chapters due to feedback from several students who wanted a concise but comprehensive overview of surgical subspecialties.

You will notice that the chapters will discuss pathophysiology and in general a lot of things that seem like they belong in a medicine book. The reason for this is that **the NBME clerkship exam covers the medicine behind surgical disease.** The exam does not ask specifics of operative technique. So, in a way, you are studying for three distinct purposes. The knowledge you need on the wards is the day-to-day management know-how. The knowledge you want in the OR involves surgical knowledge of anatomy and operative technique (see OR TIPs). The knowledge you want on the end of rotation examination is the epidemiology, risk factors, pathophysiology, diagnosis, and treatment of major diseases seen on a general surgery service.

As You See Patients, Note Their Major Symptoms and Diagnosis for Review

Your reading on the symptom-based topics above should be done with a specific patient in mind. For example, if a patient comes to the office with a thyroid mass, read about Graves' disease, Hashimoto's, thyroid cancer, and the technique of needle aspiration in the review book that night.

Select Your Study Material

We recommend:

- This review book, *First Aid for the Surgery Clerkship*
- A major surgery textbook such as *Schwartz's Principles of General Surgery* (costs about $140)
- A full-text online journal database, such as *www.mdconsult.com* (subscription is $99/year for students)
- A small pocket reference book to look up lab values, clinical pathways, and the like, such as *Maxwell Quick Medical Reference* (ISBN 0964519119, costs $7)
- A small book to look up drugs, such as *Pocket Pharmacopoeia* (Tarascon publishers, $8)

Prepare a Talk on a Topic

You may be asked to give a small talk once or twice during your rotation. If not, you should volunteer! Feel free to choose a topic that is on your list; however, realize that this may be considered dull by the people who hear the lecture. The ideal topic is slightly uncommon but not rare, for example: bariatric surgery. To prepare a talk on a topic, read about it in a major textbook or a review article not more than 2 years old, and then search online or in the library for recent developments or changes in treatment.

Procedures

During the course of the surgery clerkship, there is a set of procedures you are expected to learn or at least observe. The common ones are:

- Intravenous line placement
- Nasogastric tube placement
- Venipuncture (blood draw)
- Foley (urinary) catheter placement
- Wound closure with sutures/staples
- Suture/staple removal
- Surgical knots (hand and instrument ties)
- Dressing changes (wet to dry, saline, Vaseline gauze)
- Incision and drainage of abscesses
- Technique of needle aspiration (observe)
- Ankle–brachial index (ABI) measurement
- Evaluation of pulses with Doppler
- Skin biopsy (punch and excisional)
- Removal of surgical drains
- Transillumination of scrotum

If you have read about your core illnesses and core symptoms, you will know a great deal about the medicine of surgery. To study for the clerkship exam, we recommend:

2 to 3 weeks before exam: Read this entire review book, taking notes.

10 days before exam: Read the notes you took during the rotation on your core content list, and the corresponding review book sections.

5 days before exam: Read this entire review book, concentrating on lists and mnemonics.

2 days before exam: Exercise, eat well, skim the book, and go to bed early.

1 day before exam: Exercise, eat well, review your notes and the mnemonics, and go to bed on time. Do not have any caffeine after 2 P.M.

Other helpful studying strategies include:

Study with Friends

Group studying can be very helpful. Other people may point out areas that you have not studied enough, and may help you focus on the goal. If you tend to get distracted by other people in the room, limit this to less than half of your study time.

Study in a Bright Room

Find the room in your house or in your library that has the best, brightest light. This will help prevent you from falling asleep. If you don't have a bright light, get a halogen desk lamp or a light that simulates sunlight (not a tanning lamp).

Eat Light, Balanced Meals

Make sure your meals are balanced, with lean protein, fruits and vegetables, and fiber. A high-sugar, high-carbohydrate meal will give you an initial burst of energy for 1 to 2 hours, but then you'll drop.

Take Practice Exams

The point of practice exams is not so much the content that is contained in the questions, but the training of sitting still for 3 hours and trying to pick the best answer for each and every question.

Tips for Answering Questions

All questions are intended to have one best answer. When answering questions, follow these guidelines:

Glance the answers first. For all questions longer than two sentences, reading the answers first can help you sift through the question for the key information.

Look for the words *EXCEPT, MOST, LEAST, NOT, BEST, WORST, TRUE, FALSE, CORRECT, INCORRECT, ALWAYS,* and *NEVER.* If you find one of these words, circle or underline it for later comparison with the answer.

Evaluate each answer as being either true or false. Example:

Which of the following is *least* likely to be associated with pulmonary embolism?

    A.   Tachycardia **T**
    B.   Tachypnea **T**
    C.   Chest pain ? **F not always**
    D.   Deep venous thrombosis ? **T not always**
    E.   Back pain **F ? aortic dissection**

By comparing the question, noting LEAST, to the answers, "E" is the best answer.

Finally, as the boy scouts say, "BE PREPARED."

The following "cards" contain information that is often helpful during the surgery rotation. We advise that you make a copy of these cards, cut them out, and carry them in your coat pocket when you are on the wards.

SUTURE TECHNIQUE

I. SIMPLE INTERRUPTED

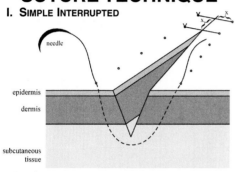

- Used to close most simple wounds
- Edges should always be everted to prevent depression of scar. Do this by entering needle at 90 degrees to skin surface and follow curve of needle through skin.
- Entrance and exit point of needle should be equidistant from laceration.
- Do not place suture too shallow, as this will cause dead space.
- Use instrument tie or surgeons knot and place knot to one side of laceration not directly over laceration.

II. RUNNING

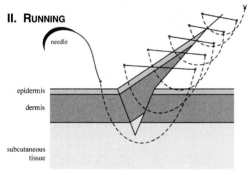

- Not commonly used in the ED
- Disadvantage: One nicked stitch or knot means the entire suture is out.
- Advantage: Done well with sturdy knots, it provides even tension across wound.

III. HORIZONTAL MATTRESS

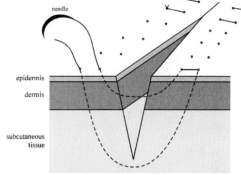

- This suture also assists in wound edge eversion and helps to spread tension over a greater area.
- This stitch starts out like a simple interrupted suture; however, after the needle exits, it then enters again on the same side that it exited from only a few millimeters lateral to the stitch and equidistant from the wound edge and exits on the opposite side.

IV. VERTICAL MATTRESS

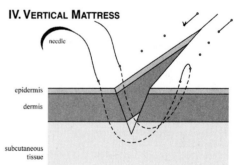

- This suture helps in reducing dead space and in eversion of wound edges.
- It does not significantly reduce tension on wound.
- The needle enters the skin farther away (more lateral) from the laceration than the simple interrupted and also exits further away on the opposite side.
- It then enters again on the same side that it just exited from but more proximal to the laceration and exits on the opposite side (where it originally entered) proximally.

V. CORNER STITCH

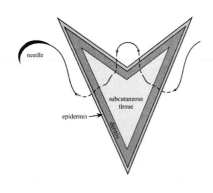

- This is used to repair stellate lacerations and help to preserve the blood supply to the tips of the skin.
- The needle enters the epidermis of the nonflap or nontip portion of the wound.
- It then enters the dermal layer of the skin tip on one side and proceeds through the dermal layer to exit the dermis on the other side of the tip (this portion will be buried).
- It then enters and exits the other side of the stellate wound. It will appear as a simple interrupted suture.

VI. DEEP SUTURES

- Absorbable
- Used for multilayered closure
- Deep sutures are absorbable because you will not be removing them.
- Use your forceps (pickups) to hold the skin from the inside of the wound.
- The first stitch is placed deep inside wound and exits superficially in dermal layer on same side of wound.
- Then it enters in the superficial dermal layer on the opposite side and exits deep.
- Tie a square knot and cut the tail of the suture close to the knot, which is called a buried knot.
- Now proceed with your superficial closure of the skin with nonabsorbable sutures.

LOCATION	SUTURE SIZE & TYPE	SUTURE TECHNIQUE	REMOVAL
Scalp	3-0 or 4-0 nylon or polypropylene	Interrupted in galea, single tight layer in scalp, horizontal mattress if bleeding not well controlled	7–12 days
Pinna	5-0 Vicryl/Dexon in perichondrium	Close perichondrium with interrupted Vicryl and close skin with interrupted nylon	3–5 days
Eyebrow	4-0 or 5-0 Vicryl (SQ) / 6-0 nylon for skin	Layered closure	3–5 days
Eyelid	6-0 nylon	Single-layer horizontal mattress or simple interrupted	3–5 days
Lip	4-0 Vicryl (mucosa) / 5-0 Vicryl (SQ or muscle) / 6-0 nylon (skin)	If wound through lip, close three layers (mucosa, muscle, skin); otherwise do two-layer closure	3–5 days
Oral cavity	4-0 Vicryl	Simple interrupted or horizontal mattress if muscularis of tongue involved	N/A
Face	6-0 nylon (skin) / 5-0 Vicryl (SQ)	Simple interrupted for single layer, layered closure for full-thickness laceration	3–5 days
Trunk	4-0 Vicryl (SQ, fat) / 4-0 or 5-0 nylon (skin)	Single or layered closure	7–12 days
Extremity	3-0 or 4-0 Vicryl (SQ, fat, muscle) / 4-0 or 5-0 nylon (skin)	Single-layer interrupted or vertical mattress; apply splint if over a joint	10–14 days
Hands and feet	4-0 or 5-0 nylon	Single-layer closure with simple interrupted or horizontal mattress; apply splint if over a joint	7–12 days
Nail bed	5-0 Vicryl	Meticulous placement to obtain even edges, allow to dissolve	N/A

SECTION II

High-Yield Facts for the Surgery Clerkship

The Surgical Patient

Ask yourself: What does the patient need in order to undergo the operation with the lowest risk possible?

Patients with aortic stenosis are at increased risk for ischemia, myocardial infarction (MI), and sudden death.

Stress test is positive if ST depressions > 0.2 mV are present or if there is an inadequate response of heart rate to stress or hypotension.

Echo is concerning when there is evidence of aortic stenosis (AS) or if the ejection fraction (EF) is < 35%.

Low-risk patients require only history and physical (H&P) and ECG. Higher-risk patients may require further workup as described above.

▶ PREOPERATIVE EVALUATION

- Thorough history and physical exam.
- Optimization of any medical problems (i.e., cardiac or pulmonary diseases).

Anesthetic History

Note any prior anesthetics and associated complications.

The ASA Physical Status Classification System

See Anesthesia chapter.

Evaluate Airway

Mallampati Classfication (Figure 1-1) predicts difficulty of intubation. Test is performed with the patient in the sitting position, the head held in a neutral position, the mouth wide open, and the tongue protruding to the maximum.

- *Class I*: Visualization of soft palate, fauces, uvula, anterior and posterior tonsillar pillars.
- *Class II*: Visualization of soft palate, fauces, uvula.
- *Class III*: Visualization of soft palate, base of uvula.
- *Class IV*: Nonvisualization of soft palate.

▶ CARDIAC RISK ASSESSMENT

- For a patient less than 35 years old with no cardiac history: Obtain electrocardiogram (ECG); if normal, no further workup required.
- For a patient of any age with cardiac history, or for an older patient: Obtain ECG; consider stress test and echocardiogram.

Goldman's risk assessment for noncardiac surgery (see Figure 1-2).

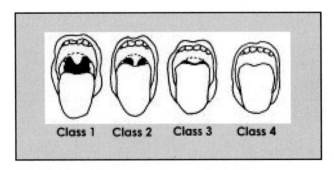

Class 1   Class 2   Class 3   Class 4

FIGURE 1-1. Mallampati Classification of ease of intubation.

Points		Probability of life-threatening complications
S3 gallop or JVD on exam	11	
MI within 6 months	10	Add points to get risk
> 5 PVCs/minute	7	0–5 = class I = 1%
Rhythm other than sinus rhythm (SR) or SR with APCs on last ECG	7	6–12 = class II = 5% 13–25 = class III = 11%
Age > 70	5	> 25 = class IV = 22%
Emergent operation	4	
Intrathoracic, intraperitoneal, or aortic surgery	3	
Significant aortic stenosis	3	
Poor general medical condition	3	

FIGURE 1-2. Goldman's risk assessment for noncardiac surgery.

(Reproduced, with permission, from Goldman L, Caldera DL, Nussbaum SR, et al. Multifactorial index of cardiac risk in noncardiac surgical procedures. *N Engl J Med* 297:845, 1977.)

▶ PULMONARY RISK ASSESSMENT

Risk Factors for Pulmonary Complications

- Known pulmonary disease.
- Abnormal pulmonary function tests (PFTs) (FEV < 11, max breathing capacity < 50% predicted).
- Smoking.
- Age > 60.
- Obesity.
- Upper abdominal or thoracic surgery.
- Long OR time.

Goals to Reduce Risks

- Decrease or cease smoking (benefit if at least 8 weeks preoperatively).
- Increase/optimize bronchodilator therapy.

Ways to Decrease Complications

1. Incentive spirometry.
2. Early postop ambulation.
3. Chest physical therapy (PT).
4. Deep vein thrombosis (DVT) prophylaxis by sequential compression device (SCD) and subcutaneous heparin.

▶ HEPATIC RISK ASSESSMENT

Child's Classification of Operative Risk for Patients with Cirrhosis

See Table 1-1.

Echocardiography:
- Sensitivity 90–100%
- Specificity 50–80%
- Fixed defects, or defects that persist with time, indicate infarcted or scarred tissue.
- Reversible defects are more concerning: Normal and fixed defects have similar negative predictive values for cardiac events.

Up to 35% of postoperative deaths are due to pulmonary complications.

Major abdominal surgery decreases vital capacity by 50% and functional residual capacity by 30%.

- FEV_1 < 70% predicted indicates increased risk.
- If VO_2 > 20, patient not likely to have pulmonary complications.

Heparin-induced thrombocytopenia (HIT).

Because of the method by which they work (accentuate systemic thrombolysis) one SCD should work as well as two if one leg is injured.

Atelectasis and/or pneumonia affect 20–40% of all postoperative patients.

Pneumonia has the highest morbidity and mortality of all pulmonary complications. The mortality of elderly patients with postoperative pneumonia is 50%.

Remember that fluid mobilization typically occurs on postoperative day 2 or 3.

TABLE 1-1. Child's Classification of Operative Risk

	A	B	C
Ascites	None	Controlled	Uncontrolled
Total bilirubin	< 2	2–3	> 3
Encephalopathy	None	Minimal	Advanced
Nutrition	Excellent	Good	Poor
Albumin	> 3.5	3–3.5	< 3
Operative mortality	2%	10%	50%

Cautions

- Watch for prolonged elevations in drug levels in patients with preoperative liver dysfunction.
- Acute hepatitis is relative contraindication with 10% increase in morbidity/mortality if viral origin.
- Recommend abstinence from alcohol; alcohol's hypermetabolic state causes increased need for amino acids (by 2×).
- Attempt to control ascites prior to elective surgery, with fluid restriction, diuretics, and nutritional therapy.

▶ RENAL RISK ASSESSMENT

Preoperative Evaluation

- Check blood urea nitrogen (BUN) and creatinine.
- Estimate preoperative creatinine clearance (Cockcroft Gault equation):

$$[(140 - \text{age}) \times \text{Ideal body weight in kilograms}]/72 \times \text{Plasma creatinine (mg/dL)}$$

- Maintain intravascular volume.
- Ensure electrolytes are repleted; correct acidosis.
- Dialysis patients should be dialyzed within 24 hours of surgery to best control creatinine and electrolytes.

Dialysis

- Overall mortality for dialysis-dependent patients: 5% (even when dialyzed within 24 hours of surgery).
- Acute renal failure that develops in perioperative period requiring dialysis is associated with a mortality of approximately 50–80%.
- Morbidity: Shunt thrombosis, pneumonia, wound infection, hemorrhage.

Preoperative Labs

- Check complete blood count (CBC).
- Blood should be typed and crossed.

Anemia

- Determine cause.
- Postpone elective operations when possible; patients who will not tolerate anemia well include those with chronic hypoxia, ischemic heart disease, or cerebral ischemia.
- Sickle cell patients have increased risk of vaso-occlusive crises with operations. (This increased risk does not generally include patients with sickle cell trait.)
- Minimize risk by maintaining euvolemia.

Thrombocytopenia

See Figure 1-3.

Coagulopathy

- Check prothrombin time (PT) and partial thromboplastin time (PTT) preoperatively.
- Note that elevated values should be expected in patients with liver disease.
- Factor abnormalities should be addressed (e.g., with hemophilia).

- Ideal body weight (IBW) = 50 kg + 2.3 kg/inch over 5 ft (male) or 45.5 kg + 2.3 kg/inch over 5 ft (female).
- Body mass index (BMI) = kg/m^2.
  - Loss of > 10% body weight in 6 months or a serum albumin level of < 3 is a poor prognostic indicator.

Platelets	Likelihood of bleed perioperatively
> 150,000	Normal
100,000–150,000	Unlikely
50,000–100,000	Unlikely with adequate hemostasis
20,000–50,000	Possible excessive surgical bleeding
10,000–20,000	Spontaneous mucosal and cutaneous bleeding
< 10,000	Major spontaneous mucosal bleed, including GI tract

FIGURE 1-3. Risk of postoperative bleeding by platelet count.

- NH$_3$ > 150: Mortality 80%
- INR > 2: Mortality 40–60%

Increased BUN and creatinine indicate a loss of at least 75% of renal reserve.
Intra- and postop hypotension must be strictly avoided in renal patients.

The risk of bleeding increases in patients with BUN > 100 due to platelet dysfunction, which can be corrected by desmopressin (DDAVP).

The most common complication in dialysis is *hyperkalemia* (in nearly one third of patients).

To determine source of a renal problem:
- FE$_{Na}$ > 1 = intrinsic damage
- Specific gravity = 1.010 in ATN
- U$_{Na}$ < 20 in prerenal

- Risk of bleeding is further increased at any platelet level if patient is septic or has a functional platelet deficit.
- One unit of platelets raises platelet count by 5,000–10,000.

- Ideal BMI = 19 – 25.
- Increased risk if < 80% or > 12% of IBW or recent change of > 10% body weight.
- Consider baseline state of patient: Well-nourished with acute illness versus chronically ill, alcoholic, obese.

Antibiotic prophylaxis: Single dose 30 minutes prior to skin incision, and again 6 hours later if operation is ongoing.

▶ ANTIBIOTIC PROPHYLAXIS

By Type of Surgery

1. In general: Cefazolin.
2. Colorectal surgery, appendectomy: Cefoxitin or cefotetan.
3. Urologic procedures: Ciprofloxacin.
4. Head and neck: Cefazolin or clindamycin and gentamicin.

▶ GENERAL POSTOPERATIVE COMPLICATIONS

- Immediate (0–24 hrs):
  - Primary hemorrhage—either starting during surgery or following postoperative increase in blood pressure: Replace blood loss, and may require return to OR to reexplore wound.
  - Basal atelectasis.
  - Shock: blood loss, acute MI, pulmonary embolism (PE).
  - Oliguria: (hypotension intra- or postoperatively).
- Early (2 days to 3 weeks):
  - Mental status changes due to electrolyte imbalance, dehydration, and sepsis.
  - Nausea and vomiting: Analgesia or anesthesia related; paralytic ileus.
  - Fever.
  - Secondary hemorrhage (infection).
  - Pneumonia.
  - Wound infection.
  - Wound or anastomosis dehiscence.
  - DVT, PE.
  - Acute urinary retention.
  - Urinary tract infection.
  - Postoperative wound infection.
  - Bowel obstruction due to fibrinous adhesions.
  - Paralytic ileus.
- Late (weeks to months):
  - Bowel obstruction due to fibrous adhesions.
  - Incisional hernia.
  - Persistent sinus.
  - Recurrence of reason for surgery (e.g., malignancy).

▶ COMMON COMPLICATIONS

Ileus

- Incidence after GI surgery: 5%.
- In general, await return of bowel function before advancing diet.

Clostridium difficile Colitis

- Variable presentation, from mild diarrhea and discomfort to severe pain, tenderness, fever, and elevated white blood count (WBC).

- Associated with age, prior residence in nursing home, renal failure, immunocompromised state, antibiotic use (especially cefoxitin), small or large bowel obstruction, gastrointestinal (GI) surgery, nasogastric tube (NGT) for > 48 hours.
- Treatment: PO metronidazole or vancomycin.

1. Atelectasis
    - Most common cause of fever within 24 hours of surgery.
    - Mediated by macrophage.
    - Reduced by early ambulation.
    - Treated by incentive spirometry and chest PT; no role of antibiotics.
2. Pneumonia
    - Characterized by fever, cough, dyspnea, pleuritic chest pain, purulent sputum.
    - Exam shows bronchial breath sounds, dullness, rales.
    - Chest x-ray shows infiltrates; sputum culture demonstrates causative organism.
    - Treated by organism-specific antibiotics.

Return of bowel function: *Small intestine,* then *stomach,* then *colon.*

To estimate when bowel function will return, allow one postoperative day per decade for major abdominal surgery.

DVT/PE

- PE presents with tachycardia, tachypnea, and hypoxia when symptomatic (see Table 1-2).

TABLE 1-2. Wells' Criteria for PE

CRITERIA	POINTS
Clinical signs and symptoms of DVT (objectively measured calf swelling and pain with palpation in the deep vein region)	3.0
An alternative diagnosis is less likely than PE	3.0
Heart rate > 100 beats per minute	1.5
Immobilization or surgery in the previous four weeks	1.5
Previous DVT or PE	1.5
Hemoptysis	1.0
Malignancy (on treatment, treated in the past 6 months, or palliative care)	1.0

INTERPRETATION OF POINT TOTAL

SCORE	MEAN PROBABILITY	RISK
< 2 points	3.6	Low
2–6 points	20.5	Moderate
> 6 points	66.7	High

From Wells PS, Anderson DR, Rodger M, et al. Excluding pulmonary embolism at the bedside without diagnostic imaging: Management of patients with suspected pulmonary embolism presenting to the emergency department by using a simple clinical model and D-dimer. *Ann Int Med* 135:98–107, 2001.

- Prevented by SCDs, subcutaneous heparin, and ambulation.
- PE diagnosed by ventilation/perfusion (V/Q) scan or chest computed tomographic (CT) angiography.
- Treated by heparin infusion for segmental, sub-segmental PE. Massive PE is treated by surgery (embolectomy).

Wound Infection

See Wounds chapter.

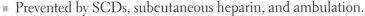

▶ **INSTRUCTIONS TO PATIENT**

NPO

- To decrease the risk of aspiration with intubation, patients should refrain from solids 6–8 hours prior, and from liquids 2–3 hours prior to surgery.
- In bowel surgery, when patients require bowel preps, the duration of NPO may be preceded by a day of clear liquids only with the prep to clear the bowel of stool and facilitate the operation.

Bowel Preparation

- Purpose: To clear bowel of stool, thereby reducing bacterial count and risk of contamination with fecal spillage.
- Types:
  - Mechanical prep: Facilitates operation.
  - Oral antibiotics (neomycin, erythromycin base): Nadir bacterial count at commencement of operation if doses given at 1 P.M., 2 P.M., 11 P.M., the day prior (for a first case).

Usual Medications

- **Aspirin:** Avoid for 10 days preoperatively to allow platelets to regenerate.
- Hold clopidogrel (Plavix) for 7 days.
- **Warfarin (Coumadin):**
  - Three options: Avoid 3 days prior to operation and resume postoperative day 2; admit preoperatively and change to heparin, which can be held only a couple of hours ahead; operate through coumadin.
- **Antihypertensives:** Continue, especially β-blockers; hold diuretics the morning of surgery.
- **Antithyroid medications:** Hold on morning of surgery.
- **Thyroid replacement:** Give on morning of surgery.
- **Oral hypoglycemics:** Avoid on day of surgery.
- **Insulin:** Give half usual dose on morning of surgery.

HIGH-YIELD FACTS IN

Wounds

By definition, the end result of any surgical case is one type of wound or another. Surgeons define a successful surgical case as one in which the patient survives, the pathology is removed and/or corrected, and the patient's wound heals. To accomplish this, it is important to understand the processes involved in wound repair, and ways in which these processes can lead to complications.

► **STEPS OF WOUND HEALING**

Phases of wound healing:
Hemostasis and
   inflammation
Proliferation
Maturation
Remodelling

- Coagulation
- Inflammation
- Collagen synthesis
- Angiogenesis
- Epithelialization
- Contraction

Coagulation

- Begins following wound formation.
- Coagulation and complement cascades are activated, and platelets create a hemostatic plug.
- Release of various inflammatory mediators from activated platelets sets the stage for the steps that follow.
- Impaired by anticoagulants, antiplatelet agents, and coagulation factor deficiency. Also may see impaired coagulation in the setting of chronic liver disease and uremia.

Inflammation

Macrophages are essential
for wound healing.

- The signs of inflammation are pain, swelling, heat, erythema, and loss of function.
- Inflammation occurs as a result of the wound's being invaded by polymorphonuclear neutrophils (PMNs, from the initial wound through the first 48 hours), and macrophages (peak numbers at 24 hours).
- Macrophages are essential for wound healing.
- Bacteria, cellular debris, dirt, and other foreign materials are also cleared from the wound site by the macrophages and PMNs.
- Impaired by steroids and other immunosuppressants, congenital or acquired immune-deficient states.

Collagen Synthesis

- Occurs by fibroblasts in the vicinity of the wound, in response to various growth factor peptides.
- The amino acids hydroxyproline and hydroxylysine are components of collagen. Their synthesis and hydroxylation is dependent on Fe, α-ketoglutarate, and ascorbate (vitamin C).

Angiogenesis (Granulation)

- Occurs in response to peptide growth factors such as vascular endothelial growth factor (VEGF).
- Presence of these new vascular networks is what gives granulation tissue its characteristic beefy-red appearance.

Epithelialization

- Occurs with the migration of epithelial cells over the wound defect.
- Integrity of the basement membrane is restored as type IV collagen and other matrix components are deposited.
- Foreign bodies, such as suture material, and necrotic tissue remain separated from the wound by the migrating epithelial cells.
- Once this step has occurred, the wound is essentially waterproofed.

Contraction and Remodelling

- Process by which the surrounding uninjured skin is pulled over the wound defect and the size of the scar is reduced.
- Made possible by the action of myofibroblasts, which possess a contraction mechanism similar to that seen in muscle cells.
- A long process that takes many months before it is complete.
- *Do not confuse wound contraction with scar contracture, as the latter occurs after wound repair has ceased.* Scar contracture can lead to undesirable effects since architecture of the surrounding tissue may become distorted.
- Maturation of the scar occurs over the next 9 months to 2 years, characterized by cross-linking of collagen and clinical flattening of the scar.

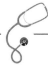

The presence of granulation tissue is reassuring evidence that the healing process is under way. At one month postinjury, the wound is at approximately 85% of its ultimate cohesive strength.

Epithelialization of surgical wounds closed primarily is usually complete by 24–48 hours.

► SURGICAL WOUND CLASSIFICATION

Clean

For a wound to be considered "clean," the following must be true:

- Wound created in a sterile and nontraumatic fashion, in an area that is free of preexisting inflammation.
- The respiratory, alimentary, genital, or urinary tract was not entered.
- All persons involved in the case maintained strict aseptic technique.

Clean-Contaminated

- The respiratory, alimentary, genital, or urinary tract was entered, but there was no significant spillage of its contents (e.g., feces), and there was no established local infection.
- There was only a minor break in aseptic technique.

Risk of infection for wounds:
Clean—2%
Clean-contaminated—5%
Contaminated—15%
Dirty—35%

Contaminated

- There was gross spillage from the gastrointestinal tract.
- The genitourinary and biliary tracts were entered in the presence of local infection (e.g., cholangitis).
- The wound was the result of recent trauma.
- There was a major break in aseptic technique.

Dirty/Infected

- The wound was the result of remote trauma and contains devitalized tissue and/or purulent material.
- There is established infection or perforated viscera prior to the procedure.

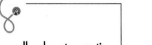

Generally, clean traumatic lacerations are closed with sutures or staples (primary intention) if less than 6–8 hours old.

▶ **TYPES OF WOUND HEALING**

Primary (First) Intention

See Figure 2-1.

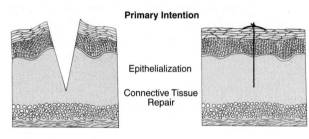

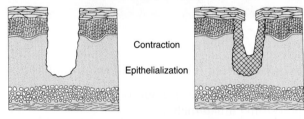

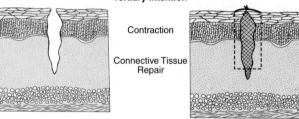

FIGURE 2-1. Different clinical approaches to the closure and healing of acute wounds.

(Reproduced, with permission, from Brunicardi FC, Andersen DK, Billiar TR, et al. *Schwartz's Principles of Surgery*, 8th ed., New York: McGraw-Hill, 2004: 235.)

- Type of healing seen following closure of clean surgical wounds, or traumatic lacerations in which there is minimal devitalized tissue, and minimal contamination.
- Edges of the incisional defect are approximated with the use of sutures or staples.
- Since the defect is very small, reepithelialization occurs rapidly, and overall healing time is short.
- Wounds closed primarily may have their dressing changed after 24–48 hours. By this time, epithelialization should be complete, and a less bulky dressing can be applied.
- Wound strength reaches its maximum at about 3 months and is generally 70–80% that of normal skin.

Second Intention

- Type of healing seen following closure of wounds that are not approximated with sutures.
- Reason for not using sutures may be (1) that the wound edges cannot be apposed because the defect is very large (e.g., donor site of skin graft) or (2) that the surgeon chooses not to close the wound primarily because of the high risk of infection.
- Wounds healing by second intention should be packed loosely with moist gauze and covered with a sterile dressing. The wound should be assessed daily for the development of granulation tissue and the presence of infection.
- Wound closes by contraction and then epithelialization. Contraction occurs from the edges of the wound inward, via contraction of myofibroblasts. Epithelialization then proceeds at 1 mm per day, also from the edges inward. Granulation tissue is generated at the center of the closing wound.

Third (Delayed Primary) Intention

- Type of healing seen following closure of wounds in which there is obvious gross contamination at the incisional site (i.e., the wound is classified as contaminated or dirty).
- An example of where delayed primary closure is often used is following removal of a ruptured appendix in which there was leakage of pus into the peritoneal cavity. In such cases, the parietal peritoneum and fascial layers are closed, and antibiotics are administered. The skin and subcutaneous tissue are not sutured until 3–5 days later after bacterial contamination has decreased.

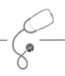

Sutures are utilized in primary and delayed primary intention healing only.

Sutures are tied to approximate, not strangulate, a healing wound!

▶ FACTORS AFFECTING WOUND HEALING

See Table 2-1.

TABLE 2-1. Factors Affecting Wound Healing

Systemic	Local
Age	Mechanical injury
Nutrition	Infection
Trauma	Edema
Metabolic diseases	Ischemia/necrotic tissue
Immunosuppression	Topical agents
Connective tissue disorders	Ionizing radiation
Smoking	Low oxygen tension
	Foreign bodies

Reproduced, with permission, from Brunicardi FC, Andersen DK, Billiar TR, et al. *Schwartz's Principles of Surgery*, 8th ed., New York: McGraw-Hill, 2004: 235.

▶ WOUND INFECTIONS

Classification

Surgical site infections (SSIs) generally occur within 30 postoperative days. Depending on their location, they may be classified as superficial incisional, deep incisional, or organ/space infections.

Infections that involve both deep and superficial tissues are classified as deep incisional SSIs.

- **Superficial incisional SSIs** exist when there is involvement by infection of the skin and subcutaneous tissue in the vicinity of the incision.
- **Deep incisional SSIs** exist when there is involvement by infection of deeper soft tissues, such as fascia or muscle, that were divided by the incision.
- **Organ/space SSIs** exist when there is infection of any anatomical structure remote from the incisional site but manipulated during the procedure.

Early surgical site infections that occur in the first 24 hours postoperatively are most commonly due to *Streptococcus* or *Clostridium*. These bacteria grow very fast because they excrete enzymes that digest local tissue and impair host defenses. Infections due to other bacteria generally become apparent later (4–5 days postoperatively) because they lack such virulence factors.

Many of the factors that impair wound healing will also increase the risk of wound infections.

Pathophysiology

Depend on:

- Factors relating to microorganism:
  - The magic number is 10^5 (dose of contaminating microorganisms required to result in an increased risk of wound infection).
- Factors relating to the patient—increased risk with:
  - Infection that is *remote* from the surgical site.
  - Diabetes.

- Smokers.
- Immunosuppressive agents, such as corticosteroids.
- Severe protein–calorie malnutrition.
- AIDS, disseminated malignancy, and any other immunocompromised state.
  - Factors relating to surgical technique:
    - Preoperative considerations:
      - Patient skin preparation, scrubbing, and the administration of antimicrobial prophylaxis.
    - Intraoperative considerations:
      - Strict attention to aseptic technique.
      - OR should be well ventilated and maintained under positive pressure to prevent the entrance of pathogens from the corridor.
      - Avoid excessive use of electrocautery and tying sutures too tightly.
    - Postoperative considerations:
      - Proper wound management and discharge instructions are key.
      - Wound management will differ depending on whether the wound is closed by primary, secondary, or delayed primary intention (see above).

Hair in the vicinity of the incision should be trimmed immediately before the procedure with clippers.

In the healthy individual, the lower respiratory tract and the upper urinary tract are essentially sterile.

▶ COMMON SURGICAL PATHOGENS

- The organism responsible for causing a surgical site infection is best identified by culturing the involved region.
- The most likely causative organism can be predicted based on the site of the operation:
  - *Staphylococcus aureus* **and coagulase-negative staphylococci** are commonly isolated from wounds that follow thoracic (cardiac and noncardiac), neurological, breast, ophthalmic, vascular, and orthopedic surgery.
  - **Gram-negative bacilli and anaerobes** are commonly isolated from wound infections that develop following appendectomy, colorectal, biliary tract, OB/GYN, and urological cases.
  - **Streptococci and oropharyngeal anaerobes** are commonly isolated from wounds that follow head and neck procedures in which the mucosa of the oral cavity is involved.
  - Animal bite infections: *Pasteurella multocida*; also *Streptococcus* and *Staphylococcus*.

Signs and Symptoms of Wound Infections

- Classic signs:
  - Calor (heat, warmth)
  - Rubor (redness)
  - Tumor (swelling)
  - Dolor (pain)
- More severe infections may produce systemic symptoms such as fever, chills, and rigors.
- Unusual for a wound infection to cause fever before postoperative day 3.
- Other causes of postoperative fever include urinary tract infection (UTI) (owing to prolonged placement of a Foley catheter), deep vein thrombosis (DVT)/thrombophlebitis, and certain medications.

The 5 W's of postoperative fever:
- **Wound** infection
- **Wind** (atelectasis) — most common cause of postop fever within 1 day after surgery (caused by macrophages)
- **Water** (UTI)
- **Walking** (DVT)
- **Wonder** drugs (direct side effects or those compromising immunity, respiration, or perfusion)

DIAGNOSTIC APPROACH

- Physical exam should be directed at the surgical wound, looking for signs of infection such as induration, warmth, erythema, or frank purulent discharge.
- Any discharge present should be sent for microbiological culture.
- The febrile patient should be evaluated with an appropriate fever workup: complete blood count (CBC), blood and urine cultures, urinalysis, and chest x-ray should be sent.
- If an intra-abdominal abscess is suspected, a computed tomographic (CT) scan of abdomen should be done.
- Lumbar puncture may be required for the patient with fever and altered mental status, especially in a patient that is status post craniotomy for a neurosurgical procedure.

Atelectasis is the most common cause of postoperative fever within the first 24 hours.

TREATMENT

- Wound abscesses (superficial SSIs) require incision and drainage followed by thorough irrigation.
- Deeper SSIs may require surgical debridement.
- Systemic antibiotic therapy is required for deep SSIs; they may or may not be required for superficial SSIs, depending on the severity of the infection.
- Peritoneal abscesses (organ/space SSI) may be treated by CT-guided percutaneous drainage; those that cannot be drained percutaneously require open drainage.

▶ ANTIMICROBIAL PROPHYLAXIS

The benefits of surgical antimicrobial prophylaxis are maximized if the chosen antibiotic:

- Provides appropriate coverage against the most probable contaminating organisms.
- Is present in optimal concentrations in serum and tissues at the time of incision.
- Is maintained at therapeutic levels throughout the operation.

General Principles

- For gram-positive cocci: First- and second-generation cephalosporins.
- For gram-negative rods: Third-generation cephalosporins.
- For anaerobes: Metronidazole or clindamycin.
- For gram-negative rods: Aminoglycosides.
- For methicillin-resistant *Staphylococcus aureus*: Vancomycin.
- All choices of antibiotics should be tailored based on the resistance profile of the community your hospital serves.

Hematoma

- Collection of blood that may form in the vicinity of a surgical wound.
- Small hematomas may be left alone and allowed to reabsorb spontaneously, while larger hematomas may require drainage.

Seroma

- Collection of fluid in the vicinity of a wound that is not blood or pus.
- Due to creation of a potential space combined with disruption of local draining lymphatic channels (e.g., mastectomy).
- Small seromas may be left alone and allowed to reabsorb spontaneously, while larger ones may require aspiration.

Wound Failure (Dehiscence and Incisional Hernia)

DEFINITIONS

- Occurs when there has been complete or partial disruption of one or more layers of the incisional site.
- Termed **dehiscence** if it occurs early in the postoperative course before all stages of wound healing have occurred (complete disruption).
- Termed **incisional hernia** when it occurs months or years after the surgical procedure (at least the skin is intact, i.e., partial disruption).

CAUSES

Poor operative techniques that may lead to wound failure include the following:

- *Suture material with inadequate tensile strength.* Since absorbable sutures lose their tensile strength rather quickly, nonabsorbable sutures should be used to close the fascia.
- *Inadequate number of sutures.* Sutures should be placed no greater than 1 cm apart; if placed greater than 1 cm apart, herniation of viscera may occur between sutures.
- *Too small bite size.* Sutures should be placed no less than 1 cm from the wound edge; if placed closer to the wound edge, the fascia may tear.

Patient factors may be divided into:

1. Systemic illnesses that impair wound healing, such as malnutrition, corticosteroid therapy, sepsis, uremia, liver failure, or poorly controlled diabetes.
2. Physical factors that place stress on the incisional site, such as coughing/retching, obesity, and the presence of ascites.

- Immediate treatment of wound dehiscence involves minimizing contamination of the operative site by the placement of sterile packing. The patient must then be brought back to the OR to reclose the incision.
- Incisional hernia must be treated promptly, especially if the patient is symptomatic (e.g., abdominal pain, nausea, vomiting). This is because strangulation of the bowel may occur, resulting in necrosis and increased morbidity. Incisional hernias are repaired by repairing the fascial defect, with or without the use of a synthetic mesh to reinforce the defect.

Complications of Excess Scar Formation

Hypertrophic scar and keloid formation (both are raised above skin level):

- Keloids spread beyond the margins of the original wound and are painful.
- Common in African-Americans (genetic predisposition).
- Commonly seen around the earlobes and the deltoid, presternal, and upper back regions.
- Hypertrophic scars usually subside spontaneously, whereas keloids need treatment with intralesional corticosteroid injection, topical application of silicone sheets, or the use of radiation or pressure. Surgery is reserved for excision of large lesions or as second-line therapy when other modalities have failed.

Acute Abdomen

Definition

Abrupt onset of abdominal pain usually accompanied by one or more peritoneal signs (i.e., rigidity, tenderness (with or without rebound), involuntary guarding). Most causes of acute abdomen are surgical.

History

Pain is the most common presenting feature of an acute abdomen. Special attention to the characteristics of the pain will aid in reaching the diagnosis.

LOCATION

Visceral pain: Poorly localized, usually dull, achy pain arising from distention or spasm in hollow organs. *Example: Crampy pain felt during early intestinal obstruction.*

> Mid-epigastrium: Stomach, duodenum, hepatobiliary system, pancreas.
> Mid-abdomen: jejunum, ileum.
> Lower abdomen: colon, internal reproductive organs.

Parietal pain: Sharp, well-localized, somatic pain arising from irritation (usually by pus, bile, urine, or gastrointestinal secretions) of the parietal peritoneum. *Example: Inflamed appendix causing sharp right lower quadrant (RLQ) pain due to irritation of nearby peritoneum.*

QUALITY OF PAIN

Steady pain is most common, but differentiating character of pain is helpful:

Gradual, steady pain	**Intermittent, colicky pain**
Acute cholecysitis	Small bowel obstruction
Acute cholangitis	Inflammatory bowel disease
Hepatic abscess	Biliary colic
Diverticulitis	

Abrupt, excruciating pain	**Rapid-onset, severe constant pain**
Perforated ulcer	Acute pancreatitis
Ruptured aneurysm	Ectopic pregnancy
Ureteral colic	Mesenteric ischemia
	Strangulated bowel
	Acute appendicitis

PRECIPITATING OR PALLIATIVE FACTORS

May include:

- Change in position.
- Association with food (better, worse).
- Pain that wakes one from sleep (significant).

RADIATION

- Biliary tract pain may radiate to the right shoulder or right scapula (due to right hemidiaphragmatic irritation).
- Splenic rupture pain may radiate to left shoulder.

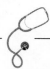

Assessment of pain should include **PQRST:**
Precipitating or palliative factors
Quality of pain: Stabbing, shooting, boring, dull
Radiation
Severity
Timing

Kehr's sign is pain referred to the left shoulder due to irritation of the left hemidiaphragm. Often seen with splenic rupture.

HIGH-YIELD FACTS

Acute Abdomen

- Kidney pain may radiate from flank to groin and genitalia (loin to groin).
- Pancreas pain may radiate to back.

ASSOCIATED SYMPTOMS

- Vomitting: Pain relieved by vomiting is supportive of small bowel obstruction (SBO), afferent loop syndrome.
  - Bilious vomiting is a clue for proximal SBO.
- Bowel habits: Constipation or obstipation (no stool or flatus) is suggestive of bowel obstruction.
- Mucoid diarrhea with blood (red currant jelly stool) is seen in intussusception.
- Anorexia: Very nonspecific symptom; however, most patients with acute appendicitis will have anorexia. Fever: seen in appendicitis, acute cholecystitis, acute pancreatitis.

MEDICAL AND SURGICAL HISTORY

- Past abdominal surgery? Any abdominal surgery increases the chance of SBO secondary to adhesions (even years later).
- Atrial fibrillation: Increased risk for mesenteric ischemia (embolism) because of emboli to mesenteric arteries.
- Menstrual and sexual history (acute salpingits vs. pelvic inflammatory disease vs. ruptured ectopic).

Serial abdominal exams and observation may be necessary in cases in which the etiology of abdominal pain is initially unclear.

▶ PHYSICAL EXAM

Things to look for:

- Vital signs: Most patients with a surgical abdomen will have vital sign abnormalities secondary to pain, inflammation, fluid and electrolyte derangements, and anxiety.
- General: Hydration status, mentation, nutritional status.
- Chest: Auscultation.
- Abdomen: See Tables 3-1 and 3-2.

Pain of perforated ulcer is severe and of **sudden onset.**
Murphy's sign is seen in cholecystitis.

TABLE 3-1. Steps in Physical Examination of the Acute Abdomen

1. Inspection	7. Punch tenderness
2. Auscultation	Costal area
3. Cough tenderness	Costovertebral area
4. Percussion	8. Special signs
5. Guarding or rigidity	9. External hernias and male genitalia
6. Palpation	10. Rectal and pelvic examination
One-finger	
Rebound tenderness	
Deep	

Reproduced, with permission, from Doherty GM. *Current Surgical Diagnosis & Treatment,* 12th ed. New York: McGraw-Hill; 2006: 484.

Most common cause by far (90%) of free air under diaphragm is perforated peptic ulcer. Other causes include hollow viscus injury secondary to trauma, mesenteric ischemia (usually under left hemidiaphragm), and large bowel perforation.

TABLE 3-2. Physical Findings in Various Causes of Acute Abdomen

Condition	Helpful Signs
Perforated viscus	Scaphoid, tense abdomen; diminished bowel sounds (late); loss of liver dullness; guarding or rigidity.
Peritonitis	Motionless; absent bowel sounds (late); cough and rebound tenderness; guarding or rigidity.
Inflamed mass or abscess	Tender mass (abdominal, rectal, or pelvic); punch tenderness; special signs (Murphy's, psoas, or obturator).
Intestinal obstruction	Distention; visible peristalsis (late); hyperperistalsis (early) or quiet abdomen (late); diffuse pain without rebound tenderness; hernia or rectal mass (some).
Paralytic ileus	Distention; minimal bowel sounds; no localized tenderness.
Ischemic or strangulated bowel	Not distended (until late); bowel sounds variable; severe pain but little tenderness; rectal bleeding (some).
Bleeding	Pallor, shock; distention; pulsatile (aneurysm) or tender (e.g., ectopic pregnancy) mass; rectal bleeding (some).

Reproduced, with permission, from Doherty GM. *Current Surgical Diagnosis & Treatment*, 12th ed. New York: McGraw-Hill; 2006: 484.

Contrast for abdominal CT:

For the most optimal imaging, both oral and IV contrast is used. In some cases (such as impaired renal function or allergy to IV contrast) this is not feasible. Noncontrast CT, although suboptimal for most cases (except nephrolithiasis), still provides lots of information.

▶ DIAGNOSIS

Initial laboratory evaluation should include:

- CBC.
- Electrolytes.
- Amylase, lipase.
- Electrocardiogram (ECG) to rule out myocardial infarction (MI) and also as a preoperative baseline cardiac assessment.
- Liver function tests (LFTs) for right upper quadrant (RUQ) pain.
- β-hCG (human chorionic gonadotropin) for all women of childbearing age.
- Chest x-ray (CXR) and abdominal x-ray (AXR) to look for free air (can detect as little as 1–2 mL); easier to see under right hemidiaphragm. Presence of stomach bubble obscures it on the left (see Figure 3-1).
- Abdominal computed tomography (CT) should be used after the above assessment is complete and the diagnosis remains elusive (e.g., young male with clinical signs and symptoms of appendicitis should not undergo CT) (see Figure 3-2).

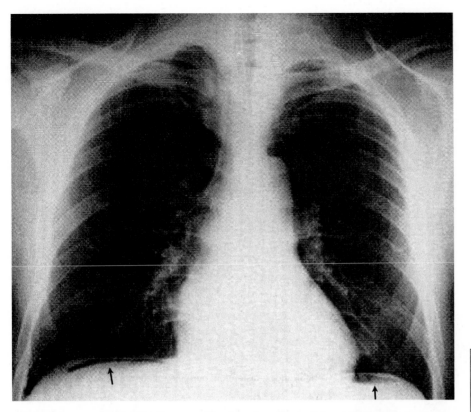

FIGURE 3-1. Upright CXR demonstrating free air under both hemidiaphragms (arrows).

(Reproduced, with permission, from Billittier et al. *Emerg Med Clin of N Amer* 14:(4); November 1996: 795.)

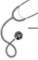

The pain of appendicitis localizes to **McBurney's point**.
Physical exam signs in appendicitis: Rovsing's, obturator, psoas (see Appendix chapter).

▶ **MANAGEMENT**

- Early diagnosis improves outcome.
- Key is deciding whether surgical intervention is needed (see Table 3-3).

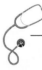

Appendicitis is still the most common surgical emergency in the pregnant woman.

▶ **SURGICAL CAUSES OF ABDOMINAL PAIN**

Right Upper Quadrant (RUQ)

Perforated duodenal ulcer
Acute cholecystitis
Hepatic abscess
Retrocecal appendicitis
Appendicitis in a pregnant woman

Patients with splenic rupture will have an elevated white count in the setting of trauma.

Right Lower Quadrant (RLQ)

Appendicitis
Cecal diverticulitis
Meckel's diverticulitis intussusception

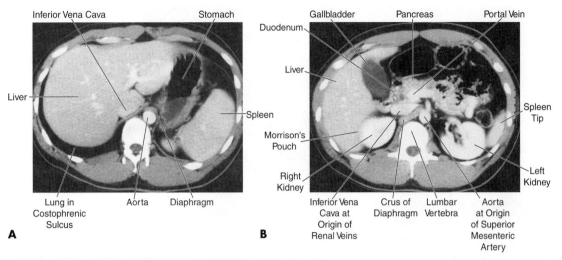

A

B

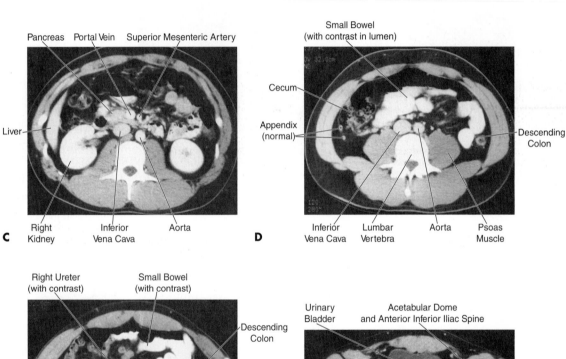

C

D

E

F

FIGURE 3-2. Abdominal CT anatomy.

Normal abdominopelvic CT scan of a 26-year-old man. Both oral and intravenous contrast was administered. **A.** Liver (right and left lobes), stomach, and spleen. **B.** Liver, gallbladder, kidneys, and pancreas. **C.** Kidneys, pancreas, and intestines. **D.** Small bowel, cecum, ascending colon, and normal appendix. **E.** Intestines and ureters at level of iliac wings. **F.** Bladder, distal ureters, and rectum at the level of the acetabular domes. (Reproduced, with permission, from Schwartz DT, Reisdorff EJ, eds. *Emergency Radiology*. New York: McGraw-Hill, 2000: 519.)

TABLE 3-3. Indications for Urgent Operation in Patients with Acute Abdomen

Physical findings

Involuntary guarding or rigidity, especially if spreading.

Increasing or severe localized tenderness.

Tense or progressive distention.

Tender abdominal or rectal mass with high fever or hypotension.

Rectal bleeding with shock or acidosis.

Equivocal abdominal findings along with—

Septicemia (high fever, marked or rising leukocytosis, mental changes, or increasing glucose intolerance in a diabetic patient).

Bleeding (unexplained shock or acidosis, falling hematocrit).

Suspected ischemia (acidosis, fever, tachycardia).

Deterioration on conservative treatment.

Radiologic findings

Pneumoperitoneum.

Gross or progressive bowel distention.

Free extravasation of contrast material.

Space-occupying lesion on scan, with fever.

Mesenteric occlusion on angiography.

Endoscopic findings

Perforated or uncontrollably bleeding lesion.

Paracentesis findings

Blood, bile, pus, bowel contents, or urine.

Reproduced, with permission, from Doherty GM. *Current Surgical Diagnosis & Treatment,* 12th ed. New York: McGraw-Hill; 2006: 491.

Left Lower Quadrant (LLQ)

Sigmoid diverticulitis
Volvulus

Left Upper Quadrant (LUQ)

Splenic rupture
Splenic abscess

Diffuse

Bowel obstruction
Leaking aneurysm
Mesenteric ischemia

Periumbilical

Early appendicitis
Pain from small bowel obstruction

Patients with bowel obstruction will initially be able to take in fluids by mouth, and vomit a short time afterward.

Abdominal aortic aneurysm (AAA): Pulsatile mass on physical exam.

Fitz-Hugh–Curtis syndrome is perihepatitis associated with chlamydial infection of cervix.

MI: Do an ECG on all patients presenting with midepigastric pain.

Pain of pancreatitis is described as boring, radiating straight to the back.

Suprapubic

Ectopic pregnancy
Ovarian torsion
Tubo-ovarian abscess
Psoas abscess
Incarcerated groin hernia

► **IMPORTANT NONSURGICAL CAUSES OF ABDOMINAL PAIN**

Myocardial infarction
Mittelschmerz
Poisoning (lead, black widow spider)
Herpes zoster
Lower lobe (RLL) pneumonia
Endocrine (Addisonian crisis, diabetic ketoacidosis)
Sickle cell crisis
Porphyrias
Psychological (hysteria)

HIGH-YIELD FACTS IN

Trauma

"Golden Hour" of Trauma

Period immediately following trauma in which rapid assessment, diagnosis, and stabilization must occur.

Primary Survey

Initial assessment and resuscitation of vital functions. Prioritization based on ABCs of trauma care.

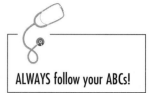

ALWAYS follow your ABCs!

ABCs

- **A**irway (with cervical spine precautions)
- **B**reathing and ventilation
- **C**irculation (and **C**ontrol of hemorrhage)
- **D**isability (neurologic status)
- **E**xposure/**E**nvironment control
- **F**oley

AIRWAY AND C-SPINE

- Assess patency of airway.
- Use jaw thrust or chin lift initially to open airway.
- Clear foreign bodies.
- Insert oral or nasal airway when necessary.
- Obtunded/unconscious patients should be intubated.
- Surgical airway = cricothyroidotomy—used when unable to intubate.

Assume C-spine injury in trauma patients until proven otherwise.

BREATHING AND VENTILATION

- Inspect, auscultate, and palpate the chest.
- Ensure adequate ventilation and identify and treat injuries that may immediately impair ventilation:
  - Tension pneumothorax
  - Flail chest and pulmonary contusion
  - Massive hemothorax
  - Open pneumothorax

All trauma patients should receive supplemental O_2.

CONTROL OF HEMORRHAGE

- Place two large-bore peripheral (14- or 16-gauge) IVs.
- Assess circulatory status (capillary refill, pulse, skin color) (see Shock section).
- Control of life-threatening hemorrhage using direct pressure.

Draw blood samples at the time of intravenous catheter placement.

DISABILITY

- Rapid neurologic exam.
- Establish pupillary size and reactivity and level of consciousness using the AVPU or Glasgow Coma Scale.

AVPU scale:
Alert
Verbal
Pain
Unresponsive

Don't forget to keep your patients warm (cover them up again as soon as possible).

Examine prostate and genitalia before placing a Foley.

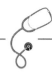

Place OGT rather than NGT when fracture of cribriform plate is suspected.

Trauma resuscitation requires teamwork with many different activities overlapping in both time and space.

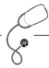

The antecubital fossae are a good place to find nice veins in which to place large-bore IVs.

Use **warmed** fluids whenever possible.

Exposure/Environment/Extras

Completely undress the patient.

Foley Catheter

- Placement of a urinary catheter is considered part of the resuscitative phase that takes place during the primary survey.
- Foley is contraindicated when urethral transection is suspected, such as in the case of a pelvic fracture. If transection suspected, perform retrograde urethrogram before Foley.

Signs of Urethral Transection

- Blood at the meatus.
- A "high-riding" prostate.
- Perineal or scrotal hematoma.
- Be suspicious with any pelvic fracture.

Gastric Intubation

Placement of nasogastric (NGT) or orogastric tube (OGT) may reduce risk of aspiration by decompressing stomach, but does not assure full prevention.

▶ RESUSCITATION

- Begins during the primary survey.
- Life-threatening injuries are tended to as they are identified.

Intravenous Fluid

- Fluid therapy should be initiated with up to 2 L of an isotonic (either lactated Ringer's or normal saline) crystalloid (see below) solution.
- Pediatric patients should receive an IV bolus of 20 cc/kg.

"3-to-1 Rule"

Used as a rough estimate for the total amount of crystalloid volume needed acutely to replace blood loss.

Shock

- Inadequate delivery of oxygen on the cellular level secondary to tissue hypoperfusion.
- In traumatic situations, shock is the result of hemorrhage until proven otherwise.

See Critical Care chapter.

Radiologic and Diagnostic Studies

- X-rays of the chest, pelvis, and lateral cervical spine usually occur concurrently with early resuscitative efforts; however, this procedure should never interrupt the resuscitative process.
- Diagnostic peritoneal lavage (DPL) and focused abdominal sonogram for trauma (FAST) are also tools used for the rapid detection of intra-abdominal bleeding that often occurs early in the resuscitative process (see Abdominal Trauma).
  - CT scans should be done only for patients who are hemodynamically stable.

Secondary Survey

TRAUMA HISTORY

- Begins once the primary survey is complete and resuscitative efforts are well under way. Whenever possible take an **AMPLE** history:
  - **A**llergies
  - **M**edications/**M**echanism of injury
  - **P**ast medical history/**P**regnant?
  - **L**ast meal
  - **E**vents surrounding the mechanism of injury
- Head-to-toe evaluation of the trauma patient; frequent reassessment is key.
- Neurologic examination including the GCS (see Table 23-2), procedures, radiologic examination, and laboratory testing take place at this time if not already accomplished.

Tetanus Prophylaxis

Immunize as needed.

▶ HEAD TRAUMA

See Neurosurgery chapter.

▶ NECK TRAUMA

General

Described in broad terms as penetrating vs. blunt injuries even though considerable overlap exists between the management of the two.

Anatomy

- The neck is divided into **zones** (see Figure 4-1):
  - Zone I lies below the cricoid cartilage.

Body water:
2/3 intracellular
1/3 extracellular:
1/4 intravascular
3/4 extravascular

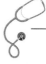
A "trauma series" consists of radiographs of the C-spine, chest, and pelvis.

"Fingers and tubes in every orifice."

The majority of the vital structures of the neck lie within the anterior triangle.

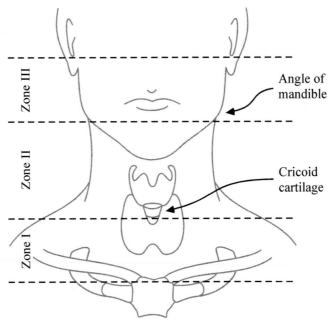

FIGURE 4-1. Zones of the neck.

- Zone II lies between I and III.
- Zone III lies above the angle of the mandible.
- These divisions help drive the diagnostic and therapeutic management decisions for penetrating neck injuries.

Penetrating Injuries

Any injury to the neck in which the platysma is violated.

VASCULAR INJURIES

- Very common and often life threatening.
- Can lead to exsanguination, hematoma formation with compromise of the airway, and cerebral vascular accidents (e.g., from transection of the carotid artery or air embolus).

NONVASCULAR INJURIES

- Injury to the larynx and trachea including fracture of the thyroid cartilage, dislocation of the tracheal cartilages and arytenoids, for example, leading to airway compromise and often a difficult intubation.
- Esophageal injury does occur and, as with penetrating neck injury, is not often manifest initially (very high morbidity/mortality if missed).

Resuscitation

- Obtain soft-tissue films of the neck for clues to the presence of a soft-tissue hematoma and subcutaneous emphysema, and a chest x-ray (CXR) for possible hemopneumothorax.

C-spine injuries are much more common with blunt neck injury.

Fracture of the hyoid bone is suggestive of a significant mechanism of injury.

Avoid unnecessary manipulation of the neck, as this may dislodge a clot.

Keep cervical in-line stabilization until C-spine fracture has been ruled out.

- Surgical exploration is indicated for:
  - Expanding hematoma
  - Subcutaneous emphysema
  - Tracheal deviation
  - Change in voice quality
  - Air bubbling through the wound
- Pulses should be palpated to identify deficits and thrills, and auscultated for bruits.
- A neurologic exam should be performed to identify brachial plexus and/or central nervous system (CNS) deficits as well as Horner's syndrome.

Management

- Zone II injuries with instability or enlarging hematoma require exploration in the OR.
- Injuries to Zones I and III may be taken to OR or managed conservatively using a combination of angiography, bronchoscopy, esophagoscopy, gastrografin or barium studies, and computed tomographic (CT) scanning.

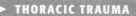

▶ SPINAL TRAUMA

See Neurosurgery chapter.

▶ THORACIC TRAUMA

Pericardial Tamponade

- Life-threatening emergency usually seen with penetrating thoracic trauma, but may be seen with blunt thoracic trauma as well.
- Signs include tachycardia, muffled heart sounds, jugular venous distention (JVD), hypotension, and electrical alternans on electrocardiogram (ECG) (see Figure 4-2).
- Diagnosis may be confirmed with cardiac sonogram (usually as part of focused assessment with sonography for trauma [FAST] ultrasound).
- Requires immediate decompression via needle pericardiocentesis, pericardial window, or thoracotomy with manual decompression.

Blunt Cardiac Trauma

- Usually secondary to motor vehicle collision (MVC), fall from heights, crush injury, blast injury, direct violent trauma.
- Screening: ECG.

Tracheostomy is the procedure of choice in the patient with laryngotracheal separation.

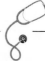
Control of hemorrhage in the emergency department is via direct pressure (no blind clamping).

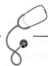
Never blindly probe a neck wound, as this may lead to bleeding in a previously tamponaded wound.

Beck's tamponade triad:
1. Hypotension
2. JVD
3. Muffled heart sounds

Clinically apparent tamponade may result from 60–100 mL of blood.

HIGH-YIELD FACTS

Trauma

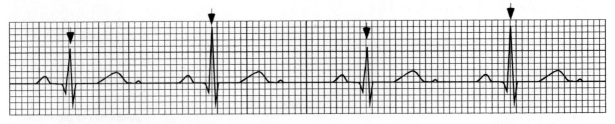

FIGURE 4-2. ECG demonstrating electrical alternans.

Note alternating heights of the R in the QRS complexes.

1. Pericardium should be opened anterior and parallel to phrenic nerve (longitudinally).
2. Lacerations are repaired with 3-0 nonabsorbable suture and pledgets.
3. A Foley catheter with inflated balloon may be used as a temporizing measure to gain control for large defects.

Typical scenario: A 19-year-old male who was stabbed in the chest with a knife presents complaining of dyspnea. Breath sounds on the left are absent. *Think:* Pneumothorax.

The neurovascular bundle runs on the inferior margin of each rib.

Pneumothorax

DEFINITION

Air in the pleural space.

SIGNS AND SYMPTOMS

- Usually asymptomatic.
  - Chest pain
- Dyspnea.
- Hyperresonance of affected side.
- Decreased breath sounds of affected side.

DIAGNOSIS

Upright chest x-ray is ~83% sensitive and demonstrates an absence of lung markings where the lung has collapsed (see Figure 4-3).

TREATMENT

Tube thoracostomy: Chest tube placement should be confirmed by chest x-ray.

Tension Pneumothorax

- Life-threatening emergency caused by air entering the pleural space (most often via a hole in the lung tissue) and unable to escape.
- Causes total ipsilateral lung collapse and mediastinal shift (away from injured lung), impairing venous return and thus decreased cardiac output, eventually resulting in shock.

SIGNS AND SYMPTOMS

Same as for pneumothorax, *plus* tracheal deviation away from affected side (in tension pneumothorax).

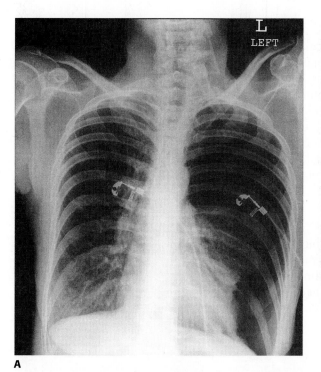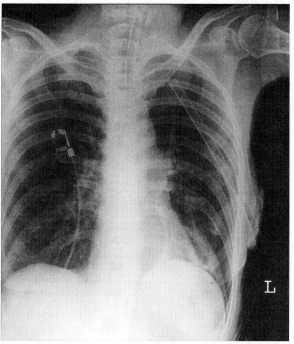

A   **B**

FIGURE 4-3. **A. CXR demonstrating left-sided pneumothorax. (Note lack of lung markings.) B. Same patient, after tube thoracostomy and endotracheal intubation.**

TREATMENT

- Requires immediate needle decompression followed by tube thoracostomy.
- Needle decompression involves placing a needle or catheter over a needle into the second intercostal space, midclavicular line, over the rib on the side of the tension pneumothorax, followed by a tube thoracostomy (chest tube).

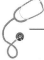

When the clamp enters the pleura, a rush of air or fluid should be obtained.

Hemothorax

The presence of blood in the chest.

- More than 200 cc of blood must be present before blunting of costophrenic angle will be seen on CXR.
- Treatment involves chest tube placement and drainage, and control of bleeding.

INDICATIONS FOR THORACOTOMY

- 1,500 cc initial drainage from the chest tube.
- 200 cc/hr for 4 hours continued drainage:
  - Thoracic great vessel injury.
  - Esophageal injury.
  - Patients who decompensate after initial stabilization.

Size of chest tube to use:
For adult large hemothorax: 36–40 French.
For adult pneumothorax: 24 French or pigtail catheter.
For children: Four times the size of appropriate endotracheal tube size:

$$ET\ tube\ size = \frac{age + 16}{4}$$

A diagnosis of tension pneumothorax via x-ray is a missed diagnosis. Do not delay treatment of a suspected tension pneumothorax in order to confirm your suspicion (i.e., tension pneumothorax is a clinical diagnosis).

Remember to confirm appropriate chest tube placement with CXR.

- One fourth of hemothorax cases have an associated pneumothorax.
- Three fourths of hemothorax cases are associated with extrathoracic injuries.

Bleeding usually stops spontaneously for low-velocity gunshot wounds and most stab wounds.

DIAGNOSTIC MODALITIES

- Angiography to localize injury and plan appropriate operation.
- CT scan for patients with normal initial CXR but suspicious mechanism and requiring CT for other reasons. If CT identifies injury, angiography still required for precise delineation of injury.
- Transesophageal echocardiogram (TEE):
  - Fast, no contrast required, concurrent evaluation of cardiac function, versatile in terms of location.
  - Contraindicated if potential airway problem or C-spine injury.
  - Not as sensitive or specific as angiography or CT scan.
  - User dependent.

DEFINITIVE TREATMENT

- Surgical: Control bleeding, reconstruction, with graft if needed.
- Control hypertension pharmacologically.
- Endovascular stenting.
- Cardiac bypass as needed.
- Nonoperative: Close observation and pharmacologic treatment.

▶ ABDOMINAL TRAUMA

General

Penetrating abdominal injuries (PAIs; see Figure 4-4) resulting from a gunshot wound create damage via three mechanisms:

1. Direct injury by the bullet itself.
2. Injury from fragmentation of the bullet.
3. Indirect injury from the resultant "shock wave."

PAIs resulting from a stabbing mechanism are limited to the direct damage of the object of impalement.

Blunt abdominal injuries (BAIs) also have three general mechanisms of injury:

1. Injury caused by the direct blow.
2. Crush injury.
3. Deceleration injury.

Physical Examination

SIGNS

- **Seat-belt sign**—ecchymotic area found in the distribution of the lower anterior abdominal wall and can be associated with perforation of the bladder or bowel as well as a lumbar distraction fracture (Chance fracture).
- **Cullen's sign** (periumbilical ecchymosis) is indicative of intraperitoneal hemorrhage.
- **Grey-Turner's sign** (flank ecchymoses) is indicative of retroperitoneal hemorrhage.
- **Kehr's sign**—left shoulder or neck pain secondary to splenic rupture. It increases when patient is in Trendelenburg position or with left upper quadrant (LUQ) palpation (caused by diaphragmatic irritation).

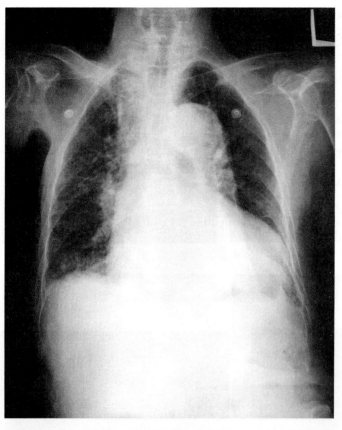

FIGURE 4-4. CXR illustrating wide mediastinum due to penetrating trauma of the ascending aorta.

GENERAL

- Inspect the abdomen for evisceration, entry/exit wounds, impaled objects, and a gravid uterus.
- Check for tenderness, guarding, and rebound.

DIAGNOSIS

- Perforation: AXR and CXR to look for free air.
- Diaphragmatic injury: CXR to look for blurring of the diaphragm, hemothorax, or bowel gas patterns above the diaphragm (at times with a gastric tube seen in the left chest).

Focused Abdominal Sonography for Trauma (FAST)

- Positive if free fluid is demonstrated in the abdomen.
- Four views are utilized to search for free intraperitoneal fluid (presumed to be blood in the trauma victim) that collects in dependent areas and appears as hypoechoic areas on ultrasound (see Figures 4-5 and 4-6):
  - Morrison's pouch (RUQ): Free fluid can be visualized between the liver and kidney.
  - Splenorenal recess (LUQ): Free fluid can be visualized between the spleen and kidney.

Potential causes of iatrogenic great vessel injury:
- Central venous pressure (CVP) line or chest tube placement
- Intra-aortic balloon pump (IABP) placement
- Overinflation of Swan–Ganz balloon

Traumatic aortic rupture is a high-mortality injury: Almost 90% die at the scene, and another 50% die within 24 hours.

- Patient should be prepped and draped from sternum to knees to allow alternate access from the groins in the event of an emergency.
- Traditional approach (i.e., left anterolateral sternotomy) is used for the unstable patient with an undiagnosed injury.
- Angiography in the stable patient may dictate an alternate operative approach based on the location of injury.

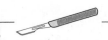

Safe margin for cross-clamping of aorta to control bleeding is < 30 minutes.

Typical scenario: A 25-year-old female presents after a high-speed MVC with dyspnea and tachycardia. There is local bruising over right side of her chest. CXR shows a right upper lobe consolidation. *Think:* Pulmonary contusion.

The most frequently injured solid organ associated with penetrating trauma is the **liver**.

ADVANTAGES

- Performed at bedside.
- Widely available.
- Highly sensitive for hemoperitoneum.
- Rapidly performed.

DISADVANTAGES

- Invasive.
- Risk for iatrogenic injury (< 1%).
- Low specificity (many false positives).
- Does not evaluate the retroperitoneum.

CT Scanning

- Useful for the hemodynamically stable patient.
- Has a greater specificity than DPL and ultrasound (US).
- Noninvasive.
- Relatively time consuming when compared with FAST.

Angiography

- May be used to identify and embolize pelvic arterial bleeding secondary to pelvic fractures, or to assess blunt renal artery injuries diagnosed by CT scan.
- Otherwise limited use for abdominal trauma.

Serial Hematocrits

Serial hematocrits (every 4–6 hours) should be obtained during the observation period of the hemodynamically stable patient.

Laparoscopy

- Usage is increasing (mainly to identify peritoneal penetration from gunshot/knife wound), especially for the stable or marginally stable patient who would otherwise require a laparotomy.
- Helpful for evaluation of diaphragm.
- May help to decrease negative laparotomy rate.
- However, may miss hollow organ injuries.

Indications for Exploratory Laparotomy

- Abdominal trauma and hemodynamic instability.
- Evisceration.

- Peritonitis.
- Diaphragmatic injury (see Figure 4-7).
- Hollow viscus perforation: Free intraperitoneal air.
- Intraperitoneal bladder rupture (diagnosed by cystography).
- Positive DPL.
- Surgically correctable injury diagnosed on CT scan.
- Removal of impaled weapon.
- Rectal perforation.
- Transabdominal missile (bullet) path (e.g., a gunshot wound to the buttock with the bullet being found in the abdomen or thorax).

Types of Injury: General Approach

Liver Injury

See Hepatobiliary System chapter.

Splenic Trauma

See Spleen chapter.

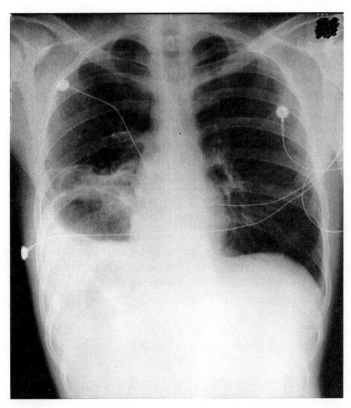

FIGURE 4-7. CXR demonstrating ruptured diaphragm. Note elevation and irregular contour of diaphragm, and viscera in chest.

The most frequently injured solid organs associated with blunt trauma are the liver and spleen.

Peritonitis and guarding in a neurologically intact patient obviate the need for much diagnostic workup. Trauma laparotomy is indicated in this setting.

In a stable patient with neurologic dysfunction, whether from drugs, alcohol, head trauma, or baseline dementia, exam findings have a limited ability to direct care. These patients often require additional diagnostic tests.

Serial abdominal examinations should be performed.

DPL should be undertaken only after gastric and urinary decompression.

DPL is especially useful in marginal or unstable patients with equivocal ultrasounds and for patients with hollow viscus injuries.

If pelvic fracture is suspected, a supraumbilical approach should be used for DPL.

Criteria for a positive DPL:
- > 10 mL gross blood on initial aspiration.
- Presence of bile, stool, or intestinal contents.
- > 100,000 red blood cells (RBCs).
- > 500 white blood cells (WBCs).
- Gram stain with bacteria or vegetable matter.
- Amylase > 20 IU/L.

Absolute contraindication for DPL: Clear indication for laparotomy (e.g., peritonitis).

CT is the most sensitive test for retroperitoneal injury.

Bowel Injury

STOMACH, JEJUNUM, AND ILEUM

- Isolated leaks from penetrating trauma lead to minimal contamination and patients usually do well if diagnosis is not delayed.
- Blunt injuries are "blowouts" resulting frequently from lap belts, and occur near the ligament of Treitz and the ileocecal valve.
- Mesentery can be significantly injured following blunt trauma.
- **Diagnosis:**
  - If the patient is awake and reliable, the exam is important to look for peritoneal irritation.
  - If the exam is not reliable, DPL or laparoscopy may be required.
  - CT scan has a high false-negative rate for small bowel injuries.
  - Look for free air on CXR.
  - Laparotomy for gastric or small bowel injury with primary repair and peritoneal lavage except in cases that have heavy soiling of the peritoneal cavity and present late, where intestinal diversion must be considered (e.g., ileostomy).
    - Small bowel resection is needed where more than 50% of the bowel circumference is transected or several penetrating injuries are present within a very short segment of bowel where resecting is a better option than individually repairing each hole.

DUODENUM

- **Mechanisms:** Three fourths of injuries result from penetrating trauma.
- **Diagnosis:**
  - Upper GI series with water-soluble contrast.
  - CT and DPL often miss duodenal injuries.
- **Treatment:**
  - Eighty percent of patients are able to undergo a primary repair.
  - Repair may be protected with an omental patch, jejunal serosal patch and/or gastric diversion.
  - More complex injuries need pyloric exclusion or rarely pancreaticoduodenectomy (Whipple procedure).

LARGE BOWEL

- Injuries generally occur via a penetrating mechanism (75% gunshot wound, 25% stab wound). Blunt injuries are rare but result from MVCs. Iatrogenic transanal injuries may also occur.
- **Signs and symptoms:** Abdominal distention, tenderness, guaiac-positive stool.
- **Diagnosis:**
  - In an awake and reliable patient, exam findings are consistent with peritonitis.
  - CXR may show free air.
  - In a patient with a flank injury but without clear peritoneal signs, consider a contrast enema.
- **Treatment:**
  - Primary repair: For small or medium-sized perforations, repair the perforation or, if needed, resect the affected segment and close with primary anastomosis. A proximal diverting stoma (e.g., ileostomy) is commonly placed.
  - Anastomosis is contraindicated in the setting of massive soiling.

RECTUM

- Two thirds are extraperitoneal.
- **Mechanism:** Majority by gunshot injury.
- **Diagnosis:**
  - DRE/guaiac: Suspicion increased by blood in stool or palpation of defect or foreign body on exam.
  - Rigid proctoscopy: May be done in OR if needed; mandatory for patients with known trajectory of knife or gunshot wound across pelvis or transanal; if patient is unstable, may be delayed until after resuscitation.
  - X-ray to look for missiles or foreign bodies.
- **Treatment:**
- Diversion via colostomy is key.
- Extraperitoneal injuries must be diverted via colostomy but may not need to be repaired (if not too big and not easily accessible).
- Colostomy may be closed in 3–4 months.

ANUS

- Reconstruct sphincter as soon as patient is stabilized.
- Divert with sigmoid colostomy.

▶ PANCREATIC INJURY

GENERAL

- **Mechanism:** Largely penetrating (gunshot wound >> stab wound).
- Seventy-five percent of patients with penetrating injury to the pancreas will have associated injuries to the aorta, portal vein, or inferior vena cava.

DIAGNOSIS

- Inspect pancreas during laparotomies performed for other indications.
- Check amylase (may be elevated).
- CT: Look for parenchymal fracture, intraparenchymal hematoma, lesser sac fluid, fluid between splenic vein and pancreatic body, retroperitoneal hematoma or fluid.
- Endoscopic retrograde cholangiopancreatography (ERCP): May be used in the stable patient if readily available or available intraoperatively; also may be used to evaluate missed injuries.

TREATMENT

- Nonoperative: May follow with serial labs and exam if patient can be reliably examined.
- Operative:
  - No ductal injury: Hemostasis and external drainage.
  - Distal transection, parenchymal injury with ductal injury: Distal pancreatectomy with duct ligation.
  - When duodenum or pancreatic head is devitalized, consider Whipple or total pancreatectomy.
  - Proximal transection/injury with probable ductal disruption:
    - If duct is spared, external drainage.
    - If duct is damaged, external drainage and pancreatic duct stenting may be considered.

Contrast use:
- Noncontrast to look for intraparenchymal hematomas.
- PO contrast to assess location and integrity of upper gastrointestinal (GI) tract.
- IV contrast to look for organ or vascular injury.
- Contrast enema to evaluate the colon and rectum.

Trauma laparotomy:
- Midline incision.
- Pack all four quadrants with laparotomy pads.
- Evacuation of gross blood and clot.
- Control bleeding.
- Resuscitate as needed.
- Systematically remove pads and inspect for source(s) of injury.
- Definitive repair based on stability of patient and type of injury.

Any wound from the nipple line to the gluteal crease can cause peritoneal or retroperitoneal injury.

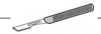

Have a low threshold for conversion to laparotomy during laparoscopy.

Because of a common mechanism, Chance fractures and blunt small bowel injury are strongly associated. If one is present, you should look for the other.

To determine viability of the bowel in the OR, inject fluorescein dye IV, and use a Wood's lamp to inspect the bowel. Nonviable bowel will have patchy or no fluorescence.

Duodenal hematoma may result from an MVC, but has been found to be associated with child abuse in the pediatric population. Patients present with signs and symptoms of small bowel obstruction and require CT/upper GI series for diagnosis. Treatment is nonoperative and includes NGT decompression, total parental nutrition (TPN), and reevaluation with upper GI series after about 1 week.

Thirty percent of patients with rectal injury will have an associated injury to the bladder.

General

- Often overlooked in the initial evaluation of the multiply injured trauma victim.
- Diagnostic evaluation of the GU tract is performed in a "retrograde" fashion (i.e., work your way back from the urethra to the kidneys and renal vasculature).

Signs and Symptoms

- Flank or groin pain.
- Blood at the urethral meatus.
- Ecchymoses on perineum and/or genitalia.
- Evidence of pelvic fracture.
- Rectal bleeding.
- A "high-riding" or superiorly displaced prostate.

Urinalysis

- The presence of gross hematuria indicates GU injury and often concomitant pelvic fracture.
- Urinalysis should be done to document presence or absence of microscopic hematuria.
- Microscopic hematuria is usually self-limited.

Retrograde Urethrogram

- Should be performed in any patient with suspected urethral disruption (before Foley placement).
- A preinjection KUB (kidneys, ureters, bladder) film should always be taken.

Retrograde Cystogram

- Should be performed on patients with gross hematuria or a pelvic fracture.
- Extravasation of contrast into the pouch of Douglas, paracolic gutters, and between loops of intestine is diagnostic for intraperitoneal rupture.
- Extravasation of contrast into the paravesicular tissue or behind the bladder is indicative of extraperitoneal bladder rupture.

Bladder Rupture

INTRAPERITONEAL

- Usually occurs secondary to blunt trauma to a full bladder.
- Treatment is surgical repair.

EXTRAPERITONEAL

- Usually occurs secondary to pelvic fracture.
- Treatment is nonsurgical management by Foley drainage.

Ureteral Injury

- Least common GU injury (mostly iatrogenic).
- Must be surgically repaired.
- Diagnosed at the time of IVP or CT scan during the search for renal injury.

Renal Injury

- Commonly diagnosed by CT scan with contrast.
- Grade IV and V operative; the rest conservative (see Table 4-1 and Figure 4-8).

TABLE 4-1. **Urologic Injury Scale of the American Association for the Surgery of Trauma**

	GRADE	INJURY DESCRIPTION
Renal Injury Scale		
I	Contusion	Microscopic or gross hematuria; urologic studies normal
	Hematoma	Subcapsular, nonexpanding without parenchymal laceration
II	Hematoma	Nonexpanding perirenal hematoma confined to the renal retroperitoneum
	Laceration	< 1 cm parenchymal depth of renal cortex without urinary extravasation
III	Laceration	> 1 cm parenchymal depth of renal cortex without collecting-system rupture or urinary extravasation
IV	Laceration	Parenchymal laceration extending through the renal cortex, medulla, and collecting system
	Vascular	Main renal artery or vein injury with contained hemorrhage
V	Laceration	Completely shattered kidney
	Vascular	Avulsion of renal hilum that devascularizes kidney

Modified, with permission, from Feliciano DV, Mattox KL, Moore EE, *Trauma*, 6th ed. New York, NY: McGraw-Hill; 2008: T. 39-1.

Minimizing the time from injury to treatment is important in minimizing morbidity and mortality associated with pancreatic injury.

Eighty percent of pancreas can be resected without endocrine or exocrine dysfunction.

Suspect GU trauma with:
- Straddle injury: Pelvic fracture.
- Penetrating injury to lower abdomen.
- Falls from height.
- Hematuria noted on Foley insertion.

Blood at the urethral meatus is virtually diagnostic for urethral injury and demands early retrograde urethrogram before Foley placement.

Do not probe perineal lacerations as they are often a sign of an underlying pelvic fracture and disruption of a hematoma may occur.

Signs of arterial insufficiency: **The 6 Ps**
Pain
Pallor
Paresthesias
Pulse deficit
Poikilothermia
Paralysis

Rhabdomyolysis causes myoglobin release, which can cause renal failure. Maintaining a high urine output together with alkalinization of the urine can help prevent the renal failure by reducing precipitation of myoglobin in the kidney.

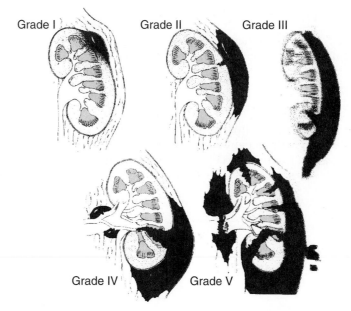

Grade I Grade II Grade III

Grade IV Grade V

FIGURE 4-8.   **Organ injury scaling system for renal trauma.**

(Reproduced, with permission, from Feliciano DV, Mattox KL, Moore EE. *Trauma*, 6th ed. New York: McGraw-Hill, 2008: Fig. 39-6).

Critical Care

Think ABCs with any patient in "shock": Secure airway, breathing, and circulation.

If the skin is warm, it is distributive shock. If the skin is cold and clammy, it is hypovolemic or cardiogenic shock. Shock with bradycardia is neurogenic unless proved otherwise.

Shock in trauma or postop patient is assumed to be hypovolemic until proven otherwise.

Of the vital organs, the first "casualty" of hypovolemic or cardiogenic shock (both "cold shocks") is the kidneys, as blood is shunted away from the constricted renal arteries. Therefore, it is crucial to monitor for renal failure. An adequate urine output is one of the crucial signs that the treatment is adequate.

HIGH-YIELD FACTS

Critical Care

Definition

Shock is defined as inadequate delivery of oxygen and nutrients to maintain normal tissue and cellular function.

Shock becomes irreversible if not treated early.

Pathophysiology and Types of Shock

Shock describes a state of imbalance between tissue substrate delivery (supply) and tissue substrate consumption (demand).

Tissue perfusion is determined by:

1. Cardiac Output (CO) = Stroke Volume (SV) × Heart Rate (HR)
2. Systemic Vascular Resistance (SVR) = [Mean Arterial Pressure (MAP) – Central Venous Pressure (CVP)] / [CO]
3. BP = CO × SVR

Deterioration in any one of these factors can cause hypotension and shock. Shock is classified into different types according to which of these factors are abnormal. The three major types of shock are **hypovolemic, distributive (includes septic, anaphylactic, and neurogenic),** and **cardiogenic.**

Note: The first step in treatment of any type of shock is control of airway and breathing, next is restoration of circulation (ABC).

HYPOVOLEMIC SHOCK—REDUCED VENOUS RETURN, ADEQUATE PUMP FUNCTION

DEFINITION

Decreased tissue perfusion secondary to rapid volume/blood loss (i.e., preload). **CO is consequently decreased.** The causes include bleeding, vomiting/diarrhea, and third spacing (e.g., from burns, bowel obstruction, pancreatitis). Most common cause in surgical or trauma patient is hemorrhagic shock.

SIGNS AND SYMPTOMS

Early on, patients will have tachycardia, orthostatic hypotension, and cool skin. As the condition progresses, they are hypotensive, have decreased pulse pressure, become confused, and have cold, clammy skin due to "clamping down" of peripheral vessels via increased sympathetic tone.

CLASSIFICATION OF SEVERITY OF HYPOVOLEMIC SHOCK

Class I—Compensated: Loss of < 15% of circulating blood volume. Little or no clinical manifestations.

Class II—Partially compensated: Loss of 15–30% of blood volume. Manifestations include mild tachycardia, tachypnea, anxiety, orthostatic hypotension, decreased pulse pressure, and oliguria. Reduced splanchnic and renal blood flow.

Class III—Uncompensated: Loss of 30–40% of blood volume. Hypotension, oliguria, marked tachycardia, and confusion.

Class IV—Life threatening: Loss of > 40% of circulating blood volume. All of the above plus lethargy, mental status change, severe hypotension, and oliguria or anuria. Needs operative control of bleeding.

- Rapid initial FLUID resuscitation! Crystalloids (normal saline [NS]/ lactated Ringer's [LR]) infusion via two large-bore peripheral IVs is best for volume repletion. Adequate resuscitation requires 3–4 mL of fluid for each 1 mL of shed blood.
  - Normal saline vs. lactated Ringer's: Large-volume NS infusion may result in hyperchloremic acidosis. Therefore, LR (containing alternative anions to Cl-) is the preferred choice.
  - Colloid vs. isotonic crystalloid: No evidence that colloid fluids improve mortality in critically ill patients.
- Replacement of blood if hemorrhage is cause.
- Treat underlying cause (i.e., surgical correction if patient has ongoing hemorrhage). Failure to respond to fluid resuscitation is usually due to persistent massive hemorrhage, hence requiring emergent surgical procedure.

DISTRIBUTIVE SHOCK

DEFINITION

A family of shock states that are caused by systemic vasodilation (i.e., severe decrease in SVR). They include septic shock (most common), neurogenic shock, and anaphylactic shock. These patients will have warm skin from vasodilation.

SEPTIC SHOCK

Infection that causes vessels to dilate and leak, causing hypotension refractory to fluid recuscitation.

LAB/PHYSICAL FINDINGS

- Physical exam findings—fever, tachypnea, warm skin and full peripheral pulses (from vasodilation), normal urine output.
- Later, delayed physical examination findings include vasoconstriction, poor urinary output, mental status changes, and hypotension.
- Positive blood cultures (negative about 50% of the time, particularly if drawn after antibiotics are started).

THE CONTINUUM

SIRS → Sepsis → Severe Sepsis → Septic Shock

Septic shock is the most severe manifestation of infection in a continuum. Milder manifestations of infection are classified as systemic inflammatory response syndrome (SIRS), sepsis, and severe sepsis (Figure 5-1 and Table 5-1).

TREATMENT

- Fluids!!
- Antibiotics: **Start broad-spectrum antibiotics early** and empirically treat until blood cultures come back!!
  - Surgical drainage of abscess or focus of infection.

Tachycardia is the first symptom in hypovolemic shock.
Factors that suppress the tachycardic response to hypovolemia:
- Beta blockers
- Atheletes
- Damage to autonomic nervous system (as in spinal shock)
- Never use dextrose-containing solution for resuscitation.

Adequate (at minimum) urine output is 0.5 cc/kg/hr = 35 cc/hr for average 70-kg person.

Poor prognostic signs in septic shock:
- Disseminated intravascular coagulation (DIC).
- Multiple organ failure.

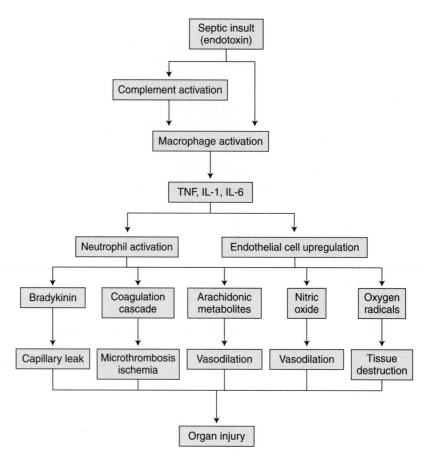

FIGURE 5-1. Schematic depiction of physiologic consequences of septic insult.

TABLE 5-1. Clinical Spectrum of Infection and Systemic Inflammatory Response Syndrome (SIRS)

Term	Definition
Infection	Identifiable source of microbial insult
SIRS	Two or more of following criteria Temperature $\geq 38°C$ or $\leq 36°C$ Heart rate ≥ 90 beats/min Respiratory rate ≥ 20 breaths/min or $Paco_2 \leq 32$ mmHg or mechanical ventilation White blood cell count $\geq 12,000/\mu L$ or $\leq 4,000/\mu L$ or $\geq 10\%$ band forms
Sepsis	Identifiable source of infection + SIRS
Severe sepsis	Sepsis + organ dysfunction
Septic shock	Sepsis + cardiovascular collapse (requiring vasopressor support)

Reproduced, with permission, from Brunicardi FC, Andersen DK, Billiar TR, et al. *Schwartz's Principles of Surgery,* 8th ed. New York: McGraw-Hill, 2004: 4.

- If blood pressure is unresponsive to fluids, use pressors, classically nor-epinephrine (Levophed).
  - Tight glycemic control (maintain blood glucose 80–150). Tight glucose management has been shown to reduce mortality and morbidity in the intensive care unit (ICU).
  - Activated protein C may have some role in patients with sepsis and dysfunction of two or more organs. Causes bleeding, so use is restricted in surgical patients.

ANAPHYLACTIC SHOCK

Systemic type I hypersensitivity reaction causing chemically mediated angio-edema and increased vascular permeability, resulting in hypotension and/or airway compromise.

SALIENT PHYSICAL FINDINGS

- Urticaria and anigoedema (especially around lips).
- Laryngeal edema (stridor), wheezing.

TREATMENT

- Epinephrine
- Antihistamines (diphenhydramine)
- Steroids

NEUROGENIC SHOCK

Central nervous system (CNS) injury causing disruption of the sympathetic system, resulting in unopposed vagal outflow and vasodilation. It is characterized by hypotension and bradycardia (absence of reflex sympathetic tachycardia and vasoconstriction). Usually secondary to spinal cord injury of cervical or high thoracic region.

TREATMENT

- IV fluids: Usually patients respond; helps to place patient in Trendelenburg position.
- Vasopressors: Used early if patient is unresponsive to fluids.

CARDIOGENIC SHOCK

Pump failure, resulting in decreased cardiac output (CO). This can be caused by myocardial infarction (MI), arrhythmias, valvular defects, cardiac contusion, or extracardiac obstruction (tamponade, pulmonary embolism, tension pneumothorax). Wedge pressure and SVR are elevated.

FINDINGS

Patients will have cold, clammy skin from peripheral vasoconstriction. Additionally, they will have jugular venous distention (JVD), dyspnea, bilateral crackles, and S3/4 gallop. Chest x-ray (CXR) will show bilateral pulmonary congestion. Echocardiography demonstrates poorly contractile left ventricle, pulmonary capillary wedge pressure (PCWP) > 20 mmHg, cardiac index (CI) < 2.0.

Gram-negative bacteria are notorious for causing septic shock.
Most common gram-negative organisms: *Escherichia coli, Klebsiella, Pseudomonas aeruginosa.*
Top three gram-positive organisms: *Staphylococcus aureus, Enterococcus,* coagulase-negative *Staphylococcus.*

Even when SIRS criteria are met, infection is present < 50% of the time.

Causes of anaphylaxis: Drugs (penicillin), radiocontrast, insect bites (honeybee, fire ant, wasp), and food (shellfish, peanut butter).

Remember, type I hypersensitivity reactions are immunoglobulin E (IgE) mediated and require prior exposure.

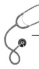

TREATMENT

- Correct electrolyte abnormalities: Most commonly hypokalemia and hypomagnesemia.
- Pain control: IV morphine sulfate or fentanyl to minimize anxiety.
- Antiarrythmics, cardiac pacing, or cardioversion for pathologic dysrhythmias or heart block.
- Treatment of cardiogenic shock is specific to cause:
  - Acute MI: Oxygen, nitroglycerin, aspirin, IV morphine, cardiology consultation.
  - Cardiac contusion: Infusion of inotropes. Intra-aortic balloon pump can provide temporary treatment.
  - Cardiac tamponade: Pericardiocentesis for aspiration of fluid or blood; surgical exploration to repair possible heart wound.
  - Massive pulmonary embolism: IV heparin (unless contraindication of bleeding), recombinant tPA, embolectomy as alternative to thrombolysis.
- **Left heart failure or biventricular failure:**
  - Isolated left ventricular failure: Pressors, and reduce afterload.
  - Congestive heart failure: Diuretics and vasodilators (nitrates) to decrease preload. May or may not use pressors.
  - Classically, the following inotropes can be used:
    - Dobutamine: Used after dopamine to increase cardiac contractility.
    - Amrinone and milrinone (phosphodiesterase inhibitors): Used in patients unresponsive to dopamine or dobutamine.
  - Intra-aortic balloon pump (IABP): Used as mechanical support in patients who do not respond to pressors or inotropes. IABP increases CO, and decreases work of heart by reducing systolic afterload and increasing diastolic perfusion to coronary arteries. Device can be inserted percutaneously via femoral artery at the ICU bedside.
- **Isolated right heart failure:**
  - Most commonly caused by right ventricular infarction or PE.
  - Give fluids (maintains preload).

See Table 5-2.

► SWAN-GANZ CATHETER

The Swan-Ganz catheter (pulmonary artery catheter) is often used with ICU and shock patients in order to obtain information relevant to fluid and volume

TABLE 5-2. Types of Shock and Their Hemodynamic Profiles

	PCWP	CO	SVR
Hypovolemic shock	↓↓	↓	↑
Cardiogenic shock	↑	↓↓	↑
Neurogenic shock	↓	↓	↓
Distributive shock	↓ or normal	↑	↓↓

status. It is threaded via the subclavian or internal jugular into superior vena cava → right atrium → right ventricle → pulmonary artery.

The following are some of the measurements obtainable through the Swan-Ganz that will allow a better understanding of the different types of shock (Table 5-3):

- **Pulmonary artery occlusion pressure (PAOP or PCWP)** (normal 6–12 mmHg). This reflects the pressures of the left ventricle (end-diastolic pressure). It can be thought of as preload.
  Clinical context: If the pump fails, pressures in the left ventricle increase and you will have an increased wedge.
- **Cardiac output (CO)** (normal 4–8 mmHg). Remember, CO = Stroke Volume × Heart Rate. The Swan-Ganz allows CO to be measured via the **thermodilutional technique:** The temperature change is measured at the distal end of the catheter when cold fluid is injected from the proximal port. The difference in temperature reflects the CO, which can also be thought of as pump function.

End points of resuscitation for shock of any etiology:
- Normalization of lactate (marker of oxygen debt), base deficit, and pH.
- Normalization of mixed venous oxygen saturation (marker of oxygen delivery and extraction) and CO.
- Urine output—most useful measure of effective fluid resuscitation (marker of renal perfusion).

TABLE 5-3. Normal Ranges for Selected Hemodynamic Parameters in Adults

PARAMETER	NORMAL RANGE
CVP	0–6 mmHg
Right ventricular systolic pressure	20–30 mmHg
Right ventricular diastolic pressure	0–6 mmHg
PAOP	6–12 mmHg
Systolic arterial pressure	100–130 mmHg
Diastolic arterial pressure	60–90 mmHg
MAP	75–100 mmHg
Q_T	4–6 L/min
Q_{T^*}	2.5–3.5 L · min^{-1} · m^{-2}
SV	40–80 mL
SVR	800–1,400 dyne · sec · cm^{-5}
SVRI	1500–2,400 dyne · sec · cm^{-5} · m^{-2}
PVR	100–150 dyne · sec · cm^{-5}
PVRI	200–400 dyne · sec · cm^{-5} · m^{-2}
Cao_2	16–22 mL/dL
Cvo_2	~15 mL 02 dL blood
$\dot{D}o_2$	400–660 mL · min^{-1} · m^{-2}
$\dot{V}o_2$	115–165 mL · min^{-1} · m^{-2}

Cao_2 = arterial oxygen content; Cvo_2 = central venous oxygen pressure; CVP = mean central venous pressure; $\dot{D}o_2$ = systemic oxygen delivery; MAP = mean arterial pressure; PAOP = pulmonary artery occlusion (wedge) pressure; PVR = pulmonary vascular resistance; PVRI = pulmonary vascular resistance index; Q_T = cardiac output; Q_{T^*} = cardiac output indexed to body surface area (cardiac index); SV = stroke volume; SVI = stroke volume index; SVR = systemic vascular resistance; SVRI = systemic vascular resistance index; $\dot{V}o_2$ = systemic oxygen utilization.

Reproduced, with permission, from Brunicardi FC, Andersen DK, Billiar TR, et al. *Schwartz's Principles of Surgery*, 8th ed. New York: McGraw-Hill, 2004: 366.

Risks of the Swan-Ganz:
- Infection.
- Arrhythmia (the guidewire can irritate the endocardium and trigger this). Injury of the pulmonary artery.

How is the wedge pressure obtained? The "wedge" pressure is obtained by inflating the distal end of the Swan-Ganz and "floating" this "balloon" down the pulmonary artery until it "wedges." The pressure measured equals the pulmonary capillary pressure, and this, theoretically, represents the left atrial pressure and ultimately the left ventricular end-diastolic pressure (LVEDP).

What is the significance of the wedge pressure? It reflects the left ventricular pressure, which will be increased with left ventricular failure.

- **Clinical context:** If you have an MI and lose wall motion, your stroke volume will be decreased. Likewise, if you hemorrhage and have no preload, your stroke volume will decrease as well.
- **Systemic vascular resistance (SVR)** (usually divided by body surface area to give systemic vascular resistance index [SVRI]): SVR reflects the vascular resistance across the systemic circulation (it can be thought of as afterload as well).
- **Clinical context:** Distributive shock causes vessels to dilate and leak, causing SVR to decrease. Cardiogenic and hypovolemic shock results in vasoconstriction, causing SVR to increase.

▶ PRESSORS AND INOTROPES

A group of vasoactive drugs that are the final line of defense in treating shock (Table 5-4).

Effects and Side Effects

Generally, pressors are used to increase CO or SVR. All of them have important side effects that can limit their use.

These side effects are easily predicted based on the drug's action. For example, in addition to stimulating β_1 receptors, dobutamine stimulates β_2 (which causes vasodilation). The β_2 stimulation causes the side effect of hypotension.

Furthermore, remember that virtually any direct stimulation of the heart (β_1) can cause the side effect of arrhythmias.

TABLE 5-4. **Relative Selectivity of Adrenoceptor Agonists**

	RELATIVE RECEPTOR AFFINITIES
Alpha agonists	
Phenylephrine, methoxamine	$\alpha_1 > \alpha_2 >>>>> \beta$
Clonidine, methylnorepinephrine	$\alpha_2 > \alpha_1 >>>>> \beta$
Mixed alpha and beta agonists	
Norepinephrine	$\alpha_1 = \alpha_2; \beta_1 >> \beta_2$
Epinephrine	$\alpha_1 = \alpha_2; \beta_1 = \beta_2$
Beta agonists	
Dobutamine	$\beta_1 > \beta_2 >>>> \alpha$
Isoproterenol	$\beta_1 = \beta_2 >>>> \alpha$
Terbutaline, metaproterenol, albuterol, ritodrine	$\beta_2 >> \beta_1 >>>> \alpha$
Dopamine agonists	
Dopamine	$D_1 = D_2 >> \beta >> \alpha$
Fenoldopam	$D_1 >> D_2$

Reproduced, with permission, from Katzung BG. *Basic & Clinical Pharmacology,* 10th ed. New York: McGraw-Hill, 2007: 124.

Dobutamine

- **Action:** Strong stimulation β_1 receptors (ionotropic/chronotropic effects on the heart) with a mild stimulation of β_2 (vasodilation).
- **Result:** ↑ CO, ↓ SVR.
- **Typical use:** Cardiogenic shock.

Isoproterenol

Similar to dobutamine.

- **Action:** Strong stimulation of β_1 receptors (ionotropic/chronotropic effects on the heart) and β_2 (vasodilation).
- **Result:** ↑ CO, ↓ SVR.
- **Typical use:** Cardiogenic shock with bradycardia.

Milrinone

Milrinone is technically not a pressor, but it is an important intrope used in the ICU.

- **Action:** Phosphodiesterase inhibitor, which results in increased cyclic adenosine monophosphate (cAMP). This has positive ionotropic effects on the heart and also vasodilates.
- **Result:** ↑ CO, ↓ SVR.
- **Typical use:** Heart failure/cardiogenic shock.

Dopamine

Dopamine has different action depending on the dose.

Low Dose (1–3 µg/kg/min): "Renal Dose"

- **Action:** Stimulation of dopamine receptors (dilates renal vasculature) and mild β_1 stimulation.
- **Typical use:** None.

Intermediate Dose (5–10 µg/kg/min): "Cardiac Dose"

- **Action:** Stimulation of dopamine receptors, moderate stimulation of β_1 receptors (heart ionotropy/chronotropy), and mild stimulation of α_1 receptors (vasoconstriction).
- **Result:** ↑ CO.
- **Typical use:** Cardiogenic shock.

High Dose (10–20 µg/kg/min)

- **Action:** Stimulates dopamine receptors, β_1 receptors (heart ionotropy/chronotropy), and strong stimulation of α_1 receptors (vasoconstriction).
- **Result:** ↑↑ SVR.
- **Typical use:** Septic shock (replaced by norepinephrine).

The concept of low-dose dopamine's being a "renal dose" and helping perfuse the kidney has been debunked. It dilates the vasculature, but no evidence shows that it is renal protective or improves renal failure.

Norepinephrine

- **Action:** Strong stimulation of α_1 receptors (vasoconstriction), moderate stimulation of β_1 receptors (heart ionotropy/chronotropy).
- **Result:** ↑↑ SVR, ↑ CO.
- **Typical use:** Septic shock.

Epinephrine

- **Action:** Strong stimulation of β_1 and β_2 receptors. Also $\alpha_{1,2}$ stimulation (vasoconstriction).
- **Result:** ↑↑ SVR, +/– ↑ CO, bronchodilation.
- **Typical use:** Anaphylaxis, septic shock, cardiopulmonary arrest.

Phenylephrine

Pressure support is an important weaning mode.

- **Action:** Strong stimulation of α_1 receptors (vasoconstriction).
- **Result:** ↑↑ SVR.
- **Typical use:** Septic shock, neurogenic shock, anesthesia-induced hypotension.

The goals of mechanical ventilation are to:

1. Improve gas exchange.
2. Decrease the work of breathing.

Indications for intubation:

Complications of mechanical ventilation:

- Ventilator-associated pneumonia.
- Barotrauma and tension pneumothorax.
- Decreased venous return (preload) and CO.

- Airway protection (patients with GCS < 8).
- Failure to oxygenate—hypoxia despite high oxygen delivery content and clinical signs of respiratory distress (excess work of breathing).
- Failure to ventilate leading to progressive hypercapnia with acidosis and signs of mental status change.

Setting the Ventilator

Several parameters have to be set for the ventilator. You need to define the mode (e.g., AC, IMV), respiratory rate, tidal volume, and the FiO_2.

- **Mode:** Choose AC, IMV, PS, or CPAP.
- **Respiratory rate** (for AC or IMV only): Usually 10–20.
- **Tidal volume** (for AC or IMV only): Usually 400–600 cc (6–8 cc/kg).
- **FiO_2:** Always start at 100% and titrate down, maintaining the pulse oximetry > 90%. Keep FiO_2 below 60% to minimize oxygen-induced free radical injury.

Strategies to improve oxygenation:

- Increase FiO_2.
- Increase positive end-expiratory pressure (PEEP).

EXAMPLE

Initial AC mode setting used in the surgical patient: AC 12–16, tidal volume 6–8 cc/kg (ideal body weight), $FiO_2 = 100\%$ (reduced after initial ABG), PEEP 5.

TABLE 5-5. Various Modes of Mechanical Ventilation

Continuous positive airway pressure (CPAP)	Noninvasive ventilation that applies constant positive pressure, with no variation in breathing cycle. Patient must breathe on his or her own. CPAP keeps inspiratory airway pressure above atmospheric pressure without increasing work of breathing; improves functional residual capacity and compliance. Can be used to help avoid intubation. Mode of choice for sleep apnea.
Synchronized intermittent mandatory ventilation (SIMV)	Patient breathes on his or her own, plus receives a preset rate of MV that is synchronized to and delivered with the patient's breath. Pressure support is often added to spontaneous breathing (gives patient initial boost of pressure to overcome airway resistance).
Assist-control ventilation (ACV) (may be volume controlled or pressure controlled)	Each breath initiated by patient triggers machine to deliver the set tidal volume (volume control) or set peak inspiratory pressure (pressure control). A set tidal volume/pressure is given a set number of times per minute, even if patient is breathing less than the preset respiratory rate.
Pressure support ventilation (PSV)	Each breath initiated by patient triggers the machine to deliver an initial "boost of pressure" with variable flow of air into lungs. The patient determines the rate, duration of inspiration, and tidal volume. This boost helps the patient overcome resistance of the endotracheal tube and reduces work of breathing. This mode can be used alone, as the only ventilator setting, or in conjunction with the IMV/SIMV modes. Pressure support is typically set at between 5 and 20. This mode is used in weaning off ventilator.

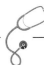

PEEP is used primarily in congestive heart failure (CHF) or acute respiratory distress syndrome (ARDS). It maintains alveoli open, allowing more time for gas exchange. It is therefore used to increase the oxygen level. Problems with PEEP include hypotension (decreases preload).

What are the causes of failure to wean off the ventilator?
1. Anxiety/agitation.
2. Drugs (usually sedatives).
3. Electrolyte abnormalities (hypophosphatemia).
4. Diaphragm dysfunction (neuromuscular dysfunction).
5. Hypothyroidism/ malnutrition.
6. Excess CO_2 production (overfeeding).

Adjusting the Ventilator

1. Based on ABG (interpretation discussed in previous chapter).
2. Minute ventilation.

$$\text{Minute Ventilation} = \text{Respiratory Rate} \times \text{Tidal Volume}$$

You can therefore adjust either the rate or the tidal volume to change the minute ventilation.

Know this simple rule: Increasing minute ventilation will decrease P_{CO_2} and increase pH. Decreasing minute ventilation will increase P_{CO_2} and decrease pH.

OXYGENATION

FiO_2 and PEEP are the ventilator parameters that adjust oxygenation.

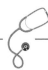

P_{CO_2} is the marker of ventilation.
P_{O_2} is the marker of oxygenation.

Try to titrate down the FiO₂ (< 50% is ideal) in order to avoid oxygen toxicity. Oxygen toxicity is thought to be caused by oxygen free radicals damaging the lung interstitium.

Acute lung injury due to inflammatory process in both lungs causing increased permeability of the capillaries and severe ventilation/perfusion mismatch. ARDS is a disease of altered lung compliance. These patients are tachypneic and hypoxic and have bilateral crackles on lung exam.
The diagnostic criteria are:

1. Bilateral, fluffy infiltrates on chest x-ray (three out of four lung fields).
2. PaO_2/FiO_2 ratio < 200.
3. No evidence of heart failure (PCWP ≤ 18 mmHg).
4. Acute onset.
5. Presence of an underlying cause.

Causes

There is a wide variety of causes of ARDS. Common causes include:

- Direct lung injury:
  - Pneumonia
  - Aspiration
  - Near drowning
- Indirect causes:
  - Sepsis (most common of all causes).
  - Massive transfusion.
  - Severe trauma, burns, toxins.
  - Pancreatitis.

The CXR does not reliably distinguish ARDS from CHF. A Swan-Ganz catheter can be useful in this matter.
- PCWP < 18 = ARDS
- PCWP > 18 = CHF

Management

1. It is necessary to intubate because of hypoxemia.
2. Treat underlying cause, especially infections.
3. **Low tidal volume ventilation (6–8 cc/kg).**
4. PEEP is often used to improve gas exchange and keep lungs open at relatively low lung volumes.
5. FiO_2 is kept at ≤ 60% to avoid free radical injury.

Fluids, Electrolytes, and Nutrition

Total Body Water

- Fifty to seventy percent of total body weight.
- Greater in lean individuals because fat contains little water, average 60%.
- Greatest percentage in newborns 70%, then decreases with age to around 50%.
  - **Example:** Average 70-kg male would be 42 L water since 1 L of water = 1 kg.
- Made up of two compartments—ICF and ECF.

Intracellular Fluid (ICF)

- Mostly in skeletal muscle mass, thus slightly lower in females (50%) than males (60%).
- Cell wall separates the ICF from the ECF and acts as a semipermeable membrane.

Extracellular Fluid (ECF)

- Made up of plasma and interstitial (extravascular) fluid.
- Capillary membrane separates plasma and interstitial fluid and acts as a semipermeable membrane.

Intracellular Compartment	Extracellular Compartment	
⅔ = 67% TBW	⅓ = 33% TBW	
	Interstitial	Plasma
	¾ ECC = 25% TBW	¼ ECC = 8% TBW
In 70-kg man (42 L TBW) = 28 L	11 L	3 L
In 45-kg woman (22.5 L TBW) = 15 L	5.6 L	1.8 L
	↑ Cell membrane	↑ Capillary wall

Water Movement Between ICF and ECF

Water flows freely between the three compartments, shifting compartments to maintain osmotic equilibrium between them (Figure 6-1). See Table 6-1.

Normal Plasma Osmolality 285–295 mmol/L

Calculated Plasma osmolality (POSMc) = 2[Na] + [glucose] / 18 + [BUN] / 2.8

Where [Na] is in mmol/L and [BUN], [glucose] in mg/dL

Osmolar Gap = measured osmolality − POSMc

Normal Osmolar Gap < 10 mmol/L

Osmolar Gap > 10 mmol/L—think lactic acid, ketones, methanol, ethanol.

Even without intake, you must excrete 800 mL/day in urine waste products.

Insensible loss increases with fever and hyperventilation.

May lose 1,500 mL/day with an unhumidified tracheostomy and hyperventilation.

HIGH-YIELD FACTS

Fluids, Electrolytes, and Nutrition

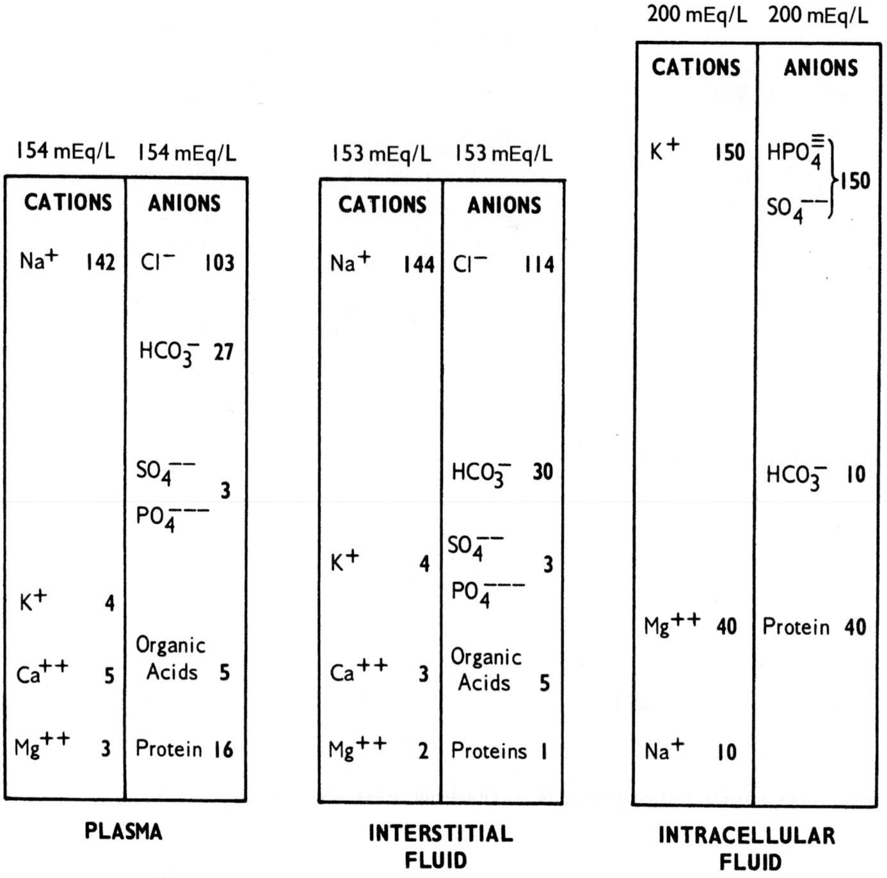

FIGURE 6-1. **Chemical composition of body fluid compartments.**

(Reproduced, with permission, from Brunicardi FC, Andersen DK, Billiar TR, et al. *Schwartz's Principles of Surgery*, 8th ed. New York: McGraw-Hill, 2004: 45.)

▶ RENAL CONTROL OF FLUIDS/ELECTROLYTES

See Figure 6-2.

- Distal tubules—reabsorption of Na in exchange for K and H secretion.
- Affected by adrenocorticotropic hormone (ACTH) and aldosterone.
- Aldosterone directly stimulates K secretion and Na reabsorption from the distal tubule.

Volume Deficit (Dehydration)

Most common fluid disorder.

CAUSES

Losses that Mimic ECF
- Hemorrhage.
- Loss of gastrointestinal (GI) fluid—vomiting, nasogastric (NG) suction, diarrhea, fistular drainage.

TABLE 6-1. **Signs and Symptoms of Volume Disturbances**

SYSTEM	VOLUME DEFICIT	VOLUME EXCESS
Generalized	Weight loss	Weight gain
	Decreased skin turgor	Peripheral edema
Cardiac	Tachycardia	Increased cardiac output
	Orthostasis/hypotension	Increased central venous pressure
	Collapsed neck veins	Distended neck veins
		Murmur
Renal	Oliguria	
	Azotemia	
Gastrointestinal	Ileus	Bowel edema
Pulmonary		Pulmonary edema

Reproduced, with permission, from Brunicardi FC, Andersen DK, Billiar TR, et al. *Schwartz's Principles of Surgery,* 8th ed. New York: McGraw-Hill, 2004: 45.

- Postoperative fluid sequestration (third spacing): Intestinal obstruction.
- Intra-abdominal and retroperitoneal inflammation (e.g., pancreatitis, peritonitis).
- Systemic inflammatory response syndrome (SIRS), burns, sepsis, pancreatitis.

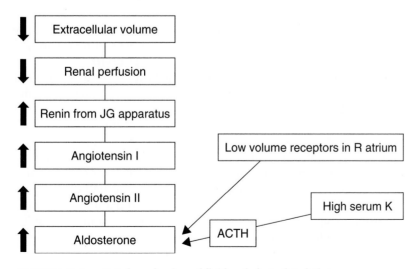

FIGURE 6-2. **Renal mechanism of fluid and electrolyte balance.**

Losses that Are Principally Water
- Fever.
- Osmotic diuresis.
- Diabetes insipidus.
- Prolonged water deprivation.
- Inadequate input during procedure.

SIGNS AND SYMPTOMS

See Table 6-1.

- Central nervous system (CNS) and cardiovascular (CV) signs occur early with acute loss.
- CV signs are secondary to a decrease in plasma volume.
- Tissue signs may be absent until the deficit has existed for 24 hours.
- Tissue signs may be difficult to assess in the elderly patient or patient with recent weight loss.
- Body temperature varies with environment—cool room may mask fever.
- After partial correction of volume deficit, the temperature will generally rise to the appropriate level.
- Severe volume depletion depresses all body systems and interferes with the clinical evaluation of the patient.
- Volume depleted patient with severe sepsis from peritonitis may be afebrile and have normal white blood count (WBC), complain of little pain, and have unremarkable findings on abdominal exam. This may change dramatically when the ECF is restored.
- History items important for evaluating fluid deficits include:
  - Weight change, intake (quantity and composition), output, general medical status.
  - Degree of dehydration dependent on acute loss of body weight and is assessed clinically:
    - Mild—3% for adults, 5% for kids
    - Moderate—6% for adults, 10% for kids
    - Severe—9% for adults, 15% for kids

TREATMENT

- Goal is to replace this deficit in most patients over the next 24 hours.
- The amount of fluid the patient is missing needs to be combined with the expected maintenance fluid for the next 24 hours.
- Rehydration is done over this period of time to try to allow continual equilibration between the reexpanded intravascular space and the contracted ECF and ICF.
- The initial intervention is to give a fairly large aliquot of fluid as a volume expander; 20 mL/kg of normal saline (NS) or Ringer's lactate (LR) is given as a bolus. During the remaining 8 hours, the expected maintenance fluid is given plus about one half of the remaining calculated loss. Over the remaining 16 hours, the other one half of the remaining calculated loss is given along with the assumed maintenance fluid.
- Volume expansion can be accomplished with crystalloid (NaCl, Ringer's lactate, etc.) or colloid (albumin, blood products).

Crystalloid
- Dextrose solutions are used to deliver free water to the body (dextrose is quickly metabolized).

- 0.9% NaCl quickly adds volume to the intravascular space.
- Goal is to expand the intravascular space.

Colloids
- Includes packed RBCs, FFP, albumin.
- Stay mainly within intravascular space if the capillary membranes are intact.
- Possible increased incidence of pulmonary embolism (PE) and respiratory failure (controversial).
- Expensive.
- Indications:
  - Patients with excess Na and water but are hypovolemic—such as ascites, congestive heart failure (CHF), postcardiac bypass patients.
  - Patients unable to synthesize enough albumin or other proteins to exert enough oncotic pressure—such as liver disease, transplant recipients, resections, malnutrition.
  - Severe hemorrhage or coagulopathy—packed red blood cells (PRBCs) and fresh frozen plasma (FFP) may increase hematocrit to help correct coagulopathy.

When replacing fluids, remember that:
- Large volumes may lead to peripheral and/or pulmonary edema.
- Large amounts of dextrose may cause hyperglycemia.
- Large amounts of NS may cause hyperchloremic metabolic acidosis.
- Ringer's lactate given when patient is hypovolemic and in metabolic alkalosis (i.e., from NG tube, vomiting) may worsen the alkalosis when the lactate is metabolized.

▶ VOLUME EXCESS

CAUSES

Isotonic
- Iatrogenic—intravascular overload of IV fluids with electrolytes.
- Increased ECF without equilibration with ICF—especially postoperative or trauma when the hormonal responses to stress are to decrease Na and water excretion by kidney.
- Often secondary to renal insufficiency, cirrhosis, or CHF.

Hypotonic
- Inappropriate NaCl-poor solution as a replacement for GI losses (most common).
- Third spacing.
- Increased antidiuretic hormone (ADH) with surgical stress, inappropriate ADH (SIADH).

Hypertonic
Most common cause: excessive Na load without adequate water intake:

- Water moves out of the cells because of increased ECF osmolarity.
- Causes an increase in intravascular and interstitial fluid.
- Worse when renal tubular excretion of water and/or Na is poor.
- Can also be caused by rapid infusion of nonelectrolyte osmotically active solutes such as glucose and mannitol.

SIGNS AND SYMPTOMS
See Table 6-2.

Third spacing is the shift of ECF from the plasma compartment to elsewhere, such as the interstitial or transcellular spaces.

- Normal: 1,000–1,200 mg—most is in the bone in the form of phosphate and carbonate.
- Normal daily intake: 1–3 g.
- Most excreted via stool (–200 mg via urine).
- Normal serum level: 8.5–10.5 mg/dL (total calcium).
- Half of this is nonionized and bound to plasma protein.

If hypocalcemia is seen on laboratory report, first correct for low albumin:

$$\text{Corrected Calcium} = 0.8\,(\text{Normal Albumin} - \text{Observed Albumin}) + \text{Observed Calcium}$$

If corrected calcium falls within normal range, no action is required.

- Ionized calcium is the most accurate measure of calcium, but labs report total calcium.
- An additional nonionized fraction (5%) is bound to other substances in the ECF.
- Ratio of ionized to nonionized Ca is related to pH (see Figure 6-5):
  - Acidosis causes increase in ionized fraction.
  - Alkalosis causes decrease in ionized fraction.

Hypocalcemia

DEFINITION

< 8 mg/dL.

CAUSES

- Acute pancreatitis.
- Massive soft-tissue infections (necrotizing fasciitis).
- Acute/chronic renal failure.
- Pancreatic/small bowel fistulas.

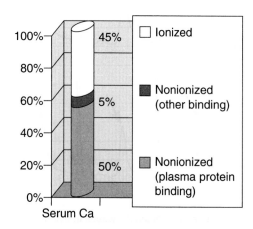

FIGURE 6-5. Concentration of ionized and nonionized calcium in serum.

- Hypoparathyroidism (common after parathyroid or thyroid surgery).
- Hypoproteinemia (often asymptomatic, corrected calcium will fall within normal range).
- Severe depletion of magnesium.
- Severe alkalosis may elicit symptoms in patient with normal serum levels because there is a decrease in the ionized fraction of total serum calcium.

SIGNS AND SYMPTOMS

- Numbness and tingling of fingers, toes, and around mouth.
- Increased reflexes.
- Chvostek's sign: Tapping over the facial nerve in front of the tragus of the ear causes ipsilateral twitching.
- Trousseau's sign: Carpopedal spasm following inflation of sphygmomanometer cuff to above systolic blood pressure for several minutes.
- Muscle and abdominal cramps.
- Convulsions.
- ECG—prolonged QT interval.

TREATMENT

- IV Ca gluconate or Ca chloride.
- Monitor QT interval on ECG.

Hypercalcemia

DEFINITION

> 15 mg/dL.

CAUSES

- Hyperparathyroidism.
- Cancer (especially breast, multiple myeloma).
- Drugs (e.g., thiazides).

SIGNS AND SYMPTOMS

- Fatigue, weakness, anorexia, weight loss, nausea, vomiting.
- Somnambulism, stupor, coma.
- Severe headache, pain in the back and extremities, thirst, polydipsia, polyuria.
- Death.

TREATMENT

- Vigorous volume repletion with salt solution—dilutes Ca and increases urinary Ca excretion:
  - May be augmented with furosemide.
  - Definitive treatment of acute hypercalcemic crisis in patients with hyperparathyroidism is immediate surgery.
- Treat underlying cause.

Enteral

- Gut works but oral intake not possible—altered mental state, ventilator, oral/pharyngeal/esophageal disorders.
- Oral intake not sufficient for metabolic requirements—anorexia, sepsis, severe trauma/burns.
- Presence of malnutrition and wasting.

Total Parenteral Nutrition (TPN)

- Enteral feeding not possible—GI obstruction, ileus.
- Enteral intake not sufficient for metabolic requirements—chronic diarrhea/emesis, malabsorption, fistulas, chemotherapy, irradiation therapy.
- The biggest danger of TPN is infection (the organic products in TPN can become infiltrated with bacteria and sent directly into the bloodstream).
- Adjunctive support necessary for managing disease—pancreatitis, hepatic failure, renal failure, chylothorax.

► NUTRIENT REQUIREMENTS

Calorie Requirements

- Harris-Benedict equation and Fick equation (in patients with Swan-Ganz catheters) used to estimate basal energy expenditure (BEE).
- General estimation of BEE:
  - Males: BEE = **25 kcal/kg/day**
  - Females: BEE = **22 kcal/kg/day**
  - Multiply this by the desired goal:
    - Nonstressed patient: BEE × 1.2
    - Postsurgery: BEE × 1.3 to 1.5
    - Trauma/sepsis/burns: BEE × 1.6 to 2.0
    - Fever: 12% increase per °C
- The caloric needs must be met by nonprotein calories (i.e., fat and carbohydrate). Usually, carbs provide 70% of calories and fat provides 30%.

Respiratory Quotient (RQ) of Individual Substrates

RQ is defined as the ratio of carbon dioxide released to oxygen consumed per unit metabolism of a substrate (i.e., VCO_2/VO_2).

- RQ for lipid: 0.7
- RQ for protein: 0.8
- RQ for carbohydrates: 1.0
- RQ for balanced diet: 0.83

Protein Requirement

- Usual protein requirement is 0.8–1 g/kg body weight.
- The requirement increases in illness and is maximal in burn patients.
- The average surgical patient needs 1.2–1.6 g/kg protein intake.
- Each gram of urinary nitrogen is equivalent to 6.25 g of degraded protein.
    - Nitrogen balance:

    N Balance (g) = (Protein Intake (g) / 6.25) – (UUN + 4)

    - UUN = Urinary urea nitrogen, 4 represents daily nitrogen loss other than UUN.
    - The goal of nitrogen balance is to maintain positive balance of 4–6 g.
- Vitamins and trace elements must be incorporated in all feeding regimens.

▶ ENTERAL NUTRITION

- Preferred over parenteral nutrition.
- Reduces incidence of infection.
- May be continuous or intermittent.
- Routes for GI feeding: PO; nasogastric feeding, gastrostomy, jejunostomy.
- Glutamine is the fuel for enterocytes.
- Short-chain fatty acids serve as fuel for the colonocytes.
- Omega-3 fatty acids and arginine serve as immune-modulating agents.

Complications

- Diarrhea.
- Aspiration.
- Obstruction of feeding tube.

▶ ACID-BASE DISORDERS

Assess the acid-base disorder step by step (Table 6-5):

- Is the primary disorder an acidosis (pH < 7.40) or alkalosis (pH > 7.40)?
- Is the disorder respiratory (pH and P_{CO_2} move in opposite directions)?
- Is the disorder metabolic (pH and P_{CO_2} move in same direction)?
- Is the disorder a simple or mixed disorder?

Use the following general rules of thumb for acute disorders:

- Metabolic acidosis: P_{CO_2} drops ~ 1.5 (drop in HCO_3).
- Metabolic alkalosis: P_{CO_2} rises ~ 1.0 (rise in HCO_3).
- Respiratory acidosis: HCO_3 rises ~ 0.1 (rise in P_{CO_2}).
- Respiratory alkalosis: HCO_3 drops ~ 0.3 (drop in P_{CO_2}).

Compensation beyond above parameters suggests mixed disorder.

Causes of elevated anion gap metabolic acidosis:
MUDPILES
Methanol/**M**etabolism (inborn errors)
Uremia
Diabetic ketoacidosis
Paraldehyde
Iron/**I**soniazid
Lactic acidosis
Ethylene glycol
Salicylates/**S**trychnine
Narrow down to four basic processes:
Ketoacidosis
Lactic acidosis
Renal failure
Intoxication

Causes of normal anion gap metabolic acidosis:
HARD UP
Hyperparathyroidism
Adrenal insufficiency/ **A**nhydrase (carbonic anhydrase) inhibitors
Renal tubular acidosis
Diarrhea
Ureteroenteric fistula
Pancreatic fistulas

TYPE OF ACID-BASE DISORDER	ACUTE (UNCOMPENSATED)			CHRONIC (PARTIALLY COMPENSATED)		
	pH	P_{CO_2} (RESPIRATORY COMPONENT)	PLASMA HCO_3^{-a} (METABOLIC COMPONENT)	pH	P_{CO_2} (RESPIRATORY COMPONENT)	PLASMA HCO_3^{-a} (METABOLIC COMPONENT)
Respiratory acidosis	↓↓	↑↑	N	↓	↑↑	↑
Respiratory alkalosis	↑↑	↓↓	N	↑	↓↓	↓
Metabolic acidosis	↓↓	N	↓↓	↓	↓	↓
Metabolic alkalosis	↑↑	N	↑↑	↑	↑?	↑

aMeasured as standard bicarbonate, whole blood buffer base, CO_2 content, or CO_2 combining power. The *base excess value* is positive when the standard bicarbonate is above normal and negative when the standard bicarbonate is below normal.

Reproduced, with permission, from Brunicardi FC, Andersen DK, Billiar TR et al. *Schwartz's Principles of Surgery,* 8th ed. New York: McGraw-Hill, 2004: 51.

Metabolic Acidosis

- Two varieties:
    - **Anion gap acidosis**—due to addition of unmeasured acid.
    - **Nonanion gap acidosis**—due to HCO_3 loss.
- Calculating the anion gap:

$$AG = Na - [Cl + HCO_3]$$

- Normal AG = 10

Metabolic Alkalosis

Two mechanisms:

- Loss of H^+ from kidneys or GI tract:
    - Renal: Mineralocorticoid excess, diuretics, potassium-losing nephropathy.
    - GI: Vomiting, gastric drainage, villous adenoma of colon.
- Gain HCO_3: Milk-alkali syndrome, exogenous $NaHCO_3$; lactated Ringer's, packed RBCs, TPN all contain substrates that metabolize to bicarbonate.

Respiratory Acidosis

Hypercapnia secondary to one of two mechanisms:

- Hypoventilation (brain stem injury, neuromuscular disease, ventilator malfunction, opiates).
- Ventilation-perfusion (V/$\underline{Q}$) mismatch (chronic obstructive pulmonary disease, pneumonia, pulmonary embolism, foreign body, pulmonary edema).

Respiratory Alkalosis

- Hyperventilation secondary to anemia, anxiety, increased intracranial pressure (ICP), salicylates, fever, hypoxemia, systemic disease (sepsis), pain, pregnancy, CHF, pneumonia, asthma, liver disease.
- Alkalosis causes decrease in serum K and ionized Ca, resulting in paresthesias, carpopedal spasm, and tetany.

Causes of respiratory alkalosis:
MIS[HAP]³S
Mechanical overventilation
Increased ICP
Sepsis
Hypoxemia/**H**yperpyrexia/ Heart failure
Anxiety/**A**sthma/**A**scites
Pregnancy/**P**ain/ Pneumonia
Salicylates

Fluids, Electrolytes, and Nutrition

HIGH-YIELD FACTS

Fluids, Electrolytes, and Nutrition

The Esophagus

The esophagus is a 25-cm-long muscular tube that begins at the pharynx (begins at lower border of C6), travels through the thorax in the posterior mediastinum, and empties into the cardia of the stomach.

- Superior third: Striated muscle only.
- Middle third: Both striated and smooth muscle.
- Inferior third: Smooth muscle only.

Three areas of narrowing (evident on barium swallow; see Figure 7-1):

1. At the beginning of the esophagus, caused by the cricopharyngeus muscle.
2. Where the left mainstem bronchus and aortic arch cross.
3. At the hiatus of the diaphragm.

Two sphincters are present, which function as control points:

- *Upper esophageal sphincter* (UES, cricopharyngeus muscle) prevents the passage of excess air into the stomach during breathing.
- *Lower esophageal sphincter* (LES) is a physiological sphincter; it relaxes with initiation of the pharyngeal swallow and prevents the reflux of gastric contents when swallowing is not occuring.
  - Esophageal peristalsis accompanying swallowing is termed primary peristalsis.
  - Secondary peristalsis can be initiated by the esophageal musculature without the pharyngeal phase to clear the esophagus of any substance left behind from primary peristalsis.

The esophagus does not have the serosal layer, so esophageal anastomoses are prone to leaks.

The distance of the gastroesopohageal (GE) junction from the incisor teeth is 40 cm and serves as an important landmark in upper gastrointestinal (GI) endoscopy.

Clinically significant motility disorders involve smooth muscle in the lower two thirds only.

Recall the vertebral levels at which the following traverse the diaphragm:
T8 = inferior vena cava (IVC).
T10 = esophagus.
T12 = aorta.
"I (IVC) ate (T8) ten (T10) eggs (esophagus) at (aorta) noon (T12)."

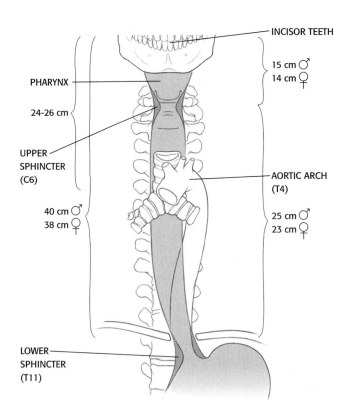

FIGURE 7-1. **Important clinical endoscopic measurements of the esophagus in adults.**

HIGH-YIELD FACTS

The Esophagus

- Barium swallow: The patient ingests a radiopaque substance; swallowing and the esophagus are analyzed fluoroscopically.
- Flexible endoscopy: A camera is passed through the oral cavity into the esophagus, with the patient under sedation. There are multiple ports in the scope to allow for biopsies, irrigation, and suction.
- Manometry: Examines the motor function.
- Twenty-four-hour ambulatory pH monitoring.

Result from abnormalities in the propulsive pump action of the esophagus or relaxation of the LES. Can be primary (achalasia, diffuse esophageal spasm [DES], nutcracker esophagus, hypertensive LES) or secondary (result of another systemic disease, including collagen vascular diseases like scleroderma and mixed connective tissue disease, neuromuscular disease, endocrine and metastatic disorders).

DEFINITION

- Dysphagia: Difficulty swallowing.
- Odynophagia: Pain on swallowing. May or may not accompany dysphagia.

Achalasia

DEFINITION

Failure of the lower portion of the esophagus to relax during swallowing is defined as achalasia. The resulting dysphagia is due to three mechanisms:

1. Complete absence of peristalsis in the esophageal body.
2. Incomplete/impaired relaxation of the LES after swallowing.
3. Increased resting tone of the LES.

These result in elevation of intraluminal esophageal pressure, esophageal dilatation, and subsequent progressive loss of normal swallowing mechanisms—a functional holdup of ingested material.

SIGNS AND SYMPTOMS

- Dysphagia for both solids and liquids.
- Regurgitation of food.
- Severe halitosis (due to the decomposition of stagnant food within the esophagus).

DIAGNOSIS

- Lateral upright chest x-ray (CXR) may reveal a dilated esophagus and the presence of air-fluid levels in the posterior mediastinum.
- Barium swallow will reveal the characteristic distal bird's beak sign due to the collection of contrast material in the proximal dilated segment and the passage of a small amount of contrast through the narrowed LES (Figure 7-2).

A complaint of dysphagia must elicit a full dietary history from a patient; what they experience, when they eat, what types of food they eat that cause it.

If the patient is immunocompromised, have a high index of suspicion for candidal esophagitis if human immunodeficiency virus (HIV)-positive, and for cytomegalovirus (CMV)/herpes simplex virus (HSV) esophagitis if non-HIV.

Achalasia: *Gr.* Failure to relax.

Classic triad of achalasia: Dysphagia, regurgitation, and weight loss.

Barium swallow:
- Bird's beak or steeple sign: Achalasia.
- Corkscrew-shaped: Diffuse esophageal spasm.

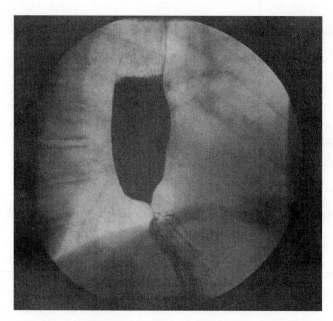

FIGURE 7-2. Barium study demonstrating a dilated esophagus and smooth, tapered gastroesophageal junction, typical of achalasia.

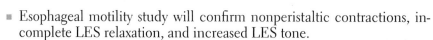

(Reproduced, with permission, from Woltman T, Oelschlager BK. Benign esophageal disorders. In Zinner MJ, Ashley SW, eds. *Maingot's Abdominal Operations*, 11th ed. New York: McGraw-Hill, 2007: 212.)

Gastroesophageal reflux produces a sour taste and a gush of saliva due to the presence of hydrochloride from the gastric acid (water brash), while achalasia does not.

Esophageal perforation is four times more likely following dilatation compared to esophagomyotomy.

- Esophageal motility study will confirm nonperistaltic contractions, incomplete LES relaxation, and increased LES tone.
- Esophagoscopy is indicated to rule out mass lesions or strictures, and to obtain specimens for biopsy.

TREATMENT

- Medical management: Drugs that relax the LES—nitrates, calcium channel blockers, and antispasmodics.
- Surgical management: Esophagomyotomy (Heller's myotomy) with or without fundoplication is the treatment of choice for achalasia.
- Esophagomyotomy: Esophagus is exposed via a transthoracic (left thoracotomy), transabdominal, thorascopic, or laparoscopic technique. The tunica muscularis of the esophagus is incised distally, with extension to the LES. Complete division of the LES necessitates the addition of an antireflux procedure such as Nissen 360° fundoplication or partial fundoplication (see later discussion of the Nissen fundoplication).
- Endoscopic dilatation: Has a lower success rate and a higher complication rate. It involves inserting a balloon or progressively larger-sized dilators through the narrowed lumen, which causes tearing of the esophageal smooth muscle and decreases the competency of the LES.

- Risk of squamous cell carcinoma is as high as 10% in patients with long-standing achalasia (duration 15–25 years).
- Patients may also develop pulmonary complications such as aspiration pneumonia, bronchiectasis, and asthma due to reflux and aspiration.

Diffuse Esophageal Spasm (DES)

DEFINITION

DES is a disorder of unknown etiology that is primarily a disease of the esophageal body. It may be a primary disease process of the muscle, or may occur in association with reflux esophagitis, esophageal obstruction, collagen vascular disease, or diabetic neuropathy. Spasm occurs in the distal two thirds of the esophagus and is caused by uncoordinated large-amplitude rapid contractions of smooth muscle. By definition, the LES tone is normal.

SIGNS AND SYMPTOMS

- Dysphagia for both solids and liquids.
- Substernal chest pain, similar to that seen in a myocardial infarction: Acute onset of severe retrosternal pain that may radiate to the arms, jaw, or back. The chest pain may occur at rest, or it may follow swallowing. The degree of chest pain depends on the duration and severity of the contractions.
- No regurgitation (unlike achalasia); no water brash (unlike gastroesophageal reflux disease).

Due to the fact that DES produces cardiac-like complaints, the diagnosis is often delayed until an extensive cardiologic workup is performed.

DIAGNOSIS

- Barium swallow may reveal the characteristic "corkscrew" appearance of the esophagus, due to the ripples and sacculations that are visible as a result of uncoordinated esophageal contraction. Barium swallow may be entirely normal, however, because the esophagus may not be in spasm at the time of the study. In contrast to achalasia, the LES appears to be a normal diameter.
- Esophageal manometry studies will reveal the presence of large, uncoordinated, and repetitive contractions in the lower esophagus. Alternatively, manometry may appear normal when the patient is asymptomatic. LES manometry will show normal resting pressure with LES relaxation upon swallowing (again, unlike achalasia).
- Esophagoscopy should be performed to rule out mass lesions, strictures, or esophagitis.

Patients with DES often have other functional intestinal disorders such as irritable bowel syndrome and spastic colon.

TREATMENT

- Nitrates or calcium channel blockers to relax smooth muscle.
- Surgical treatment via an esophageal myotomy is *not as successful* in relieving symptoms as it is for achalasia, and is therefore not recommended unless dysphagia is severe and incapacitating (see Table 7-1).

Nutcracker esophagus, another hypermotility disorder, involves more focal segments of the esophagus.

TABLE 7-1. Achalasia vs. Diffuse Esophageal Spasm

	ACHALASIA	**DIFFUSE ESOPHAGEAL SPASM**
Signs and symptoms	Dysphagia, regurgitation of undigested food, severe halitosis, weight loss, cough, diffuse chest pain.	Dysphagia, diffuse chest pain.
Pattern of contraction	Failure of LES to relax on swallowing.	Swallow-induced large wave of esophageal contraction, normal LES pressure.
Barium swallow findings	Absence of gastric bubble, narrowing of terminal esophagus that looks like a bird's beak.	Corkscrew appearance.
Treatment	Nitroglycerin, local botulinum toxin, balloon dilatation, sphincter myotomy (Heller's myotomy)	Nitroglycerin, nifedipine; surgery only if symptoms are severe and persistent.

Esophageal Diverticula

DEFINITION

EPiPhrenic and Pharyngoesophageal = caused by Elevated Pressure (Pulsion) and are Pseudo (false).

- Outpouching of the esophageal mucosa that protrudes through a defect in the muscle layer. Often occur when there are coexistent motility disorders.
- May be either a *true* diverticulum, which involves all three layers of the esophagus (e.g., midesophageal diverticulum), or a *false* diverticulum, involving only the mucosa and submucosa (e.g., Zenker's diverticulum).
- Characterized by its location: *Pharyngoesophageal* (Zenker's diverticulum), *midesophageal*, or *epiphrenic* (terminal third of the esophagus).
- *Pharyngoesophageal*/Zenker's and *epiphrenic* diverticula are called pulsion diverticula, since they are caused by increased esophageal pressure; they are *false* diverticula.

Zenker's Diverticulum

SIGNS AND SYMPTOMS

Pharyngoesophageal (Zenker's) type is the most likely to be symptomatic. Typical symptoms include dysphagia along with spontaneous regurgitation of undigested food, halitosis, choking, aspiration, repetitive respiratory infections, and, eventually, debilitation and weight loss.

DIAGNOSIS

A barium swallow will reveal the presence of all types of diverticula. Endoscopy is difficult and potentially dangerous due to the risk of perforation through the diverticulum.

TREATMENT

Treatment of Zenker's diverticulum is recommended to relieve symptoms and to prevent complications.

- The most common procedure is a cervical pharyngocricoesophageal myotomy (incising the cricopharyngeus) and is done in all cases needing operative intervention.
- Diverticulopexy (suturing the diverticulum in the inverted position to the prevertebral fascia) is added to myotomy for larger diverticula.
- Diverticulectomy (endoscopic stapling of the diverticulum), along with myotomy, is performed for the largest diverticulae.

When **Z**enker's causes **Z**ymptoms it requires **Z**urgery. Asymptomatic Zenker's is treated only if it is > 2 cm size.

► ESOPHAGEAL VARICES

PATHOPHYSIOLOGY

- Occur as a result of portal hypertension, most commonly a result of alcoholic cirrhosis.
- As elevated portal system pressure impedes the flow of blood through the liver (increased intrahepatic resistance), various sites of venous anastomosis become dilated secondary to retrograde flow from the portal to systemic circulations. Varices are portosystemic collaterals.
- Clinically significant portal-systemic sites:
  - *Cardio-esophageal junction*—dilatation leads to esophageal varices.
  - *Periumbilical region*—dilatation leads to caput medusae.
  - *Rectum*—dilatation leads to hemorrhoids.
    - Accounts for 10–30% of upper GI bleeds; up to 30% are fatal, 70% rebleed.

SIGNS AND SYMPTOMS

- Painless hematemesis.
- Unprovoked (i.e., not postemetic).
- Hemodynamic instability is common.
  - Risk for rebleeding is high.
  - Peripheral stigmata of liver disease.

TREATMENT

- Identifying high-risk patients and preventing the first bleeding episode are critical (i.e., screening endoscopy to determine varices in cirrhotic patients). This includes pharmacological therapy to reduce portal pressure and consequently intravariceal pressure—reduce collateral portal venous flow with vasoconstrictors (somatostatin, vasopressin and octreotide decrease portal flow) and intrahepatic resistance with vasodilators (beta blockers, especially propranolol and nitrates, decrease portal pressure).
  - Variceal bleeding ceases spontaneously in ~50% of cases.
- Management of ruptured varices causing an acute bleed:
  1. Stabilization of hemodynamics: Volume replacement with normal saline (NS) or lactated Ringer's and packed red blood cells (RBCs), nasogastric (NG) suction and lavage.
  2. Continuous vasopressin/somatostatin/octreotide to reduce splanchnic blood flow and portal pressure.

Endoscopic sclerotherapy or band ligation for control of ruptured esophageal varices has a 90% success rate. Patients are usually intubated prior to the procedure to prevent aspiration of blood.

3. Urgent endoscopic therapy: Endoscopic sclerotherapy (injection of the bleeding vessel(s) with a sclerosing agent via a catheter that is passed through the endoscope) stops bleeding in 80–90%; endoscopic band ligation (small elastic band is placed around the bleeding varix resulting in hemostasis) is equivalent to sclerotherapy initially, with fewer complications.
4. Balloon tamponade (Sengstaken-Blakemore tube) to apply direct pressure and hemostasis to the varix with an inflatable balloon.
5. For refractory acute bleeding, TIPSS procedure (transjugular intrahepatic portosystemic shunt).
6. Intraoperative placement of a portocaval shunt. Surgical therapy is considered when there is continued hemorrhage or recurrent rebleeding with poor control.
7. Liver transplant.

▶ ESOPHAGEAL STRICTURE

DEFINITION

Local, stenotic regions within the lumen of the esophagus; usually a result from an inflammatory or neoplastic process.

RISK FACTORS AND CAUSES

- Long-standing GERD.
- Radiation esophagitis.
- Infectious esophagitis.
- Corrosive/caustic esophagitis.
- Sclerotherapy for bleeding varices.

SIGNS AND SYMPTOMS

- While small strictures may remain asymptomatic, those that obstruct the esophageal lumen significantly will induce progressive dysphagia for solids.
- Odynophagia may or may not be present.

DIAGNOSIS

- Initial evaluation via barium swallow may reveal the presence of stricture.
- Esophagoscopy is necessary in all cases, since the stricture should be evaluated for malignancy; also useful to determine the appropriate treatment.

TREATMENT

- The esophagus is visualized endoscopically, and bougie dilators are carefully passed through the stricture; each successful dilatation is done with a progressively larger dilator.
- Dysphagia is relieved in most cases following adequate dilatation of the esophageal lumen.
- The most feared complication of dilatation is esophageal rupture.

DEFINITION

- Trauma to the esophagus that may result in leakage of air and esophageal contents into the mediastinum.
- A surgical emergency.
- Carries a 50% mortality.

ETIOLOGY

- The most common cause of esophageal perforation is iatrogenic. Occurs following endoscopy, dilatation, tamponade tubes (Blakemore, Minnesota).
- Boerhaave syndrome (15% of cases): A spontaneous perforation and *full-thickness* tear. Usually occurs in the area of the left pleural cavity or just above the GE junction, due to transmission of abdominal pressure to the esophagus. Can result from forceful vomiting, retching coughing, labor, lifting, or trauma.
- Mallory-Weiss syndrome: A *partial-thickness* mucosal tear. Usually occurs in the right posterolateral wall of the distal esophagus and results in bleeding that generally resolves spontaneously. Due to forceful vomiting.
- Foreign body ingestions (14% of cases): Objects usually lodge near anatomic narrowings and then perforate through:
    - Above the upper esophageal sphincter.
    - Near the aortic arch.
    - Above the LES.

SIGNS AND SYMPTOMS

- Severe, constant cervical, substernal, or back pain (depending on the location of the perforation).
- Dysphagia.
- Dyspnea.
- Subcutaneous emphysema.
- Mediastinal emphysema heard as a "crunching" sound (Hamman's sign).
    - Sepsis/fever.
    - Pneumothorax.

DIAGNOSIS

- CXR: Left-sided pleural effusion; mediastinal, cervical, or subcutaneous emphysema; mediastinal widening.
- Esophagogram with **water-soluble contrast** (gastrografin): Shows extravasation of contrast in 90% of patients.
- Other studies: Endoscopy, computed tomography (CT), and thoracentesis (check fluid for low pH and high amylase).

TREATMENT

Resuscitation and stabilization of patient.

- Primary surgical closure of full-thickness tears within 24 hours: 80–90% survival rate.
- Drain the contaminated mediastinum.
- Monitor for recovery from sepsis.

Typical scenario: A man presents severe retrosternal and upper abdominal pain after an episode of retching. *Think:* Boerhaave syndrome (full-thickness) or Mallory-Weiss syndrome (partial-thickness) tears in the esophagus.

A patient who recently underwent an endoscopic procedure develops fever and chest pain. *Think:* Iatrogenic esophageal rupture.

In Boerhaave syndrome, the most common site of rupture is the left lateral wall of the esophagus, just above the esophageal hiatus. Iatrogenic perforation occurs most commonly following esophagogastroduodenoscopy (EGD) in the cervical esophagus near the cricopharyngeus muscle.

Subcutaneous and mediastinal emphysema require a full-thickness tear.

- Conservative nonoperative management: If the perforation is well contained in the mediastinum (with the barium draining back into the esophagus) and the patient has mild symptoms with minimal signs of sepsis, then the perforation can be managed with hyperalimentation, antibiotics, and gastric acid inhibition. Oral intake can be resumed within 1–2 weeks.

▶ CAUSTIC INJURY

- Caused by acid (in household cleaning agents) or alkali (lye, sodium hydroxide tablets).
- Alkali burns are worse than acidic, as acid substances usually burn the mouth immediately and are less frequently swallowed; alkaline substances are more frequently ingested. Acidic substances also cause coagulative tissue necrosis, which limits their penetration, whereas alkaline substances cause injury deep into the tissue as they dissolve the tissue.
- Caustic injury has both an *acute phase*—controlling immediate tissue injury and perforation potential—and a *chronic phase*—managing structures and swallowing disturbances that have developed.
- Acute damage is dependent on nature of substance, quantity, and time in contact with tissue.

SIGNS AND SYMPTOMS

- Oral and substernal pain in the initial phase; pain on swallowing and dysphagia.
- Hypersalivation.
- Fever—strongly correlated with an esophageal lesion.
- Vomiting and hemoptysis.
- Systemic hypovolemia and acidosis.
- Laryngospasm, laryngedema.
- Dysphagia reappears in the chronic phase due to fibrosis, retraction, and narrowing of the esophagus. Strictures develop in 80% of patients within 2 months.

TREATMENT

- Careful inspection of both the oral cavity and esophagus; however, there is poor correlation between the appearance of one and damage to the other.
- Early esophagoscopy (< 24 hrs) to establish the presence of esophageal injury with exquisite care not to perforate the already damaged esophagus.
- Limiting the burn by administering neutralizing agents, preferably within the first hour. Lye/alkali can be neutralized with half-strength vinegar, lemon juice, or orange juice; acid with milk, egg white, or antacid.
- Broad-spectrum antibiotics to prevent infectious complications.
- Dilatations are controversial as they can traumatize the esophagus, but some start them early after injury to preserve the esophageal lumen and remove adhesions. They are done with a *bougie* in order to prevent and manage strictures.
- Extensive necrosis leading to perforation is best managed by resection; if the esophagus is viable, it can be managed with an intraluminal esophageal stent.

Emetics are **contraindicated**— forceful vomiting can cause perforation.

- Surgical intervention is indicated if there is complete stenosis with failure to establish a lumen, marked irregularity on barium swallow, development of severe mediastinitis with dilatation, fistula formation, or if the patient is unable to undergo prolonged periods of dilatation.
- Currently, the stomach, jejunum, and colon are organs used to replace the esophagus.

DEFINITION

- Defined by symptoms, presence of endoscopic esophagitis, or by measuring the increased exposure of the esophagus to gastric juice.
- Common disease, accounts for ~75% of esophageal pathology.

PATHOPHYSIOLOGY

- Loss of the normal gastroesophageal barriers results in reflux. The primary barrier is the LES, and it is usually secondary to low or reduced LES resistance with reflux of acidic gastric contents into the esophagus.
- Causes include a structurally defective sphincter; hiatal hernia; transient loss of the GE barrier (with a structurally normal LES) secondary to gastric abnormalities such as distention with air or food; delayed gastric emptying; and increased intra-abdominal pressure.
- Prolonged exposure to a low pH from gastric contents (acid, pepsin, and duodenal contents, including biliary and pancreatic secretions) will cause irritation of the esophageal mucosa (as well as the respiratory epithelium) and the development of complications including esophagitis, stricture, Barrett's esophagus (see next section) and risk of aspiration.

SIGNS AND SYMPTOMS

- Patients with GERD may report a range of symptoms from heartburn to angina-like chest pain.
  - Atypical symptoms include nausea, vomiting, postprandial fullness, choking, chronic cough, wheezing, and hoarseness.
- Minimal or transient reflux may cause asymptomatic esophagitis, while severe reflux may cause severe esophagitis accompanied by laryngitis, aspiration pneumonitis/recurrent pneumonia, idiopathic pulmonary fibrosis, or asthma.
- The presence of dysphagia may indicate peptic stricture formation.

DIAGNOSIS

- Patients presenting with vague symptoms of chest pain must be evaluated for cardiac and pulmonary disease as deemed necessary (thorough physical exam, electrocardiogram [ECG], cardiac enzymes, and admission as appropriate).
- A barium study is useful to look for an anatomical cause for reflux, such as a hiatal hernia; can also elucidate pathology resulting from longstanding reflux, such as a stricture or ulcer formation.
- Twenty-four-hour ambulatory pH monitoring of the esophagus: A probe with pH electrodes is inserted into the patient's esophagus for 24 hours. The probe continuously records the esophageal pH; useful in determining the severity of reflux (gold standard for diagnosing GERD).

Twenty-four-hour pH monitoring of the esophagus is the gold standard for diagnosing GERD.

- Esophageal manometry is useful in evaluating the competence of the LES.
- Esophagoscopy should be performed to evaluate the esophageal mucosa to rule out Barrett's esophagus, and to obtain specimens for biopsy and *Helicobacter pylori* testing.

TREATMENT

Initial treatment of GERD involves medications that decrease gastric acid production along with lifestyle modification, including:

If multiple modalities are available for evaluating and treating the patient, always begin with the least expensive one (i.e., digital rectal exam for suspected prostate cancer, medication trial for suspected reflux disease).

- Elevation of head end of bed.
- Antacids (symptomatic relief).
- H_2 antagonists (e.g., ranitidine).
- Proton pump inhibitors (PPIs; e.g., omeprazole).
- Education to avoid alcohol, coffee, chocolate, and peppermint, as they may aggravate symptoms; avoid nicotine, as it decreases LES tone.
- Instruct and educate the patient to eat small, frequent meals, elevate the head of the bed, avoid tight clothing, and to not go to sleep within 3–4 hours of a meal.
- Medications that promote gastric emptying (e.g., metoclopromide) may be beneficial early in the disease.
- The patient undergoes a trial of medical therapy for 6–12 weeks before further investigations.
- If medical management fails and the patient develops complications like chronic esophagitis or stricture, surgical intervention should be considered.
- Surgery should be limited to those patients who have persistent or progressive disease despite maximal medical therapy or with a structurally defective LES. The primary goal of surgery is to return normal sphincter length and function and return the physiologic swallowing functions of the esophagus. The procedure of choice is a fundoplication (Figure 7-3)—wrapping the fundus of the stomach around the distal portion of the esophagus to create a sphincter, called the Nissen procedure, can be open or laparoscopic, transabdominal or transthoracic.
- Treatment of GERD is important in order to prevent the progression to Barrett's esophagus. In addition, chronic reflux predisposes the patient to pulmonary complications as mentioned above.

► BARRETT'S ESOPHAGUS

DEFINITION

A condition in which the distal portion of the tubular esophagus becomes lined by columnar epithelium as opposed to the normal squamous epithelium—histological appearance of intestinal metaplasia (the appearance of goblet cells).

This new region is susceptible to ulceration, bleeding, stricture, and adenocarcinoma formation.

SIGNS AND SYMPTOMS

- Usually similar to patients with GERD.
- Bleeding, hematemesis.
- Signs of esophageal perforation (see previous discussion).

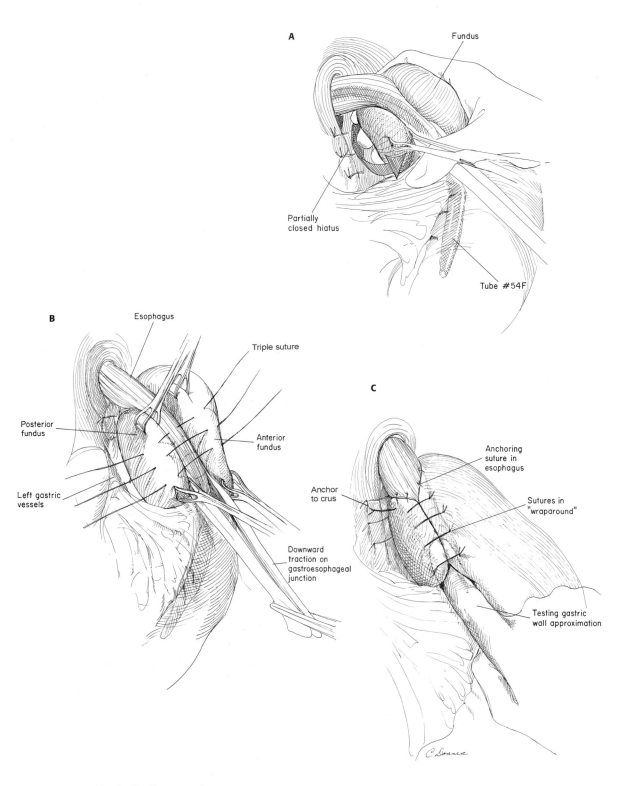

A. Fundus

Partially
closed hiatus

Tube #54F

B. Esophagus

Triple suture

Posterior
fundus

Anterior
fundus

Left gastric
vessels

Downward
traction on
gastroesophageal
junction

C. Anchoring
suture in
esophagus

Anchor
to crus

Sutures in
"wraparound"

Testing gastric
wall approximation

FIGURE 7-3. Fundoplication procedure.

A. A large gastric tube or rubber esophageal dilator is inserted into the esophagus to prevent undue compression of the esophageal lumen. The right hand is introduced behind the fundus of the stomach to test the adequacy of the gastric mobilization.
B. One or more long Babcock forceps are applied to the gastric wall on either side of the esophagus. The anterior and posterior gastric walls are approximated with interrupted silk sutures. **C.** After the traction drain and esophageal dilator are removed, the surgeon introduces the index finger or thumb upward under the plicated gastric wall. (Reproduced, with permission, from Zollinger RM Jr, Zollinger RM Sr. *Zollinger's Atlas of Surgical Operations*, 8th ed. New York: McGraw-Hill, 2003: 97.)

DIAGNOSIS

- Endoscopy for evaluation. Suspect when there is difficulty visualizing the squamocolumnar junction in the lower esophagus or an appearance of a redder mucosa.
- Multiple biopsies should be taken for a definitive or histologic diagnosis.

MANAGEMENT

- The same as those patients with GERD—require long-term PPI therapy for symptom relief and management of esophageal mucosal injury.
- Monitor and prevent disease progression to malignancy (risk 1% per year).
- Antireflux surgery when there are associated complications (stricture, ulceration, metaplastic progression).
- Surgical resection for refractory cases with high-grade dysplasia.

▶ ESOPHAGEAL CARCINOMA

EPIDEMIOLOGY

- More than 90% are squamous cell carcinomas (SCCs) and adenocarcinomas. The increasing prevalence of adenocarcinomas (due to Barrett's) as compared to what was mostly SCCs is shifting the epidemiology of esophageal cancer. Other tumors of the esophagus are less common (including leiomyomas, melanomas, carcinoids, lymphomas).
- Most cases occur in patients over the age of 50, but there is an increase in cases in younger patients with disease detected at an earlier stage.
- Males are affected more frequently than females.
- Over 50% of patients have unresectable or metastatic disease at the time of presentation.
- Five-year survival rate is poor, but increased to 14% toward the end of the 20th century.

RISK FACTORS

- Environmental:
  - Tobacco.
  - Alcohol.
  - Food additives (nitrates in smoked and pickled meats).
- Esophageal disorders:
  - GERD/Barrett's esophagus.
  - Achalasia.
  - Damage from caustic ingestion/strictures:
    - Chronic esophagitis.
    - Plummer-Vinson syndrome.
- History of radiation therapy to the mediastinum.

SIGNS AND SYMPTOMS

- Physical exam is usually entirely normal.
  - Patients may present with nonspecific GI complaints.
  - Gradual development of dysphagia (74% of patients) due to invasion of serosal layer, first for solids and later for both solids and liquids (mechanical dysphagia), may be present as well.

Dysphagia does not usually develop until > 60% of the esophageal lumen is obstructed.

- Decreased PO intake and pain on swallowing result in profound weight loss, easy fatigability, and weakness.
- With advanced disease, the patient will appear cachectic; supraclavicular lymphadenopathy may be present, as may signs of distant metastasis. May develop symptoms depending on local invasion (stridor, coughing, aspiration pneumonia, hemoptysis, vocal cord/recurrent laryngeal nerve paralysis).

DIAGNOSIS

- Population screening is untenable due to relatively low incidence, often absent early symptoms, rarity of a genetic cause.
- Asymptomatic patients are occasionally identified by surveillance endoscopy, especially patients with Barrett's esophagus.
- Barium esophagram is the initial diagnostic test—may show stricture, ulceration, or mass.
- EGD is useful to both visualize the mass and to retrieve specimens for biopsy.
  - Three fourths of adenocarcinoma is found in the distal esophagus; most SCCs are found in the middle and lower third. The cervical esophagus is an uncommon site for disease.
- CT scan of the thorax, abdomen, and pelvis is useful to define the extent of disease and thereby determine appropriate treatment.
- Endoscopic ultrasound (EUS) is useful to measure the depth of tumor invasion and presence of lymphadenopathy for preoperative staging and surgical planning.
- Positron emission tomographic (PET) scan for lymphatic spread.
- Staging according to TNM (tumor, node, mestastases) classification.

TREATMENT

Surgical therapy vs. palliative surgical therapy vs. nonsurgical palliation.

- Management of localized disease:
  - Surgical resection, especially for symptom control (right thoracic or transhiatal approach, gastric pull-up, or colonic interposition can be used to reconstruct the GI tract).
  - Radiotherapy for avoidance of perioperative morbidity and mortality (can shrink tumor but may predispose to local complications and not palliate dysphagia and odynophagia).
  - Pre/postoperative chemotherapy.
  - Combination therapy of these three modalities is becoming increasingly common.
- Treatment for advanced stage IV disease: Chemotherapy to promote tumor shrinkage and palliate symptoms; poor survival rate nonetheless.
- Postoperative complications are common and include fistulae or abscesses and respiratory complications.
- Other options include endoscopic laser therapy, endoscopic dilatation and stent placement, or placement of a gastrostomy or jejunostomy.

The 5-year survival rate for esophageal carcinoma is ~5%.

► **MISCELLANEOUS ESOPHAGEAL DISORDERS**

- Schatzki's ring: A thin, submucosal circumferential ring in the lower esophagus often associated with a hiatal hernia. Some believe it to be congenital, others due to infolding of redundant esophageal mucosa, and others due to stricture result from inflammation from chronic reflux.

- Symptoms include brief episodes of dysphagia during hurried ingestion of solid foods.
- Treatment ranges from dilatation (usually once) +/– antireflux measures to incision of the ring and excision.

- Plummer-Vinson syndrome (Patterson-Kelly syndrome): An uncommon clinical syndrome characterized by dysphagia, atrophic oral mucosa, spoon-shaped and brittle fingernails, and chronic iron deficiency anemia. More common in perimenopausal women of Scandinavian origin. Not all patients exhibit the classic picture.

  - An esophageal web, which is usually the cause of dysphagia was often thought to be a main component of the syndrome, but evidence has shown that it develops as a response to ingesting ferrous sulfate for the treatment of the anemia. Ferrous sulfate has been known to cause esophageal injury.
  - The web is usually below the cricopharyngeus muscle. Treatment consists of dilatation and iron therapy.

See Pediatric Surgery chapter for discussion of esophageal embryology and tracheoesophageal fistulas.

The Stomach

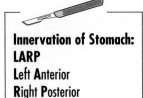

Innervation of Stomach: LARP
Left Anterior
Right Posterior

Causes of Vitamin B$_{12}$ deficiency:

- **Gastrectomy:** Loss of intrinsic factor-secreting tissue.
- **Disease or resection of terminal ileum:** Causing malabsorption of B$_{12}$.
- **Pernicious anemia:** Autoimmune destruction of parietal cells.
- **Insufficient dietary intake** (B$_{12}$ is found in most foods of animal origin).

See Figure 8-1.

Blood Supply

- Greater curvature: Right and left gastroepiploic arteries.
- Lesser curvature: Right and left gastric arteries.
- Pylorus: Gastroduodenal artery.
- Fundus: Short gastric arteries.

Innervation

See Figure 8-2.

- Anterior gastric wall: Left vagus nerve (gives branch to liver).
- Posterior gastric wall: Right vagus nerve (gives celiac branch and the "criminal nerve of Grassi").
- Gastroduodenal pain: Sensation via sympathetic afferents from level T5 (below nipple line) to T10 (umbilicus).

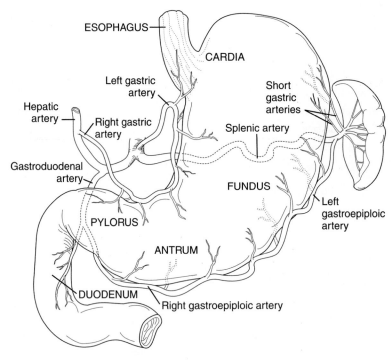

FIGURE 8-1. Anatomy of the stomach.

Histology and Physiology

- Proximal cardiac glands: Secrete mucus.
- Fundus and body:
  - Parietal (oxyntic) cells: Secrete hydrochloride (HCl), accounting for the acidic pH of stomach; secrete intrinsic factor for absorption of vitamin B_{12} in the terminal ileum.
  - Chief (peptic) cells: Secrete pepsinogen, a proenzyme activated by gastric HCl to form pepsin, which digests protein.
- Antrum: G cells—secrete gastrin, which stimulates gastric acid secretion, pepsin secretion, and mucosal growth of the gastrointestinal (GI) tract (trophic action).
- Acid secretion by parietal cells is stimulated by the vagus nerve, (acetylcholine via muscarinic M3 receptors), histamine (via H_2 receptors), and gastrin (via gastrin receptors); the final common pathway is through the proton pump (H^+/K^+ ATPase).
- Gastrin release is stimulated by gastrin-releasing peptide (GRP) and the presence of digested protein products (amino acids) in the stomach; it is inhibited by somatostatin and low antral pH (< 2.5).
- Gastric mucosal barrier (protective gel layer) is enhanced by prostaglandin E (PGE) and damaged by nonsteroidal anti-inflammatory drugs (NSAIDs).
- Gastric bicarbonate secretion into the mucous gel is inhibited by NSAIDs, acetazolamide, alpha blockers, and alcohol.

▶ PEPTIC ULCER DISEASE (PUD)

PUD is classified by location; most commonly duodenal ulcers (DUs) vs. gastric ulcers (GUs).

EPIDEMIOLOGY

- Environmental factors: *Helicobacter pylori* infection, NSAID use, smoking.
- Other risk factors: Family history of ulcers, Zollinger-Ellison (gastrinoma), corticosteroids (high dose and/or prolonged course).
- Ulcer incidence increases with age for both GU and DU; DU emerges two decades earlier than GU, particularly in males.

COMPLICATIONS

- Bleeding: 20% incidence (most common complication).
  - Hemorrhage: Dizziness, syncope, hematemesis, melena.
- Perforation (7% incidence): Sudden, severe midepigastric pain radiating to right shoulder, peritoneal signs, free peritoneal air.
  - Posterior penetration of a duodenal ulcer will cause pain that radiates to the back and can cause pancreatitis or cause GI bleeding (erosion of gastroduodenal artery). A chest or abdominal film may not show free air because the posterior duodenum is retroperitoneal.
  - Anterior perforation will show free air under the diaphragm in 70% of cases (see Figure 3-1 in Acute Abdomen chapter).
- Obstruction: Due to scarring and edema; early satiety, anorexia, vomiting, weight loss.

Typical scenario: A patient with known PUD presents with sudden onset of severe epigastric pain. Physical exam reveals guarding and rebound tenderness. *Think:* Perforation.

Alarm symptoms that indicate need for esophagogastroduodenoscopy (EGD):
- Weight loss
- Recurrent vomiting
- Dysphagia
- Bleeding
- Anemia

Typical scenario: A 52-year-old woman presents due to 3 months of early satiety, weight loss, and nonbilious vomiting. *Think:* Gastric outlet obstruction.

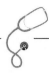

ZE accounts for 0.1–1% of patients with ulcer, but over 90% of patients with ZE have PUD (can see jejunal ulcers).

H. pylori may colonize 90% of the population — infection does not necessitate disease.

Typical scenario: A 33-year-old female smoker presents with burning epigastric pain that is improved after eating a meal. *Think:* Duodenal ulcer.

Most common location for DU: Posterior duodenal wall within 2 cm of pylorus.

▶ DUODENAL ULCER (DU)

PATHOPHYSIOLOGY

Increased acid production (in contrast to gastric ulcers); also, *H. pylori* infection may weaken mucosal defenses.

ETIOLOGY

- *H. pylori:* A bacterium that produces urease, which breaks down the protective mucous lining of the stomach; 10–20% of persons with *H. pylori* develop PUD.
- NSAIDs/steroids: Inhibit production of prostaglandin E, which stimulates mucosal barrier production.
- Zollinger-Ellison (ZE) syndrome: Gastrinoma (gastrin-secreting tumor in or near the pancreas; two thirds are malignant); 20% of ZE patients have associated multiple endocrine neoplasia type 1 (MEN-1: parathyroid hyperplasia, pancreatic islet tumors, pituitary tumors); diarrhea is common.

CLINICAL FEATURES

- Burning, gnawing epigastric pain that occurs with an empty stomach and is relieved by food or antacids (in contrast to gastric ulcers).
- Nighttime awakening (when stomach empties).
- Nausea, vomiting.
- Associated with blood type O.

DIAGNOSIS

- DU: Endoscopy; however, most symptomatic cases of DU are easily diagnosed clinically.
- *H. pylori:*
  - Endoscopy with biopsy—allows culture and sensitivity for *H. pylori* (organism is notoriously hard to culture—multiple specimens required during biopsy).
  - Serology: Anti–*H. pylori* immunoglobulin G (IgG) indicates current or prior infection.
- Urease breath test: $C^{13/14}$ labeled urea is ingested. If gastric urease is present, the carbon isotope can be detected as CO_2 isotopes in the breath.
- ZE: A fasting serum gastrin level > 1,000 pg/mL is pathognomonic for gastrinoma. Secretin stimulation test: Secretin (a gastrin inhibitor) is delivered parenterally (usually with Ca^{2+}) and its effect on gastrin secretion is measured. In ZE syndrome, there is a paradoxical astronomic rise in serum gastrin.

TREATMENT

Medical
- Risk modification:
  - Discontinue NSAIDs, steroids, smoking.
  - Prostaglandin analogues (e.g., misoprostol).
- Acid reduction:
  - Proton pump inhibitor (PPI): Omeprazole, lansoprazole, pantoprazole; 90% cure rate after 4 weeks.

- H$_2$ blockers (cimetidine, ranitidine, famotidine, nizatidine): 85–95% cure rate after 8 weeks.
- Antacids: Over the counter, good for occasional use for all causes of dyspepsia, but better drugs are available for active ulcer disease.
- Eradication of *H. pylori*:
    - Triple therapy (2-week regimen with bid dosing): PPI + amoxicillin + clarithromycin.
    - If patient is penicillin allergic, can substitute metronidazole for amoxicillin.
    - If patient fails one course of therapy, can try an alternate regimen using a different combination of drugs or quadruple therapy (2-week regimen of PPI + bismuth + tetracycline + metronidazole).

Triple therapy has 70–85% eradication rate (many regimens come prepackaged, e.g., PrevPac® = lansoprazole + amoxicillin + clarithromycin).
Quadruple therapy has 75–90% eradication rate.

Surgical

- Since the advent of highly effective medical therapy, elective surgery for PUD is quite rare.
- Surgery is indicated when ulcer is refractory to 12 weeks of medical treatment or if hemorrhage, obstruction, or perforation is present.
- Truncal vagotomy and selective vagotomy are not commonly performed anymore due to associated morbidity (high rate of dumping syndrome) despite good protection against recurrence.
- Procedure of choice is highly selective vagotomy (parietal cell vagotomy, proximal gastric vagotomy) (see Figure 8-2).
- Individual branches of the anterior and posterior nerves of Latarjet in the gastrohepatic ligament going to the lesser curvature of the stomach

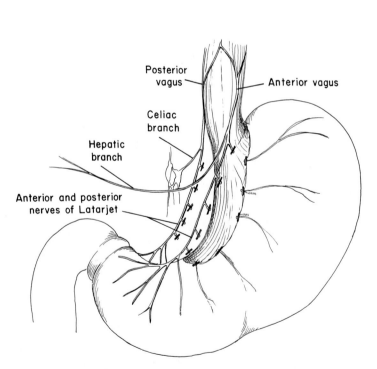

FIGURE 8-2. Highly selective vagotomy.

(Reproduced, with permission, from Zollinger RM Jr, Zollinger RM Sr. *Zollinger's Atlas of Surgical Operations*, 8th ed. New York: McGraw-Hill, 2003: 45.)

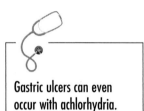

Common complications specific to surgery for peptic ulcer disease:
GAME PAD
Gallstones
Afferent loop syndrome
Marginal ulcer
Efferent loop obstruction
Postvagotomy diarrhea (most common)
Alkaline reflux gastritis
Dumping syndrome

Gastric ulcers can even occur with achlorhydria.

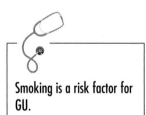

Smoking is a risk factor for GU.

are divided from a point 6 cm proximal from the pylorus to a point 6 cm proximal to the esophagogastric junction. The terminal branches to the pylorus and antrum are spared, preserving pyloroantral function and thus obviating the need for gastric drainage.

- Preferred due to its lowest rate of dumping; however, it does have the highest rate of recurrence.
- Recurrence depends on site of ulcer preop: Prepyloric ulcers have the highest recurrence rate at 30%. Least recurrence rate is with vagotomy + antrectomy.
- Laparoscopic option: A posterior truncal vagotomy coupled with an anterior seromyotomy is being done laparoscopically.
- For ZE: The tumor is resected. Occasionally, when focus of tumor cannot be found, a total gastrectomy may be considered in severe cases refractory to medical management.

▶ GASTRIC ULCER (GU)

PATHOPHYSIOLOGY

- Decreased protection against acid; acid production may not be elevated (in contrast to duodenal ulcers).
- Can be caused by reflux of duodenal contents (pyloric sphincter dysfunction) and decreased mucus and bicarbonate production.

ETIOLOGY

- NSAIDs and steroids inhibit production of prostaglandins (PGE stimulates production of protective gastric mucosal barrier).
- *H. pylori* produces urease, which breaks down the gastric mucosal barrier.

CLASSIFICATION

- Location determines classification and is important in determining treatment (Table 8-1).
- Aid to memory: One is Less, Two has Two, Three is Pre, Four is by the Door.

TABLE 8-1. Classification, Pathogenesis, and Surgical Treatment Options for Gastric Ulcer

TYPE	LOCATION OF ULCER	PATHOGENESIS	SURGICAL TREATMENT
I	Most common; near angularis incisura on lesser curvature	Normal or decreased acid secretion; decreased mucosal defense	Distal gastrectomy with ulcer excision
II	Associated with DU (active or quiescent)	Normal or increased acid secretion	Antrectomy with truncal vagotomy and ulcer excision
III	Prepyloric		
IV	Near gastroesophageal junction	Normal or subnormal acid secretion; decreased mucosal defense	Distal gastrectomy with ulcer excision and esophagogastrojejunostomy

TABLE 8-2. **Surgical Options in the Treatment of Duodenal and Gastric Ulcer Disease**

INDICATION	DUODENAL	GASTRIC
Bleeding	1. Oversew[a] 2. Oversew, V + D 3. V + A	1. Oversew and biopsy[a] 2. Oversew, biopsy, V + D 3. Distal gastrectomy[b]
Perforation	1. Patch[a] 2. Patch, HSV[b] 3. Patch, V + D	1. Biopsy and patch[a] 2. Wedge excision, V + D 3. Distal gastrectomy[b]
Obstruction	1. HSV + GJ 2. V + A	1. Biopsy; HSV + GJ 2. Distal gastrectomy[b]
Intractability/nonhealing	1. HSV[b] 2. V + D 3. V + A	1. HSV and wedge excision 2. Distal gastrectomy[a]

[a]Unless the patient is in shock or moribund, a definitive procedure should be considered.

[b]Operation of choice in low-risk patient.

GJ = gastrojejunostomy; HSV = highly-selective vagotomy; V + A = vagotomy and antrectomy; V + D = vagotomy and drainage.

Reproduced, with permission, from Brunicardi FC, Andersen DK, Billiar TR, et al. *Schwartz's Principles of Surgery,* 8th ed. New York: McGraw-Hill, 2004: 967.

SIGNS AND SYMPTOMS

- Burning, gnawing epigastric pain that occurs with anything in the stomach; pain is worst after eating (in contrast to duodenal ulcer).
- Anorexia/weight loss.
- Vomiting.
- Associated with blood type A.

DIAGNOSIS

- Endoscopy.
- All GUs are biopsied—3% are associated with gastric cancer.

TREATMENT

- Medical options: Same as for duodenal ulcers.
- Surgical options: See Tables 8-1 and 8-2.

▶ SPECIAL GASTRIC ULCERS

- Curling's ulcers: Gastric stress ulcers in patients with severe burns.
- Cushing's ulcers: Gastric stress ulcer related to severe central nervous system (CNS) damage.

Signs of duodenal perforation:
Bleeding from the **B**ack (posterior duodenal erosion/perforation, involving gastroduodenal artery).
Free **A**ir from **A**nterior duodenal perforation.
Note: Anterior perforation is more common than posterior.

Typical scenario: A 45-year-old Japanese male smoker presents with weight loss and epigastric pain exacerbated by eating. *Think:* Gastric ulcer.

- Burnt paper CURLS.
- CusHing's ulcer (think: **Head** = CNS trauma/tumor).

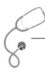

Etiologies of gastritis:
GNASHING
Gastric reflux (bile or pancreatic secretions)
Nicotine
Alcohol
Stress
Helicobacter pylori and other infections
Ischemia
NSAIDs
Glucocorticoids (long-term use)

Cimetidine is a p450 inhibitor, and therefore prolongs the action of drugs cleared by this system.

Two types of chronic gastritis and their associations:
Type **A** (fundal) — pernicious **A**nemia, parietal cell **A**ntibodies, **A**chlorhydria, **A**utoimmune disease.
Type **B** (antral) — **B**ug (*H. pylori* infection in almost all cases).

▶ GASTRITIS

DEFINITION

Acute or chronic inflammation of the stomach lining.

ETIOLOGY, SIGNS, AND SYMPTOMS

Similar to PUD; endoscopy needed to differentiate.

DIAGNOSIS

Diagnosis is made by endoscopy.

TREATMENT

Same as medical treatment of gastric ulcers.

COMPLICATIONS

Chronic gastritis leads to:

- Gastric atrophy.
- Gastric metaplasia.
- Pernicious anemia (decreased production of intrinsic factor from gastric parietal cells due to idiopathic atrophy of the gastric mucosa and subsequent malabsorption of vitamin B_{12}).

▶ POSTGASTRECTOMY COMPLICATIONS

Postvagotomy Diarrhea

- Most common complication of vagotomy.
- Usually self-limited.
- Symptomatic treatment with motility-reducing agents (kaolin-pectin, loperamide, or diphenoxylate).
- Refractory cases may respond to cholestyramine (bile-salt binding agent).

Dumping Syndromes

- Complication of gastric surgery thought to result from unregulated movement of gastric contents from stomach to small intestine.
- Symptoms typically occur 5–15 minutes postprandially (early dumping syndrome) due to high osmolar load reaching the small intestine or 2–4 hours postprandially (late dumping syndrome) due to hypoglycemia.
- Nausea, vomiting, belching, diarrhea, tachycardia, palpitations, flushing, diaphoresis, dizziness, syncope.
- Treated by dietary modification: Small, multiple low-carbohydrate/fat meals; avoid excessive liquid intake.
- Severe cases (1%) that do not respond to dietary modifications can be treated with octreotide (synthetic somatostatin—helps delay gastric emptying time and transit through small intestine).

Alkaline Reflux Gastritis

- Diagnosis of exclusion after recurrent ulcer has been ruled out; nonspecific EGD and biopsy findings (edematous, inflamed gastric mucosa).
- Presents with postprandial pain and bilious vomiting.
- Medical treatment is difficult.
- Surgical management: Roux-en-Y gastrojejunostomy with a long (~50-cm) Roux limb. Bilious vomiting may improve, but symptoms (early satiety, bloating) may persist.

Afferent Loop Syndrome

- Obstruction of afferent limb following gastrojejunostomy (Bilroth II); two thirds present in postop week 1.
- **Symptoms:** Postprandial right upper quadrant (RUQ) pain, bilious vomiting, steatorrhea (with concomitant malabsorption of fats, B_{12}), anemia.
- **Diagnosis:** Afferent loop will be devoid of contrast of UGI series.
- **Treatment:** Endoscopic balloon dilatation or surgical revision of loop if that fails.

Nutritional Deficiencies

- Vitamin B_{12} deficiency anemia.
- Iron deficiency anemia.
- Osteoporosis (due to reduced calcium absorption).

▶ **GASTRIC OUTLET OBSTRUCTION**

COMMON CAUSES

- Malignant tumors of stomach and head of pancreas.
- Obstructing gastric or duodenal ulcers.
- Usually with duodenal ulcer.
- Chronic ulcer causes secondary edema or scarring, which occludes lumen.

SYMPTOMS

Early
- Early satiety.
- Gastric reflux.
- Abdominal distention.

Late
- Vomiting.
- Dehydration.
- Hypochloremic, hypokalemic metabolic alkalosis with paradoxical aciduria.
- Weight loss.

DIAGNOSIS

Endsocopy or barium swallow x-ray.

Typical scenario: A 58-year-old woman who is 6 days postop from a gastrojejunostomy for PUD presents with postprandial RUQ pain and nausea. She reports that vomiting relieves her suffering. *Think:* Afferent loop syndrome.

CAUSES:
Mallory's Vices Gave (her) An Ulcer.
Mallory-Weiss tear
Varices
Gastritis
AV malformation
Ulcers

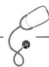

CONTRAST:
Mallory-Weiss syndrome: Postemetic *tears* in gastric mucosa (near gastroesophageal junction).
Boerhaave syndrome: Postemetic esophageal *rupture*.

Coffee grounds is the term used to describe old, brown digested blood found on gastric lavage. It usually indicates a source of bleeding proximal to the ligament of Treitz.

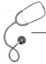

A bleeding scan detects active bleeding by infusing technetium-labeled autologous red blood cells (^{99m}Tc-labeled RBCs) and watching for their collection in the GI tract. It can be completed in ~1 hour and can detect bleeds as slow as 0.1 mL/min, but location specificity is only 60–70%. CT angiography is faster and detects bleeds up to 0.5 mL/min.

Risk of ulcers rebleeding:
- In-hospital: One third.
- GUs are three times more likely to rebleed than DUs.

TREATMENT

- Truncal vagotomy and pyloroplasty or gastrojejunostomy after 7 days of nasogastric decompression and antisecretory treatment.
- Nasogastric decompression is necessary to normalize the size of the dilated stomach.

▶ GASTROINTESTINAL HEMORRHAGE

Upper GI Hemorrhage

ETIOLOGY

- Ulcer (peptic)
- Varices
- Gastritis
- Arteriovenous malformation
- Mallory-Weiss tear

SIGNS AND SYMPTOMS

- Hematemesis (bright red or coffee grounds).
- Hypotension.
- Tachycardia.
- Bleeding that produces 60 cc of blood or more will produce black, tarry stool (melena).
- Very brisk upper GI bleeds can be associated with bright red blood per rectum (hematochezia) and hypotension.

DIAGNOSIS

- Gastric lavage with normal saline or free water to assess severity of bleeding (old vs. new blood).
- Rectal exam.
- Complete blood count (CBC).
- Endoscopy.
- Bleeding scan.
- Arteriography.

TREATMENT

- Depends on etiology and severity.
- Bleeding varices are ligated, or sclerosed via endoscopy (see Hepatobiliary System chapter).
- Most Mallory-Weiss tears resolve spontaneously.
- For severe bleeds:
  - Intravenous fluids and blood products as needed.
  - Somatostatin (inhibits gastric, intestinal, and biliary motility, decreases visceral blood flow).
  - Consider balloon tamponade for esophageal varices.
- Surgery:
  - About 5% of the time, upper GI bleeding cannot be controlled via endoscopic or other methods and emergent laparotomy will be necessary.

- For duodenal ulcers, a longitudinal incision is made across the pylorus and proximal duodenum. Bleeding is controlled by undersewing the vessel on either side of the hemorrhage.

▶ BARIATRIC SURGERY

INDICATION

BMI (body mass index) = weight in kg / (height in M)^2:

- BMI > 35 with comorbitiy (e.g., hypertension, diabetes mellitus).
- BMI ≥ 40 with or without comorbidity.

Prerequisite: Participation in supervised dietary program without success.

TYPES

- Restrictive: Reduction of the quantity of food intake.
  - Vertical banded gastroplasty (VBG): Partitioning of the stomach into a small proximal pouch (< 20 mL) and a more distal one (see Figure 8-3).
  - Sleeve gastric resection.
  - Laparoscopic adjustable band placement (Figure 8-4).
- Malabsorptive: Limit nutrient absorption by bypassing duodenum and small intestine.
  - Biliopancreatic diversion with or without duodenal switch (Figure 8-5).
  - Roux-en-Y gastric bypass (also has a restrictive component; see Figure 8-6).

Medical conditions commonly associated with morbid obesity: Diabetes mellitus, coronary artery disease, hypertension, sleep apnea, arthritis, sex hormone abnormalities, breast cancer, colon cancer.

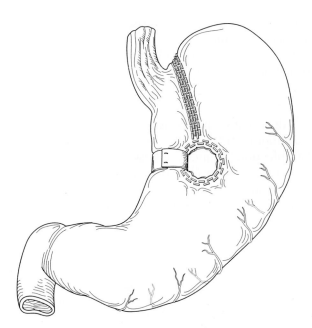

FIGURE 8-3. Vertical banded gastroplasty.

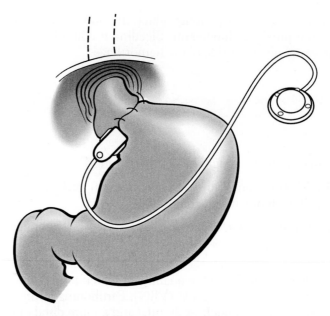

FIGURE 8-4. **Adjustable gastric banding with gastropexy.**

(Reproduced, with permission, from Miller K. Laparoscopic restrictive procedures: adjustable gastric banding. In Pitombo C, Jones KB Jr, Higa KD, Pareja JC, eds. *Obesity Surgery: Principles and Practice.* New York: McGraw-Hill, 2008: 170.)

▶ MALIGNANT TUMORS

Adenocarcinoma

EPIDEMIOLOGY

- In general, gastric cancer is a disease of the elderly (age > 60), men > women, blacks > whites.
- Adenocarcinoma comprises 95% of malignant gastric cancer.
- Leading cause of cancer-related death in Japan.

RISK FACTORS

- Familial adenomatous polyposis.
- Chronic atrophic gastritis.
- *H. pylori* infection (6× increased risk).
- Post–partial gastrectomy (15+ years).
- Pernicious anemia.
- Diet (foods high in nitrites—preserved, smoked, cured).
- Cigarette smoking.

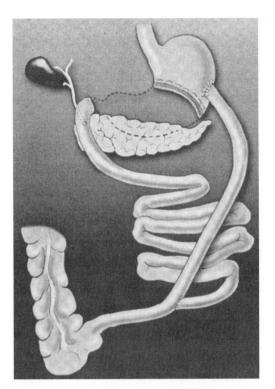

FIGURE 8-5. **Biliopancreatic diversion procedure before the gallbladder is removed.**

(Reproduced, with permission, from Jacobs DO, Robinson MK. Morbid obesity and operations for morbid obesity. In Zinner MJ, Ashley SW, eds. *Maingot's Abdominal Operations*, 11th ed. New York: McGraw-Hill, 2007: 470.)

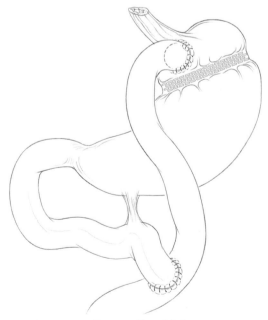

FIGURE 8-6. **Roux-en-Y gastric bypass.**

PATHOLOGY

- Polypoid: 25–50%, no substantial necrosis or ulceration.
- Ulcerative: 25–50%, sharp margins.
- Superficial spreading: 3–10%, involves mucosa and submucosa only, best prognosis.
- Linitis plastica: 7–10%, "leather bottle" type, involves all layers, extremely poor prognosis.

SIGNS AND SYMPTOMS

- Early: Mostly asymptomatic.
- Late: Anorexia/weight loss, nausea, vomiting, dysphagia, melena, hematemesis; pain is constant, nonradiating, exacerbated by food.
- Anemia—from blood loss, pernicious.
- Krukenberg's tumor—metastasis to ovaries.
- Blumer's shelf—metastasis to pelvic cul-de-sac, felt on digital rectal exam.
- Virchow's node—metastasis to lymph node palpable in left supraclavicular fossa.
- Sister Mary Joseph's nodule—periumbilical metastatic nodules.

DIAGNOSIS

- Upper GI endoscopy: Best method, allows for biopsy, definitive > 95% sensitivity and specificity.
- Upper GI series: With double contrast; 80–96% sensitivity, 90% specificity (operator dependent); excellent method in skilled hands.
- Abdominal CT: Good for detecting distant metastases; also used for preop staging, but suboptimal.
- Endoscopic ultrasound: Good for detecting depth of invasion.

STAGING

See Table 8-3.

TREATMENT

- Radical subtotal gastrectomy can be curative in early disease confined to the superficial layers of the stomach (less than one third of all patients due to typical late presentation).
- Chemotherapy: Sometimes used palliatively for nonsurgical candidates; no role for adjuvant chemotherapy.

PROGNOSIS

- Treatment is a major prognostic factor for gastric cancer—patients who are not resected have a poor prognosis.
- Location: Proximal gastric cancer has less favorable prognosis than distal lesions.
- Tumor markers: High preop serum levels of carcinoembryonic antigen (CEA) and CA 19-9 have been associated with less favorable outcomes.
- Other factors: Histologic grade, regional lymphatic spread.

TABLE 8-3. Gastric Cancer Staging

	STAGE GROUPING			5-YEAR SURVIVAL RATE
Stage 0	Tis	N0	M0	> 90%
Stage IA	T1	N0	M0	70–80%
Stage IB	T1	N1	M0	55–70%
	T2a/b	N0	M0	
Stage II	T1	N2	M0	40–50%
	T2a/b	N1	M0	
	T3	N0	M0	
Stage IIIA	T2a/b	N2	M0	10–20%
	T3	N1	M0	
	T4	N0	M0	
Stage IIIB	T3	N2	M0	
Stage IV	T1–3	N3	M0	< 1%
	T4	N1–3	M0	
	Any T	Any N	M1	

TUMOR (T) STAGE

TX	Primary tumor cannot be assessed
T0	No evidence of primary tumor
T1s	Carcinoma in situ: Intraepithelial tumor without invasion of lamina propria
T1	Tumor invades lamina propria or submucosa
T2a/b	2a–tumor invades muscularis propria 2b–tumor invades subserosa
T3	Tumor penetrates serosa (visceral peritoneum) without invasion of adjacent structures
T4	Tumor invades adjacent structures (includes spleen, colon, liver, diaphragm, pancreas, abdominal wall, adrenal gland, kidney, small intestine, retroperitoneum)

(continued)

TABLE 8-3. **Gastric Cancer Staging** *(continued)*

NODAL (N) STAGE	
Nx	Regional lymph node(s) cannot be assessed
N0	No regional lymph node metastasis
N1	Metastasis in 1–6 regional lymph nodes
N2	Metastasis in 7–15 regional lymph nodes
N3	Metastasis in > 15 regional lymph nodes

METASTASIS (M) STAGE	
Mx	Presence of distant metastasis cannot be assessed
M0	No distant metastasis
M1	Distant metastasis

Reproduced, with permission, from Greene FL, Page DL, Fleming ID, et al. *AJCC Cancer Staging Manual,* 6th ed. New York: Springer, 2002.

Gastric Lymphoma

- Second most common malignant gastric cancer.
- Stomach is most common site for primary GI lymphoma (majority are B-cell non-Hodgkin's type) but lymphoma comprise only 4% of all gastric tumors.
- Increased risk with *H. pylori* infection.

SIGNS AND SYMPTOMS

Nonspecific; include abdominal discomfort, nausea, vomiting, anorexia, weight loss, and hemorrhage; occult bleeding and anemia (50% of patients).

DIAGNOSIS

- Made by endoscopic biopsy, not readily distinguishable from adenocarcinoma by simple inspection.
- Bone marrow aspiration and gallium bone scans can diagnose metastases.

TREATMENT

- MALT (low grade)—treat *H. pylori.*
- MALT (high grade) or non-MALT—radiation/chemo ± surgical resection.
- Resection reserved for patients with bleeding or perforation.

Poor prognostic factors include:

- Involvement of the lesser curvature of the stomach.
- Large tumor size.
- Advanced stage.

Gastrointestinal Stromal Tumor (GIST)

- Mesenchymal tumors arising from the gastric stroma; submucosal and slow growing.
- Stomach is the most common site.
- Variable histology—from spindle cell tumors to epithelioid to pleomorphic.
- Approximately 95% of GISTs have c-kit (CD117) expression.
- All GISTs are regarded as malignant.
- Treated by surgical resection and Gleevec (imatinib).
- Prognosis depends on completeness of resection, presence of metastases, and the mitotic index.

▶ BENIGN LESIONS

Benign Tumors/Adenomatous Polyps

- Account for 10–20% of all gastric polyps.
- Are the only ones with any real malignant potential; others are mostly asymptomatic and uncommon.
- Biopsy lesions > 5 mm to check for neoplasia.

Ménétrier's Disease

DEFINITION

- Hypertrophic gastropathy (enlarged, tortuous gastric rugae).
- Protein-losing enteropathy.
- Mucosal thickening secondary to hyperplasia of glandular cells replacing chief and parietal cells.
- Low-grade inflammatory infiltrate—not a form of gastritis.

SIGNS AND SYMPTOMS

- Most common: Middle-aged man who presents with epigastric pain, weight loss, diarrhea, hypoproteinemia.
- Less common: Nausea, vomiting, anorexia, occult GI bleed.
- Gastric acid secretion can be high, normal, or low.

DIAGNOSIS

- Endoscopy with deep mucosal biopsy is definitive.
- Barium swallow will reveal large gastric folds and thickened rugae.

COMPLICATIONS

- Gastric ulcer
- Gastric cancer

Ménétrier's can look like gastric cancer on barium study.

Monitor closely as there may be increased incidence of gastric cancer (adenocarcinoma).

TREATMENT

- Anticholinergics, H_2 blockers to reduce protein loss.
- High-protein diet.
- Treatment of ulcers/cancer if present and eradication of *H. pylori*.
- Severe disease may require gastrectomy.

Bezoars

DEFINITION

- Concretions of nondigestible matter that accumulate in stomach.
- May consist of hair (trichobezoar), vegetable matter (phytobezoar) (especially in patients who may have eaten persimmon), or charcoal (used in management of toxic ingestions).
- May develop after gastric surgery.

SYMPTOMS

- Similar to gastric outlet obstruction.
- Occasionally causes ulceration and bleeding.

DIAGNOSIS

Upper GI endoscopy.

TREATMENT

- Proteolytic enzymes—papain.
- Mechanical fragmentation with endoscope.
- Surgical removal.

Dieulafoy's Lesion

DEFINITION

Mucosal end artery that causes pressure necrosis and erodes into stomach and ruptures.

SYMPTOMS

Massive, recurrent painless hematemesis.

DIAGNOSIS

Upper GI endoscopy.

TREATMENT

- Endoscopic sclerosing therapy or electrocoagulation.
- Wedge resection.

Gastric Volvulus

DEFINITION

Torsion/twisting of stomach typically along long axis. Often associated with paraesophageal hernia. May be acute, but most often chronic.

Brochardt's triad:

- Intermittent severe epigastric pain and distention.
- Inability to vomit.
- Difficult passage of nasogastric (NG) tube.

Diagnosis

Upper GI contrast study.

Treatment

- Surgical repair of accompanying hernia.
- Gastropexy—fixes stomach to anterior abdominal wall.
- Gastric resection if there is necrosis.

HIGH-YIELD FACTS

The Stomach

All of the small intestine is derived from the midgut except for the proximal duodenum, which is derived from the foregut. The junction between the foregut and midgut is immediately distal to the opening of the common bile duct.

Initially, the primitive gut tube communicates with the yolk sac. This communication narrows by the sixth week to form the vitelline duct. If the vitelline duct fails to obliterate by the end of gestation, it persists as a Meckel's diverticulum seen in 2% of the population.

The midgut loop rotates a total of 270° around the axis of the superior mesenteric artery (SMA) before it reaches its final fixed position in the abdomen.

▶ INTRODUCTION

The small bowel is the principal site for the absorption and digestion of nutrients, as well as for the maintenance of fluid homeostasis in the gastrointestinal system. It also serves as a major component of both the endocrine and immune systems.

▶ GASTROINTESTINAL (GI) EMBRYOLOGY

Fourth Week

The primitive gut tube, formed from the endoderm, begins to develop into the foregut, midgut, and hindgut.
- Endoderm becomes intestinal epithelium and glands.
- Mesoderm becomes connective tissue, muscle, and wall of intestine.

Fifth Week

- Intestine elongates and midgut loop herniates through umbilical ring.
- Midgut loop continues to lengthen extracoelomically until approximately week 10.

Tenth Week

Midgut loop rotates 270° counterclockwise and returns back into the abdominal cavity.

▶ GROSS ANATOMY

General

- Total length: 5–10 m (average 6 m).
- Consists of three parts: Duodenum, jejunum, ileum (~25 cm duodenum, 100–110 cm jejunum, 150–160 cm ileum).
- Aside from the first 2 cm, the duodenum is a retroperitoneal structure, while the jejunum and ileum are intraperitoneal structures.

Duodenum

- Extends from the pylorus to the duodenojejunal junction.
- Consists of four parts:
    - Superior (first) part—duodenal bulb: 5 cm long; site of most ulcers.
    - Descending (second) part—10 cm long; curves around the head of pancreas.
    - Transverse (third) part—10 cm long; crosses anterior to aorta and inferior vena cava (IVC) and posterior to the SMA and superior mesenteric vein (SMV).
    - Ascending (fourth) part—5 cm long; ascends past left side of aorta, then curves anteriorly to meet with jejunum, forming the duodenojejunal junction, which is suspended by the ligament of Treitz.

- Duodenum ends and jejunum begins at the ligament of Treitz.
- Since the duodenum is retroperitoneal, it is tethered to the posterior abdominal wall and has no mesentery at its posterior aspect.
- Plicae circulares (transverse mucosal folds in the lumen of the small bowel) are most prominent in the proximal small bowel (duodenum and jejunum) than in the distal small intestine (ileum).

Duodenal Blood Supply

- Arterial supply:
  - Proximal (up to ampulla of Vater): Gastroduodenal artery (first branch of proper hepatic artery) bifurcates into the anterior and posterior superior pancreaticoduodenal arteries.
  - Distal (beyond ampulla of Vater): Inferior pancreaticoduodenal artery (first branch of superior mesenteric artery [SMA]) bifurcates into the anterior and posterior inferior pancreaticoduodenal arteries.
- Venous drainage:
  - Anterior and posterior pancreaticoduodenal veins drain into the SMV, which joins the splenic vein behind the neck of the pancreas to form the portal vein.
  - Prepyloric vein of Mayo is landmark for pylorus.

Jejunum and Ileum

- No anatomical boundary between the two.
- Jejunum is the proximal 40% of small intestine distal to ligament of Treitz.
- Ileum is the distal 60% of small intestine.
- Combined length is 5–10 m (average 6 m).
- Mesentery tethers the jejunum and ileum to posterior abdominal wall.
- Arterial supply:
  - Both jejunum and ileum supplied by branches of SMA, which runs in the mesentery.
  - The arteries loop to form arcades that give rise to straight arteries— vasa recta.
- Venous drainage: The SMV drains both the jejunum and ileum.

Lymphatics

- Drainage: Bowel wall → mesenteric nodes → lymphatic vessels parallel the corresponding arteries → cisterna chyli (a retroperitoneal structure between the aorta and IVC) → thoracic duct (also between the aorta and IVC) → left subclavian vein.
- Participate in absorption of fat.

Innervation

Parasympathetic System

- Source: Fibers originate from vagus and celiac ganglia.
- Function: Enhances bowel secretion, motility, and other digestive processes.

Various congenital anomalies are associated with either failure of midgut loop to rotate properly (i.e., malrotation) or failure of retraction of midgut loop back into the abdominal cavity (i.e., omphalocele and gastroschisis). (See Pediatric Surgery chapter for more details.)

Anterior ulcers tend to perforate, causing leakage of duodenal contents into the peritoneal cavity, leading to peritonitis. Ulcers that result in massive bleeding are posterior ulcers that have penetrated the gastroduodenal artery.

Typical scenario: A patient with a history of duodenal ulcers presents with massive GI bleeding. Upper GI endoscopy shows an ulcer that penetrates the posterior wall of the duodenal bulb (first part of the duodenum). What is the most likely vascular structure responsible for the bleeding? *Think:* The gastroduodenal artery courses behind the first part of the duodenum and is the most likely culprit.

HIGH-YIELD FACTS

Small Bowel

HIGH-YIELD FACTS

Small Bowel

HIGH-YIELD FACTS

Small Bowel

There are no clinical or laboratory parameters that can reliably differentiate between simple obstruction and strangulated obstruction before the onset of ischemia.

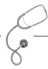

"Never let the sun rise or set on a small bowel obstruction."
While this adage was strictly adhered to in the past, currently, stable patients, particularly those with partial obstruction, are more likely to be treated nonoperatively. As with any patient, if symptoms worsen, or signs of strangulation develop, the patient should be brought to the OR.

- Upright abdominal x-ray: Multiple air-fluid levels in a "stepladder" (Figure 9-1).
- Upright chest radiograph: Can detect presence of free air under the diaphragm and thus possible bowel perforation.
- Abdominal computed tomographic (CT) scan more sensitive and specific than x-rays (Figure 9-2).
- Findings: Transition zone, with dilation of bowel proximally and decompression of the bowel distally, no contrast present distal to transition point, and paucity of gas and fluid in colon.
- Useful in acute setting to rule out other diagnoses as well.

TREATMENT

- If the patient is stable or has partial SBO, give a trial of nonoperative management:
  - NPO.
  - IV hydration to counter effects of third spacing.
  - Nasogastric tube (NGT) for gastric decompression; decreases nausea, vomiting, distention.
  - Foley catheter to monitor urine output.
  - Monitor electrolytes for signs of hypokalemia, base deficit/metabolic acidosis (signs of ischemia).
- Patients with suspected strangulation need to be resuscitated with fluids prior to surgery.

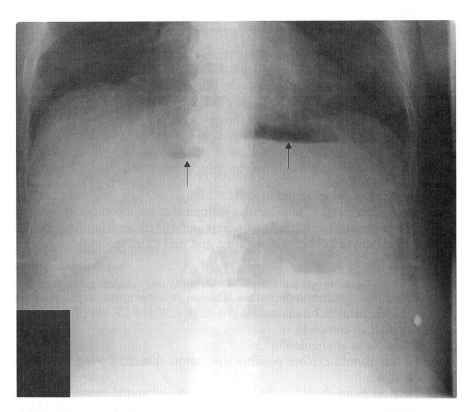

FIGURE 9-1. **AXR demonstrating loops of dilated small bowel in the midabdomen, suggestive of small bowel obstruction.**

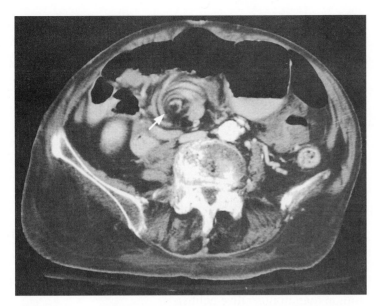

FIGURE 9-2. Contrast abdominal CT scan demonstrating midgut volvulus as a cause of small bowel obstruction.

- If the patient fails conservative management (24 hrs without improvement, abdominal tenderness worsens, fever, other signs of clinical deterioration), then laparotomy should be performed.
- The surgical procedure depends on the cause of the obstruction:
  - Adhesions call for lysis of adhesions (LOA).
  - Hernias should be reduced and repaired or, if contents of sac are strangulated, needs intestinal resection.
  - Cancer requires en bloc resection with lymph node sampling.
  - Crohn's disease requires resection or stricturoplasty of affected area only.
- Whatever the cause, the entire small bowel should be examined, and nonviable intestine should be resected.
- Primary anastomosis should be performed in hemodynamically stable patients who have had small segments of bowel resected.

Typical scenario: A 5-year-old child presents with increasing irritability, colicky abdominal pain, and rectal bleeding with stools that have a currant jelly appearance. A tubular mass is palpated in the right lower quadrant. Upright abdominal x-ray shows air-fluid levels with a stepladder pattern. *Think:* Intussusception. Barium enema is both diagnostic and therapeutic.

Crohn's Disease

DEFINITION

Inflammatory bowel disease characterized by transmural inflammation involving any part of the GI tract, from mouth to anus, of unknown etiology. The inflammation is discontinuous, resulting in skip lesions, and often leads to fibrosis and ultimately obstruction, as well as to the formation of fistulae.

EPIDEMIOLOGY

- Eighty percent of patients have involvement of small bowel, usually the distal ileum (one third of these patients just have ileitis).
- Fifty percent of patients have involvement of both the ileum and colon.
- Twenty percent of patients have involvement of the colon only. Differentiate from ulcerative colitis because Crohn's disease patients tend to have rectal sparing.

- One third of patients have perianal disease as well.
- Diagnosis most common between ages 15 and 40, although there is a second peak between 50 and 80 years of age (bimodal distribution).

RISK FACTORS

- Jewish descent.
- Positive family history.
- Urban dwelling.
- Smoking.

SIGNS AND SYMPTOMS

Typical symptoms include:

- Crampy abdominal pain (typically right lower quadrant [RLQ]), diarrhea, weight loss most common symptoms.
- Fever, fatigue.
- Bleeding (hemoccult + stools common, but gross lower GI bleeding less common than in ulcerative colitis).
- Perianal disease including skin tags, anal fissures, perirectal abscesses, and anorectal fistulae.
- Signs and symptoms of intestinal perforation and/or fistula formation (e.g., combination of localized peritonitis, fever, abdominal pain, tenderness, and palpable mass on physical exam).
- Extraintestinal manifestations include oral involvement (e.g., aphthous ulcers), joint involvement (e.g., arthritis), ocular involvement, dermatologic involvement (e.g., erythema nodosum, pyoderma gangrenosum), hepatobiliary involvement (e.g., sclerosing cholangitis).

DIAGNOSIS

- Typical history of prolonged diarrhea with abdominal pain, weight loss, and fever with or without gross bleeding.
- Physical exam can be nonspecific or suggestive of Crohn's disease, such as perianal skin tags, sinus tracts, or a palpable abdominal mass.
- Colonoscopy (with biopsy), visualization of the terminal ileum may reveal focal ulcerations adjacent to areas of normal mucosa along with a cobblestone appearance to the intestinal mucosa.
- Esophagogastroduodenoscopy (EGD) for proximal disease.
- Imaging (small bowel contrast studies) is helpful in characterizing length of involvement and areas of stricture, especially in parts of small bowel that are inaccessible via colonoscopy.
- Radiographic appearance: Mucosal nodularity, narrowed lumen, ulceration, string sign, presence of abscesses and fistulae.

TREATMENT

- Medical: Corticosteroids, aminosalicylates (sulfasalazine, 5-ASA), immune modulators (azathioprine, 6-mercaptopurine, cyclosporine), infliximab (anti-TNF-α), metronidazole.
- Many patients require surgery to relieve symptoms that do not respond to drugs, or to treat complications such as obstruction, abscesses, fistulae, perforation, perianal disease, or cancer.
- Surgery should be avoided if possible, since Crohn's disease is not curable by surgery as opposed to ulcerative colitis.

Differential diagnosis of RLQ pain:
- Appendicitis.
- Crohn's disease.
- Infectious colitis — *Yersinia, Campylobacter.*
- Gynecologic pathology in females (ovarian torsion, abscess, ectopic pregnancy).
- Ischemic colitis.

Unlike ulcerative colitis, which can be cured with surgical resection, Crohn's disease is incurable surgically.

- Surgical resection of an affected area does not preclude future disease development in adjacent or distant parts of the bowel.
- Surgical procedure depends on indication:
  - One third of patients require surgery to relieve intestinal obstruction by strictures, either via segmental small bowel resection or stricturoplasty (Figures 9-3 and 9-4).
  - For fistulae: Seton placement and drainage, fistulotomy, fistulectomy.
  - For extensive disease: Total colectomy with end ileostomy can be done.
  - For cancer: En bloc resection with lymph node dissection.

PROGNOSIS

- Typical course is one of intermittent exacerbations followed by periods of remission.
- Ten to twenty percent of patients experience prolonged remission after initial presentation.
- Approximately 80% of patients ultimately require surgical intervention.
- Like ulcerative colitis, there is an increased risk of colon cancer in patients with long-standing Crohn's colitis.

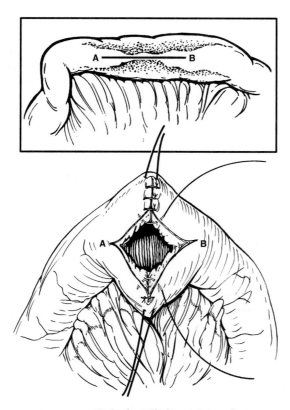

FIGURE 9-3. **Heineke-Mikulicz strictureplasty.**

(Reprinted, with permission, from Michelassi F, Hurst RD, Fichera A. Crohn's disease. In Zinner MJ, Ashley SW, eds. *Maingot's Abdominal Operations*, 11th ed. New York: McGraw-Hill, 2007: 533.)

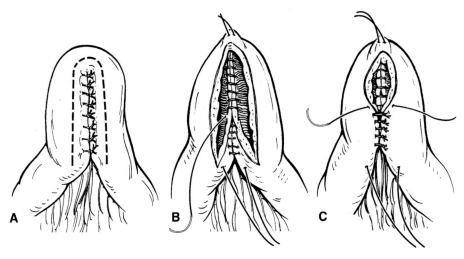

FIGURE 9-4. Finney strictureplasty.

(Reprinted, with permission, from Michelassi F, Hurst RD, Fichera A. Crohn's disease. In Zinner MJ, Ashley SW, eds. *Maingot's Abdominal Operations*, 11th ed. New York: McGraw-Hill, 2007: 534.)

- Resection with anastomosis has 10–15% clinical recurrence rate per year.
- Total colectomy with ileostomy has 10% recurrence rate over 10 years in remaining small bowel.

Benign Neoplasms of Small Intestine

INCIDENCE

- Adenomas > leiomyomas > lipomas (but leiomyomas most likely to cause symptoms).
- Most small intestinal benign neoplasms are found in the duodenum.
- Most common cause of adult intussusception.
- Most patients in 5th or 6th decade of life.

RISK FACTORS

- Hereditary syndromes:
  - Peutz-Jeghers syndrome (hamartomatous polyps).
  - Gardner syndrome (adenoma).
  - Familial adenomatous polyposis (adenoma).
- Consumption of red meat and salt-cured foods.

SIGNS AND SYMPTOMS

- Most are asymptomatic until they become large.
- Intermittent obstruction: Crampy abdominal pain, distention, nausea, and vomiting.
- Occult or overt bleeding.
- Palpable abdominal mass.
- Obstructive jaundice (periampullary lesion).

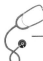

Intermittent obstruction is the most common presentation in a symptomatic patient with a small bowel neoplasm. It can be caused by either narrowing of the small bowel lumen or secondary to intussusception, with the neoplasm serving as the lead point.

- Endoscopy:
  - EGD: Can visualize proximal duodenum; most duodenal neoplasms are found incidentally on EGD.
  - Endoscopic ultrasound (EUS): Can offer more information such as the depth of intestinal wall involved.
- Radiographic:
  - Small bowel series—low sensitivity.
  - CT scan.
  - Enteroclysis: Test of choice; high sensitivity; used to detect tumors in distal small intestine.
- Majority of patients: Small bowel series with follow-through followed by enteroclysis.
- High-risk patients: Enteroclysis.

TYPES

See Table 9-3.

TREATMENT

- All symptomatic lesions should be resected, either surgically or endoscopically.
- Tumors located in proximal duodenum, even asymptomatic lesions, should be removed either endoscopically (< 1 cm) or surgically (> 2 cm).
- Tumors in second portion of duodenum, near ampulla, may require pancreaticoduodenectomy (Whipple procedure).

Malignant Neoplasms of Small Intestine

- Rare.
- Adenocarcinoma > carcinoid > gastrointestinal stromal tumor (GIST) > lymphoma.
- Risk factors, signs and symptoms, and diagnosis essentially the same as benign neoplasms of small intestine (see Table 9-4):
  - Adenocarcinoma: Crohn's disease, celiac disease, familial adenomaous polyposis (FAP), Peutz-Jeghers syndrome.
  - Lymphoma: Celiac disease, immunodeficiency states, autoimmune disorders.

TREATMENT

- Wide en bloc resection of involved intestine.
- For adenocarcinomas, wide local excision of the intestine with its accompanying mesentery is performed along with regional lymph nodes.
- GISTs usually treated with segmental resection of affected intestine and Gleevec (imatinib), a tyrosine kinase inhibitor.
- Patients with duodenal lesions may require a Whipple procedure.
- Bypass may be required for palliation.
- Localized lymphoma is treated with segmental resection of the intestine, and neighboring mesentery.
- Diffuse lymphoma is the only situation where chemotherapy, rather than surgical resection, should be the primary therapy.

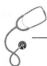

Enteroclysis is a double-contrast study that involves passing a tube into the proximal small intestine and injecting barium and methylcellulose. It can detect tumors missed on conventional small bowel follow-through. **Extended small bowel enteroscopy** (Sonde enteroscopy) is much like push enteroscopy, but involves advancement of the enteroscope by peristalsis. It visualizes up to 70% of the small bowel mucosa and detects tumors missed by enteroclysis.

Typical scenario: A patient presents with pigmented spots on his lips and a history of recurrent colicky abdominal pain. What is the cause of his abdominal pain? *Think:* Peutz-Jeghers syndrome. The hamartomatous polyps are likely causing intermittent intussusception.

Small bowel is frequently affected by metastasis or invasion from cancers originating in other organs, particularly melanoma.

HIGH-YIELD FACTS

Small Bowel

TABLE 9-3. Benign Neoplasms of the Small Intestine

Type	Risk Factors	Signs and Symptoms	Location	Treatment
Adenoma (35% of benign small bowel tumors)	Gardner's syndrome (GS)	Obstruction	Duodenum (20%)	Endoscopic or surgical excision For GS and familial adenomaous polyposis (FAP): ■ Screening EGD 2nd–3rd decade ■ Adenomas resected endoscopically ■ Adenoma recurrence requires pancreaticoduodenectomy (risk of ampullary carcinoma)
		Bleeding	Jejunum (30%)	Excision
	FAP		Ileum (50%)	Excision
Leiomyoma		Obstruction Bleeding	Jejunum	Excision
Lipoma		Obstruction Incidental finding	Duodenum Ileum	Excision is required only if symptomatic
Hamartoma	Peutz-Jeghers syndrome	■ Recurrent colicky abdominal pain (from intermittent intussusception) ■ Obstruction ■ Bleeding		■ Resection of segment responsible for symptoms
Hemangioma (3–4% of benign small bowel tumors)		Bleeding		
Fibroma		Obstruction Asymptomatic mass		

PROGNOSIS

- Overall five-year survival: ≤ 20%.
- Five-year survival by tumor type:
  - Complete resection of duodenal adenocarcinoma: 50–60%.
  - Complete resection of jejunal/ileal adenocarcinoma: 5–30%.
  - GIST: 30–40%.
  - Localized lymphoma: 60%.

TABLE 9-4. Malignant Neoplasms of the Small Intestine

TYPE	RISK FACTORS	SIGNS AND SYMPTOMS	LOCATION (IN SMALL GUT)
Adenocarcinoma (25–50% of primary small bowel malignancies)	Crohn's disease, celiac disease, FAP, Peutz-Jeghers syndrome	Obstruction	Duodenum (most found in duodenum)
		Bleeding	Ileum (in Crohn's disease most adenocarcinomas found in ileum)
		Mass	
Carcinoid (up to 40% of primary small bowel malignancies)		Often asymptomatic	Ileum
		Obstruction Carcinoid syndrome	
GIST (CD 117 [c-kit])		Hemorrhage	No regional preference
Lymphoma	Celiac disease	Obstruction Perforation	Ileum
	Immunosuppression	Weight loss	
	Autoimmune disease	Pain Fatigue Mass Bleeding	
Sarcoma (most common leiomyosarcoma)		Pain	Jejunum
		Bleeding	Ileum
		Obstruction (late symptom)	Meckel's diverticulum
Neuroendocrine		Mass	Proximal small intestine
		Hormone-specific symptoms	
Metastatic	History of melanoma, breast, lung, ovarian, colon, or cervical cancer	Obstruction; bleeding	

Carcinoid

DEFINITION

- Malignant tumor of enterochromaffin cell origin, part of amine precursor uptake and decarboxylation (APUD) system.
- Most common in appendix.

HIGH-YIELD FACTS

Small Bowel

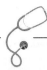

Small bowel and colonic carcinoids are associated with the highest degree of malignant potential.

The carcinoid syndrome develops when the tumor produces amines and peptides outside of the portovenous circulation. Classically, appendiceal and small intestinal carcinoids cause the carcinoid syndrome only after they have metastasized to the liver.

Patients who present with carcinoid syndrome are typically not surgical candidates since they already have extensive metastatic disease.

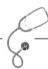

Typical scenario: A 60-year-old male presents with a history of cutaneous flushing, diarrhea, wheezing, and an unintentional 15-lb weight loss. *Think:* Carcinoid syndrome; the wheezing is a clue that the lesion may be endobronchial. Order a 24-hour urine 5-HIAA level to confirm the diagnosis.

INCIDENCE

- Carcinoid tumors represent between 29–40% of primary small bowel malignancies.
- Peak incidence between 50 and 70 years of age.
- More than 90% diagnosed in GI system:
- The appendix is the most common site of GI carcinoid followed by small bowel followed by the rectum.

SIGNS AND SYMPTOMS

- Slow growing; therefore, frequently asymptomatic, and are usually found incidentally.
- In symptomatic patients, vague abdominal pain is the most common symptom.
- Intermittent obstruction—25% of patients.
- Rectal bleeding (from rectal carcinoid), pain, weight loss.
- Carcinoid syndrome: Approximately 10% of cases:
  - Due to production of serotonin, bradykinin, or tryptrophan by tumor and exposure of these products to systemic circulation prior to break-down by the liver.
  - Characterized by cutaneous flushing, sweating, watery diarrhea, wheezing, dyspnea, valvular lesions (right > left).

DIAGNOSIS

- Most found incidentally during radiographic studies, appendectomy, or surgery for intestinal obstruction.
- If patient has carcinoid syndrome:
  - 5-HIAA (hydroxyindolacetic acid) in 24-hour urine collection.
  - Plasma chromogranin A—independent predictor of prognosis.
  - Pentagastrin provocation test: Pentagastrin administration induces flushing (used in patients with only marginally elevated 5-HIAA, but who describe flushing symptoms).
  - Otherwise diagnosed as any other small bowel neoplasm.

TREATMENT

- Medical: Serotonin antagonists (e.g., cyproheptadine) or somatostatin analogues (e.g., octreotide) for symptoms of carcinoid syndrome.
- Surgical:
  - Appendiceal carcinoid < 2 cm: Appendectomy.
  - Appendiceal carcinoid > 2 cm: Right hemicolectomy.
  - Small intestinal carcinoid: Resect tumor with mesenteric lymph nodes, as well as inspection of entire small bowel for synchronous lesions.
  - Otherwise, resect tumor and any solitary liver metastasis considered resectable.

PROGNOSIS

- Overall survival roughly 54%.
- Five-year survival after palliative resection is 25%; after curative resection is 70%.

Fistula

DEFINITION

A communication between two epithelialized surfaces. It can form between two parts of the GI or genitourinary (GU) tract, an internal fistula (e.g., choledocho-duodenal or colo-vescical), or between an internal organ and an outer epithilialized surface (e.g., enterocutaneous), an external fistula.

RISK FACTORS

- Previous abdominal surgery (most common—80%).
- Diverticular disease.
- Crohn's disease.
- Colorectal cancer.

SIGNS AND SYMPTOMS

- Iatrogenic fistulae usually appear 5–10 days postoperatively.
- If associated with an abscess, can be accompanied by fever and leukocytosis.
- Drainage of succus entericus (bowel contents) from skin (enterocutaneous fistula).
- Diarrhea, usually secondary to malabsorption (entero-enteric; especially if between proximal and distal small bowel or colon since a large portion of the small bowel absorptive surface is bypassed).
- Pneumaturia and symptoms of urinary tract infection (colovesicular fistula).

DIAGNOSIS

- CT with enteral contrast shows leakage of contrast from intestinal lumen.
- Small bowel series.
- Enteroclysis.
- Fistulogram: Contrast is injected directly into fistula tract.

TREATMENT

- Stabilization: Manage electrolyte abnormalities, fluid losses, and nutritional status.
- Drainage of abscesses (if present).
- Allow time for spontaneous closure:
  - Bowel rest.
  - Provide nutrition (usually total parental nutrition [TPN]).
  - Consider octreotide (somatostatin analogue) for high-output and pancreatic fistulas.
- If 6–8 weeks pass without improvement, then surgery should be performed to resect the fistula tract, together with the segment of small bowel from which it originates.

PROGNOSIS

- Enterocutaneous fistulas have 15–20% mortality related to complications of sepsis and underlying disease.
- Surgery is associated with considerable morbidity and a high recurrence rate.

If there is no preceding iatrogenic injury, fistula formation is most likely due to the progression of Crohn's disease or cancer.

Proximal fistulas cause more problems than distal fistulas because the draining contents are more acidic, more fluids and electrolytes are lost, and more absorptive area is lost.

High output fistulas drain > 500 mL/24 hrs and are proximal (stomach, duodenum, proximal small bowel).
Low output fistulas drain < 500 mL/24 hrs and are distal (distal small bowel and colon).

SMA is the most common
vessel involved in AMI.
Most emboli that cause AMI
originate in the heart (left
atrial or left ventricular
thrombi). Ninety-five
percent of patients with
AMI will have a history of
cardiovascular disease
(atrial fibrillation or
myocardial infarction).

■ CT has somewhat of a
  low sensitivity for
  detecting **arterial** AMI.
  Therefore, if a patient
  has high suspicion for
  AMI, then patient should
  undergo angiography
  despite negative CT
  results.
■ CT has high sensitivity
  (> 90%) for detecting
  acute mesenteric
  venous thrombosis.

Mesenteric Ischemia

DEFINITION

■ Reduction in blood flow to the small bowel secondary to a variety of mechanisms.
■ Can result in two distinct conditions: acute mesenteric ischemia and chronic mesenteric ischemia.

ACUTE MESENTERIC ISCHEMIA (AMI)

■ Rapid onset of intestinal hypoperfusion.
■ Can be caused by arterial occlusion (usually single artery):
   ■ Superior mesenteric artery *embolism*—50% of all AMI.
   ■ Superior mesenteric artery thrombosis (acute)—15–25% of all AMI.
   ■ Vasospasm (nonocclusive mesenteric ischemia)—20–30% of all AMI.
   ■ Venous obstruction (either thrombosis or strangulation usually of SMV)—5% of all AMI.
■ Regardless of cause, AMI can lead to mucosal sloughing within 3 hours of onset, and to intestinal infarction 6 hours after onset.

RISK FACTORS

■ Cardiac: Low cardiac output states, cardiac arrhythmias, severe cardiac valvular disease, recent myocardial infarction.
■ Age.
■ Atherosclerosis.
■ Hypercoagulable states.

SIGNS AND SYMPTOMS

■ Abdominal *pain out of proportion to tenderness* on physical exam (hallmark).
■ Pain is colicky and diffuse, typically in mid-abdomen.
■ Can be associated with nausea, vomiting, and diarrhea.
■ Following infarction, peritonitis (rebound and rigidity), abdominal distention, and passage of bloody stools occur.

DIAGNOSIS

■ High clinical suspicion especially if *history of cardiac disease* or hypercoagulability.
■ No lab test is sensitive for diagnosis of AMI. Findings may include leukocytosis, acidosis, hemoconcentration, and occult blood in stool.
■ If there are peritoneal signs, then patient should undergo emergent laparotomy.
■ Otherwise, pursue diagnostic tests:
   ■ Mesentric angiography: Most sensitive and specific method for diagnosing AMI, albeit invasive.
   ■ CT scan:
      ■ Good initial test for most patients with possible AMI.
      ■ Can rule out other causes of abdominal pain.
      ■ Can reveal evidence of ischemia of intestine and mesentery.
      ■ Can reveal occlusion/stenosis of vasculature.

THERAPY

■ Stabilization of patient:
   ■ Hemodynamic monitoring and fluid resuscitation.

- Correction of electrolyte abnormalities, acidosis.
- Broad-spectrum antibiotics.
- Placement of a nasogastric tube for gastric decompression.
- Patient with peritoneal features: Midline laparotomy with assessment of intestinal viability.
  - For embolic causes: *Intraoperative embolectomy.*
  - For CA/SMA thrombosis: *Bypass of site of obstruction* using a saphenous vein graft (from supraceliac aorta to distal SMA).
- Therapy via angiography includes intra-arterial vasodilators (papaverine) or thrombolytic agents (streptokinase, urokinase, tPA), angioplasty, placement of a stent, and embolectomy.
- Venous thrombosis requires immediate anticoagulation (heparin).

Thrombolytic therapy for intra-arterial emboli is most successful when initiated within 8–12 hours of symptom onset.

PROGNOSIS

- Acute arterial mesenteric ischemia mortality rate: 59–93%.
- Acute mesenteric venous thrombosis mortality rate: 20–50% (30% recurrence rate if not anticoagulated).

Patients with acute mesenteric venous thrombosis should be evaluated for hereditary and acquired thrombophilias.

CHRONIC MESENTERIC ISCHEMIA (CMI)

- Insidious, episodic, or constant state of intestinal hypoperfusion.
- Rarely leads to infarction of small bowel due to development of collateral circulation over time.
- Can be caused by:
  - Arterial ischemia (most common): Associated with atherosclerosis of more than one mesenteric and splanchnic vessels.
  - Venous thrombosis: Thrombosis of portal or splenic veins, leading to portal hypertension with subsequent development of esophageal varices and splenomegaly.
  - Vasculitis.

RISK FACTORS

- Atherosclerotic vascular disease (half of patients have history of peripheral vascular disease or coronary artery disease).
- Smoking.

SIGNS AND SYMPTOMS

- "Intestinal angina": Dull, crampy, postprandial abdominal pain leading to food aversion and weight loss (hallmark).
- Patients with chronic venous thrombosis may be asymptomatic due collateral formation, or may present with esophageal variceal bleeding.

DIAGNOSIS

- High clinical suspicion.
- Must rule out other causes of chronic abdominal pain, weight loss, and food aversion, particularly malignancy.
- Diagnosis is supported by demonstration of high-grade stenoses in multiple mesenteric vessels.
- Diagnostic tests:
  - Angiography: Gold standard.
  - CT and magnetic resonance (MR) angiography: Good initial tests since they can identify whether a stenosis is present and serve as a guide for angiography.

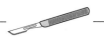

CMI can occur due to compression of celiac artery by diaphragm — celiac artery compression syndrome or median arcuate ligament syndrome. Treatment is release of the arcuate ligament and bypass of persistent stricture.

- Mesenteric duplex ultrasonography: Can be used as a screening test to detect stenoses of the celiac and superior mesenteric arteries.

THERAPY

- Arterial CMI:
  - Surgical revascularization:
    - Aortomesenteric bypass graft
    - Mesenteric endarterectomy
  - Percutaneous transluminal angioplasty (PTA) with or without placement of a stent:
    - Less relief of symptoms and less durability than surgery.
    - Serves as alternative to surgery for those patients who are not optimal surgical candidates due to considerable comorbidities.
  - Chronic venous mesenteric thrombosis: Anticoagulation (heparin).

PROGNOSIS

- Perioperative mortality rates range from 0–16%.
- Initial relief of symptoms with surgery: 90%.
- Recurrence rate:
  - Following surgery: < 10%.
  - Following PTA: 10–67%.

Short Bowel Syndrome

DEFINITION

- Presence of < 200 cm of small bowel in adult patients.
- Results in decreased small bowel absorption, leading to diarrhea, malnutrition, and dehydration.

ETIOLOGIES

- Adults: Acute mesenteric ischemia, Crohn's disease, malignancy.
- Pediatrics: Volvulus, intestinal atresia, necrotizing enterocolitis.

PATHOPHYSIOLOGY

- Malabsorption occurs following resection of 50–80% of small bowel.
- Presence of intact colon, as well as an ileocecal valve, also decreases severity of malabsorption.
- Resection of ileum is associated with increased malabsorption secondary to inability to absorb bile salts and vitamin B_{12}.
- Small bowel adaptation period lasts approximately 1–2 years following surgery.

Typical scenario: A 70-year-old male with a history of peripheral vascular disease and hyperlipidemia presents to the emergency department with severe, diffuse abdominal pain. His blood pressure is 170/100 and his pulse is 90 bpm. Supine abdominal radiograph shows free air in the abdomen and within the wall of the small intestine. What is the most likely diagnosis? *Think:* Small bowel infarction.

THERAPY

- Medical:
  - Repletion of fluid and electrolytes: Initially, most patients require TPN.
  - Proton pump inhibitors/H_2 blockers to decrease gastric acid secretion.
  - Antimotility agents to decrease transit through small bowel.
  - Octreotide may be used to decrease intestinal secretions.

TPN is associated with considerable morbidity including catheter sepsis, liver and kidney failure, and venous thrombosis.

- Surgical:
  - Restoration of intestinal continuity in patients with stomas, in order to increase absorptive capacity.
- Surgeries aimed at slowing transit through the small intestine include:
  - Segmental reversal of the small bowel.
  - Placement of a segment of colon between two segments of small bowel.
  - Creation of artificial small bowel valves.
- Surgeries aimed at lengthening the small bowel include:
  - Longitudinal intestinal lengthening and tailoring (LILT).
  - Serial transverse enteroplasty procedure (STEP).
  - Small bowel transplantation:
    - One hundred performed in United States each year.
    - Indicated for patients with life-threatening intestinal failure, or complications from TPN.
    - Eighty percent of survivors have full intestinal function without need for TPN.
    - Significant risks including acute or chronic rejection, as well as CMV infection.

PROGNOSIS

- Fifty to seventy percent of patients who initially require TPN can eventually be completely weaned off of TPN.
- Pediatric patients are more likely than adults to gain independence from TPN.

Colon, Rectum, and Anal Canal

Embryology

- Origin: Embryonic midgut (up to mid-transverse colon) and hindgut (rest of colon, and proximal anus). Distal anus derived from ectoderm.
- The dentate line marks the transition between hindgut and ectoderm.

Gross Anatomy

See Figure 10-1.

Colon

- Extends from the ileocecal valve to the rectum; consists of: right colon, transverse colon, left colon, sigmoid colon.
- Three to five feet in length.
- Cecum is widest; the colon progressively narrows distally.
- Unlike the small intestine, the colon has taenia coli, haustra, and appendices epiploicae (fat appendages that hang off antimesenteric side of colon).
  - Taenia coli—three distinct bands of longitudinal muscle—converge at the appendix and spread out to form a longitudinal muscle layer at the proximal rectum.
  - Retroperitoneal attachments of ascending and descending colon fix it to the posterior abdominal wall.
- Retroperitoneal: Ascending colon, descending colon, posterior hepatic and splenic flexures.
- Intraperitoneal: Cecum, transverse colon, sigmoid colon.
- One end of omentum attaches to anterior-superior aspect of transverse colon; other end attaches to stomach.

In development, the midgut loop rotates 270° counterclockwise around the axis of the superior mesenteric artery (SMA). Developmental anomalies include malrotation or failure of right colon to elongate.

The blood supply is based on embryology:
- Midgut: SMA
- Hindgut: Inferior mesenteric artery (IMA)
- Distal anus: Internal pudendal artery branches

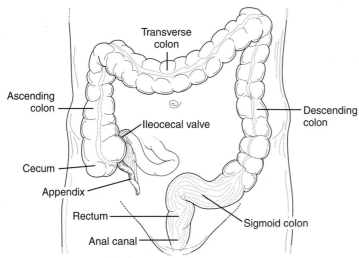

FIGURE 10-1. Bowel anatomy.

The ileocecal valve functions to prevent reflux of bowel contents from the cecum back to the ileum.

The anatomy and physiology of the colon affect how colon cancers typically present. Because the colon progressively narrows distally and functions physiologically to absorb water, left-sided colon cancers tend to present with a change in bowel habits (e.g., small-caliber stools, obstruction, and hematochezia). Right-sided colon cancers tend to present in a more indolent fashion with microcytic anemia, fatigue, and melena (dark, tarry stools) because the proximal colon has a larger circumference and the stool is less solid.

The splenic flexure represents a "watershed" area between the areas supplied by the superior and inferior mesenteric arteries. This watershed area is particularly susceptible to ischemic injury as seen in ischemic colitis. The other two watershed zones are the ileocecal area and the junction of descending and sigmoid colon.

Rectum

- 12–15 cm in length.
- Rectum has distinct peritoneal covering.
- Fascia:
  - Waldeyer's fascia: Rectosacral fascia that extends from S4 vertebral body to rectum.
  - Denonvilliers' fascia: Anterior to lower third of rectum.
- Pelvic floor: Levator ani (composed of pubococcygeus, iliococcygeus, and puborectalis muscles); innervated by S4 nerve.

Anus

- Anal canal runs from pelvic diaphragm to anal verge (junction of anoderm and perianal skin).
- Dentate line: A mucocutaneous line that separates proximal, pleated mucosa from distal, smooth anoderm (1–1.5 cm above anal verge).
- Anal mucosa proximal to dentate line lined by columnar epithelium; mucosa distal to dentate line (anoderm) lined by squamous epithelium and lacks glands and hair.
- Columns of Morgagni: 12–14 columns of pleated mucosa superior to the dentate line separated by crypts. Perianal glands discharge their secretions at the base of the columns.
- Anal sphincter:
  - Internal: Consists of specialized rectal smooth muscle (from inner circular layer); involuntary, contracted at rest, responsible for 80% of resting pressure.
  - External: Consists of three loops of voluntary striated muscle; a continuation of puborectalis muscle; responsible for 20% of resting pressure and 100% of voluntary pressure.

Blood Supply

ARTERIAL

- **Superior mesenteric artery (SMA):** Supplies the cecum, ascending colon, and proximal two thirds of the transverse colon via the ileocolic, right colic, and middle colic arteries, respectively.
- **Inferior mesenteric artery (IMA):** Supplies the distal two thirds of the transverse colon, sigmoid colon, and superior rectum via the left colic, sigmoidal, and superior rectal (hemorrhoidal) arteries, respectively.
- **Internal iliac artery:** Supplies the middle and distal rectum via the middle rectal and inferior rectal arteries, respectively (the inferior rectal artery is a branch of the internal pudendal artery).
- **Internal pudendal artery:** Supplies the anus; is a branch of the internal iliac artery.

VENOUS

- **Superior mesenteric vein (SMV):** Drains the cecum and ascending and transverse colon before joining the splenic vein.
- **Inferior mesenteric vein (IMV):** Drains the descending colon, sigmoid colon, and proximal rectum before joining the splenic vein.
- **Internal iliac vein:** Drains the middle and distal rectum.

- **Middle rectal vein:** A branch of the internal iliac vein; drains upper anus.
- **Inferior rectal vein:** A branch of the internal pudendal vein; drains lower anus.
- **Hemorrhoidal complexes:** Three complexes within the anus that drain into the superior rectal veins and one external complex that drains into the pudendal veins.

Lymphatic Drainage

Lymphatics of the colon, rectum, and anus generally follow the arterial supply, with several levels of nodes as one moves centrally toward the aorta (e.g., ileocolic nodes, superior mesenteric nodes, etc.).

Innervation

- Derives primarily from autonomic nervous system.
- Sympathetic nerves: Inhibit peristalsis.
- Parasympathetic nerves: Stimulate peristalsis.

Histology

From inner lumen to outer wall:

- Colon: Mucosa, submucosa, inner circular muscle layer, outer longitudinal muscle (taenia coli).
- Rectum: Mucosa, submucosa, inner circular muscle, outer longitudinal muscle (confluent).
- Anus: Anoderm (epithelium that is richly innervated, but without secondary skin appendages).

Microbiology

- Colon sterile at birth; normal flora established shortly thereafter.
- Normal flora: 99% anaerobic (predominantly *Bacteroides fragilis*); 1% aerobic (predominantly *Escherichia coli*).

▶ **PHYSIOLOGY**

General

The colon and rectum has three primary physiologic functions:

1. Absorption of water and electrolytes from stool
2. Storage of feces
3. Motility

Motility

Characterized by three types of contractions:

1. Retrograde movements: From transverse colon to cecum, these

The rectum has two major angles that play a significant role in continence. The first angle is formed at the origin of the rectum at the sacral promontory as it bends posteriorly and inferiorly, following the curve of the sacrum. The second angle, the anorectal angle, is formed by the puborectalis muscle as it joins the anus, pulling the rectum forward. A Valsalva maneuver enhances these angles, closing off the rectum.

Anal canal above dentate line drains to inferior mesenteric nodes or to internal iliac nodes. Lower anal canal drains to inguinal nodes.

The rectum can store approximately 500 cc of feces.

movements slow the transit of luminal contents, thereby prolonging their exposure to absorptive epithelium.

2. Segmental contractions: The most common variety, these are localized simultaneous contractions of the longitudinal and circular muscles of the colon.
3. Mass movements:
   - Contractions of long segments of colon that are 30 seconds in duration and result in antegrade propulsion of luminal contents at a rate of 0.5–1 cm/sec.
   - Occur 3–4 times each day, especially after waking up or after eating, and may result in bowel movements.
   - Neuronal control of colon:
     1. Extrinsic: Parasympathetic and sympathetic (as described above).
     2. Intrinsic (from mucosa to bowel wall): Mucosa, submucosal (Meissner's) plexus, circular muscle layer, myenteric (Auerbach's) plexus, longitudinal muscle layer, subserosal plexus, serosa.

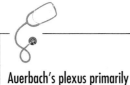

Auerbach's plexus primarily inhibits colonic activity.

Defecation

1. Mass movement causes feces to move into rectal vault.
2. Sampling reflex: Rectal distention leads to involuntary relaxation of internal sphincter, allowing descent of rectal contents and sensation of feces at transitional zone.
3. Voluntary relaxation of external sphincter pushes contents down anal canal.
4. Voluntary increase in intra-abdominal pressure assists in propelling rectal contents out of anus.

Constipation consists of the ability to pass flatus but the inability to pass stool. **Obstipation** refers to the inability to pass flatus or stool.

Flatus

Voluntary contraction of pelvic floor muscles (puborectalis and external sphincter) causes selective passage of gas with retention of stool.

Irritable Bowel Syndrome (IBS)

- **Definition:** Abnormal state of intestinal motility modified by psychosocial factors for which no anatomic cause can be found.
- IBS is often regarded as a wastebasket diagnosis for a change in bowel habits along with complaints of abdominal pain after other causes have been excluded.

Constipation

- **Definition:** < 3 stools/week.
- **Diagnosis:** By history; differentiate between acute constipation (persistent change in bowel habits for < 3 months), and chronic constipation (persistent change in bowel habits > 3 months). Total constipation with absence of flatus is a hallmark of obstruction and is termed *obstipation*.
- **Common causes:** Diet related (fluid, fiber), lack of physical activity, medications (especially opiates and anticholinergics), medical illness

(irritable bowel syndrome, diabetes, hypothyroidism), depression, neurologic disease (Parkinson's disease, multiple sclerosis), fecal impaction.

- **Treatment:** Depends on cause.
    - Short-term: Stool softeners; enema if suppository fails. Fecal disimpaction (if present).
    - Long-term: Encourage dietary changes (increasing fiber and fluid consumption).
    - If dietary changes fail, assess colonic transit time. Defecography or anometry may prove helpful.

Diarrhea

DEFINITION

- Passage of > 3 loose stools/day.
- In the hospitalized patient, a workup may be indicated to rule out infectious or ischemic etiologies.
- In the outpatient follow-up setting, diarrhea may occur due to extensive small bowel resection (short bowel syndrome), due to disruption of innervation, or even as an expected outcome (gastric bypass).

DIAGNOSIS

- Stool sample for enteric pathogens and *Clostridium difficile* toxin.
- Check stool for white blood cells (WBCs) (IBD or infectious colitis), red blood cells (RBCs) without WBCs (ischemia, invasive infectious diarrhea, cancer).

TREATMENT

Individualized based on the treatable cause, and is addressed with the specific problems that may cause diarrhea (colitis, ischemia).

Postvagotomy diarrhea occurs in 20% of patients after truncal vagotomy. Denervation of the extrahepatic biliary tree and small intestine leads to rapid transit of unconjugated bile salts into the colon, impeding water absorption and causing diarrhea. Cholestyramine is the medical treatment. If that fails, surgical reversal of a segment of the small intestine to prolong transit time and increase absorptive capacity may be considered.

▶ **COLITIS**

Pseudomembranous Colitis

- **Definition:** An acute colitis characterized by formation of an adherent inflammatory exudate (pseudomembrane) overlying the site of mucosal injury. Most commonly due to overgrowth of *Clostridium difficile*, a gram-positive, anaerobic, spore-forming bacillus.
- Typically occurs after broad-spectrum antibiotics (especially clindamycin, ampicillin, or cephalosporins) eradicate the normal intestinal flora.
- **Signs and symptoms:** Vary from a self-limited diarrheal illness to invasive colitis with megacolon or perforation as possible complications.
- **Diagnosis:** Detection of *C. difficile* toxin in stool; proctoscopy or colonoscopy if diagnosis uncertain.
- **Treatment:** Stop offending antibiotic; give flagyl or vancomycin PO (if patient unable to take PO, give flagyl IV).
- **Prognosis:** High rate of recurrence (20%) despite high response rate to treatment.

Patients with *C. difficile* colitis should be placed on contact isolation, as infection is associated with a high morbidity and is contagious.

DIAGNOSIS

- Flexible sigmoidoscopy with histolopathologic evaluation of biopsies.
- Barium enema: "Lead pipe" appearance of colon due to loss of haustral folds, but no longer test of choice.

TREATMENT

- Medical: Similar to Crohn's (see Table 10-2):
  - Mild/moderate disease: 5-ASA, corticosteroids PO or per rectum.
  - Severe disease: IV steroids.
  - Proctitis: Topical steroids.
  - Refractory disease: Immunosuppression.
- Surgical:
  - Indications: Failure of medical therapy, increasing risk of cancer in long-standing disease, bleeding, perforation.
  - Procedure: Proctocolectomy (curative).
  - If patient is acutely ill and unstable due to perforation, a diverting loop colostomy is indicated. Once stabilized, the patient may undergo a more definitive operation.
  - In Crohn's disease the treatment is stricturoplasty and segmental resections because recurrence is the rule and the goal is to preserve as much healthy intestine as possible.

PROGNOSIS

Approximately 1–2% risk of cancer at 10 years, and 1%/year thereafter.

Unless all the colonic and rectal mucosa is removed, the patient is still at risk for cancer.

TABLE 10-2. Ulcerative Colitis vs. Crohn's Disease

	ULCERATIVE COLITIS	CROHN'S DISEASE
Pathology	▪ Inflammation of the mucosa only (exudate of pus, blood, and mucus from the "crypt abscess") ▪ Always starts in rectum (up to one third don't progress) ▪ Limited to colon and rectum	▪ Inflammation involves all bowel wall layers, which is what may lead to fistulas and abscess ▪ Rectal sparing in 50% ▪ May affect mouth to anus
Diagnosis	▪ Continuous lesions ▪ Rare ▪ Lead pipe colon appearance due to chronic scarring and subsequent retraction and loss of haustra	▪ Skip lesions: Interspersed normal and diseased bowel ▪ Aphthous ulcers ▪ Cobblestone appearance from submucosal thickening interspersed with mucosal ulceration
Complications	▪ Perforation ▪ Stricture ▪ Megacolon ▪ Cancer	▪ Abscess ▪ Fistulas ▪ Obstruction ▪ Cancer ▪ Perianal disease

DEFINITION

- Herniation of the mucosa through the muscular layers of the bowel wall at sites where arterioles penetrate, forming small outpouchings or diverticula.
- Are generally numerous, collectively referred to as **diverticulosis**.
- **Diverticulitis** refers to the inflammation of diverticula.

INCIDENCE

- > 50% of Americans over 70 years of age.
- Men and women equally affected.
- Sigmoid colon most commonly involved with progressively decreasing frequency of involvement as one proceeds proximally.

RISK FACTORS

- Old age
- Low-fiber diet

SIGNS AND SYMPTOMS

Diverticulosis
- Eighty percent of patients are asymptomatic.
- **Massive, painless lower GI bleeding is classic** (notably absent in diverticulitis).

Diverticulitis
- Persistent abdominal pain initially diffuse in nature that often becomes localized to the left lower quadrant (LLQ) with development of peritoneal signs.
- LLQ and/or pelvic tenderness.
- Ileus/abdominal distention.
- Anorexia, nausea, vomiting, and change in bowel habits (usually constipation).
- Large bowel obstruction.
- Fever.
- Elevated WBC.

DIAGNOSIS

Diverticulosis
- Characteristic history and physical exam confirmed by diverticula identified on CT/barium enema and/or colonoscopy.
- Treatment: High-fiber diet, stool softeners.
- See section on lower GI bleed (LGIB) for management of patients who present with acute LGIB.

Diverticulitis
- Characteristic history and physical exam.
- Elevated WBCs.
- CT scan (test of choice): Pericolonic inflammation with or without abscess formation.
- Barium enema and colonoscopy may induce perforation and are contraindicated in the acute setting but should be obtained in follow-up (see Figure 10-2).
- Abdominal x-ray: Ileus, distention, and/or free intraperitoneal air.

The diverticula of common diverticulosis are false diverticula; all the layers of the bowel wall would need to herniated to be a "true" diverticula.

Pathophysiology of diverticulitis: A peridiverticular inflammation caused by microperforation of the diverticulum secondary to increased pressure or obstruction by inspissated feces. Feces extravasate onto the serosal surface but infection is usually well contained in a patient with normal immune function.

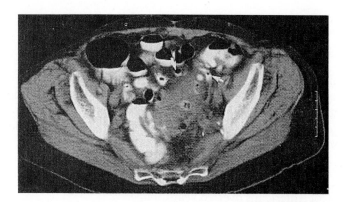

FIGURE 10-2. CT scan demonstrating multiple small sigmoid diverticuli (arrows).

(Reproduced, with permission, from Gupta H, Dupuy DE. *Surg Clin North Am* 6(77); December 1997.)

TREATMENT

- **Uncomplicated diverticulitis:**
  - Outpatient management: Clear liquid diet, PO antibiotics, and non-opioid analgesics with close follow-up.
  - Follow-up includes colonoscopy and dietary recommendations once acute infection has subsided.
  - If outpatient therapy fails, admit for IV antibiotics and IV hydration with bowel rest. Nasogastric tube (NGT) is placed when there is evidence of ileus or small bowel obstruction (SBO), with nausea and vomiting.
- The *Hinchey staging system* is often used to describe the severity of **complicated diverticulitis:**
  - Stage I includes colonic inflammation with an associated pericolic abscess.
  - Stage II includes colonic inflammation with a retroperitoneal or pelvic abscess.
  - Stage III is associated with purulent peritonitis.
  - Stage IV is associated with fecal peritonitis.
    - Stage I and II are treated by IV antibiotics and CT-guided aspiration.
  - If the abscess is inaccessible to drainage and not responding to antibiotics, then it is treated surgically (drainage with Hartmann pouch or sigmoid colectomy).
    - Stage III and IV need operative management.
  - In the emergent setting, a Hartmann's procedure is usually performed (i.e., resection with proximal colostomy and distal pouch with reversal later—two-stage procedure).
  - If patient is very unstable, then a diverting colostomy may be performed.
  - Elective resection of affected bowel must be considered in the patient who has recurrent episodes of diverticulitis requiring treatment.
  - All patients with diverticulitis *must* undergo a full colonoscopy 4–6 weeks after the attack to rule out malignancy, as sometimes colonic malignancy presents as diverticulitis.

PROGNOSIS

One third of patients remain asymptomatic, one third have episodic pain, and one third progress to have a recurrence.

▶ LOWER GI BLEED (LGIB)

DEFINITION

- GI bleeding distal to the ligament of Treitz.
- LGIB is considered massive when the patient requires 3 or more units of blood within 24 hours.
- Most common causes are diverticulosis and angiodysplasia. Other causes include cancer, IBD, ischemic colitis, hemorrhoids.
- Anticoagulation treatment increases the risk for LGIB.

MANAGEMENT

See Table 10-3.

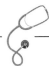

Ten to twenty-five percent of LGIBs eventually require surgery, despite the fact that 85% of bleeds initially stop spontaneously.

▶ LARGE BOWEL OBSTRUCTION

INCIDENCE

Most commonly occurs in elderly patients; much less common than small bowel obstruction.

SIGNS AND SYMPTOMS

Abdominal distention, cramping abdominal pain, nausea, vomiting, obstipation, and high-pitched bowel sounds.

DIAGNOSIS

- Supine and upright abdominal films: Distended proximal colon, air-fluid levels, and no distal rectal air.
- Establish 8- to 12-hour history of obstipation; passage of some gas or stool indicates partial small bowel obstruction, a nonoperative condition.
- Barium enema: May be necessary to distinguish between ileus and pseudo-obstruction.

TREATMENT

1. Correction of fluid and electrolyte abnormalities.
2. Nasogastric tube for intestinal decompression (as gastric emptying is reflexly inhibited).
3. Broad-spectrum IV antibiotics (e.g., cefoxitin).
4. Relieve obstruction surgically (colonic obstruction is a surgical emergency since a nasogastric tube will not decompress the colon).

An extensive operation is indicated when no site is identified in an unstable patient because although < 10% will rebleed, the mortality for those 10% is approximately 30%.

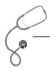

The three most common causes of obstruction of the large bowel are adenocarcinoma (65%), scarring secondary to diverticulitis (20%), and volvulus (5%).

TABLE 10-3. Management of Lower GI Bleeding (LGIB)

	DIVERTICULOSIS	ANGIODYSPLASIA
Incidence	50% of patients are > 60	25% of patients are > 60; men > women
Character	Painless, > 60% site of bleeding proximal to splenic flexure	Cecum and ascending colon
Quantity and rate	Massive and rapid	Slow
Signs and symptoms	Melena and/or hematochezia often with symptoms of orthostasis	
Diagnosis	■ First rule out upper GI bleeding with nasogastric lavage ■ To identify site of bleed: 1. Colonoscopy 2. ≥ 0.5 mL/min: Bleeding scan with Tc-sulfur colloid identifies bleeding; label lasts for up to 24 hours so a patient can be easily rescanned when rebleeding occurs after a negative initial scan 3. ≥ 1 mL/min: Angiography (selective mesenteric angiography best method to diagnose angiodysplasia)	
Treatment	1. Resuscitation 2. Therapeutic options if site identified: Octreotide, embolization, vasoconstriction with epinephrine, vasodestruction with alcohol or sodium compounds, or coagulation/cautery with heat 3. If site identified but bleeding massive or refractory, segmental colectomy 4. Without identification of bleeding site and persistent bleeding in an unstable patient, an exploratory laparotomy is performed with possible total abdominal colectomy with ileostomy	
Cause	Disruption of arteriole at either dome or antimesenteric neck of diverticulum (almost always on mucosal side, so bleed occurs into lumen rather than into peritoneal cavity)	Chronic intermittent obstruction of submucosal veins secondary to repeated muscular contractions results in dilated venules with incompetent precapillary sphincters and thus arteriovenous communication
Prognosis	10% overall mortality	

▶ VOLVULUS

DEFINITION

Rotation of a segment of intestine about its mesenteric axis; characteristically occurs in the sigmoid colon (75% of cases) or cecum (25%).

INCIDENCE

More than 50% of cases occur in patients over 65.

RISK FACTORS

- Elderly (especially institutionalized patients).
- Chronic constipation.

- Pyschotropic drugs.
- Hypermobile cecum secondary to incomplete fixation during intrauterine development (cecal volvulus).

SIGNS AND SYMPTOMS

See Large Bowel Obstruction.

DIAGNOSIS

- Clinical presentation.
- Abdominal films: Markedly dilated sigmoid colon or cecum with a "kidney bean" appearance.
- Barium enema: Characteristic "bird's beak" at areas of colonic narrowing.

TREATMENT

- Cecal volvulus: Right hemicolectomy if vascular compromise; cecopexy otherwise adequate (suturing the right colon to the parietal peritoneum).
- Sigmoid volvulus (see Figure 10-3):
  - Sigmoidoscopy with rectal tube insertion to decompress the volvulus.
  - Emergent laparotomy if sigmoidoscopy fails or if strangulation or perforation is suspected.
  - Elective resection in same hospital admission to prevent recurrence (nearly 50% of cases recur after nonoperative reduction).

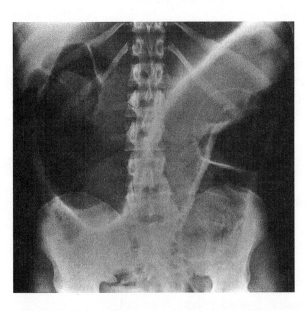

FIGURE 10-3. Abdominal x-ray shows a grossly distended coffee bean–shaped loop of bowel in the right upper quadrant, findings that are typical of a sigmoid volvulus.

(Reproduced, with permission, from Rozycki GS et al. *Annals of Surgery* 5(235); May 2002. Lippincott Williams & Wilkins.)

Ogilvie syndrome is associated with any severe acute illness, neuroleptics, opiates, malignancy, and certain metabolic disturbances.

In Ogilvie syndrome, pharmacologic decompression of the bowel with neostigmine is particularly useful because diagnosis with contrast enema or colonoscopy can be exceedingly difficult without bowel decontamination.

Malignant potential of a polyp is determined by: size, histologic type, and epithelial dysplasia.

SIZE	RISK OF CA
< 1 cm	1–3%
1–2 cm	10%
>2 cm	40%

HISTOLOGY	RISK
Tubular	5%
Tubulovillous	20%
Villous	40%

ATYPIA	RISK
Mild	5%
Moderate	20%
Severe	35%

▶ PSEUDO-OBSTRUCTION (OGILVIE SYNDROME)

DEFINITION

Massive colonic dilation without evidence of mechanical obstruction.

INCIDENCE

More common in older, institutionalized patients.

RISK FACTORS

Severe infection, recent surgery or trauma.

SIGNS AND SYMPTOMS

Marked abdominal distention with mild abdominal pain and decreased or absent bowel sounds.

DIAGNOSIS

- Abdominal radiograph with massive colonic distention.
- Exclude mechanical cause for obstruction with water-soluble contrast enema and/or colonoscopy.

TREATMENT

- NGT and rectal tube for proximal and distal decompression, respectively.
- Correction of electrolyte abnormalities.
- Discontinue narcotics, anticholinergics, or other offending medications.
- Consider pharmacologic decompression with neostigmine (a cholinesterase inhibitor).
- If peritoneal signs develop, the patient should undergo prompt exploratory laparotomy to treat possible perforation.
- Refractory cases may need total colectomy.

▶ BENIGN TUMORS OF THE LARGE BOWEL

Colorectal Polyps

MORPHOLOGY

Can be classified into sessile (flat) and pedunculated (on a stalk).

HISTOLOGIC TYPES

- Inflammatory (pseudopolyp): Seen in UC.
- Lymphoid: Mucosal bumps containing intramucosal lymphoid tissue; no malignant potential.
- Hyperplastic: Overgrowth of normal tissue; no malignant potential.
- Adenomatous: Premalignant; are classified (in order of increasing malignant potential) as tubular (75%), tubulovillous (15%), and villous (10%).
- Hamartomatous: Normal tissue arranged in abnormal configuration; juvenile polyps, Peutz-Jeghers polyps.

INCIDENCE

Thirty to forty percent of individuals over 60 in the United States.

SIGNS AND SYMPTOMS

- Asymptomatic (most common)
- Melena
- Hematochezia
- Mucus
- Change in bowel habits

DIAGNOSIS

Flexible endoscopy (sigmoidoscopy or colonoscopy).

TREATMENT

- Attempt colonoscopic resection if pedunculated, well or moderately well differentiated, no venous or lymphatic invasion, invades only into stalk, margins negative.
- Otherwise, a segmental colon resection is indicated.

Polyposis Syndromes

See Table 10-4.

▶ COLORECTAL CARCINOMA (CRC)

INCIDENCE

- Second most common cause of cancer deaths overall (behind lung cancer).
- 130,000 new cases and 55,000 deaths each year.
- Incidence increases with increasing age starting at age 40 and peaks at 60–79 years of age.
- See Table 10-5 for screening recommendations from the U.S. Preventative Services Task Force.

RISK FACTORS

- Age > 50.
- Personal history of resected colon cancer or adenomas.
- Family history of colon cancer or adenomas.
- Low-fiber, high-fat diet.
- Inherited colorectal cancer syndrome (familial adenomatous polyposis [FAP], hereditary nonpolyposis colon cancer [HNPCC]).
- Long-standing UC or Crohn's disease.

Adenoma-Carcinoma Sequence

Normal → hyperproliferative → early adenoma → intermediate adenoma → late adenoma → carcinoma (→ metastatic disease).

1. APC gene loss or mutation
2. Loss of DNA methylation
3. Ras (gene) mutation

At diagnosis of CRC: 10% in situ disease; one third local disease; one third regional disease; 20% metastatic disease.

Rule out metastases from colorectal cancer with chest x-ray (CXR), CT of abdomen and pelvis, and liver function tests. Measure carcinoembryonic antigen (CEA) to establish a baseline level.

TABLE 10-4. Polyposis Syndromes of the Bowel

Syndrome	Inheritance Pattern	Risks/Associated Findings
Familial polyposis coli (FAP)	Autosomal dominant	■ Hundreds to thousands of polyps develop between the second and fourth decades; colon cancer inevitable without prophylactic colectomy ■ Caused by abnormal gene on chromosome 5, APC gene ■ Indication for operation: Polyps ■ Operations: 　1. Proctocolectomy with ileostomy 　2. Colectomy with ileorectal anastomosis 　3. Proctocolectomy with ileal pouch—anal anastomosis
Gardner's syndrome	Autosomal dominant	Innumerable polyps with associated osteomas, epidermal cysts, and fibromatosis; colon cancer inevitable without surgery
Turcot's syndrome	Autosomal dominant	Multiple adenomatous colonic polyps with central nervous system (CNS) tumors (especially gliomas)
Peutz-Jeghers syndrome	Autosomal dominant	Hamartomatous polyps of the entire GI tract with melanotic pigmentation of face, lips, oral mucosa, and palms; increased risk for cancer of the pancreas, cervix, lung, ovary, and uterus
Hereditary nonpolyposis colon cancer syndrome (HNPCC or Lynch syndrome)	Autosomal dominant	Lynch syndrome I: Patients without multiple polyps who develop predominantly right-sided colon cancer at a young age. Lynch syndrome II: Same as Lynch I but additional risk for extracolonic adenocarcinomas of the uterus, ovary, cervix, and breast

Microcytic anemia in an elderly male or postmenopausal woman is colon cancer until proven otherwise.

CRC 5-year survival by stage:
Stage I: T1N0M0/T2N0M1 (90%)
Stage II: T3N0M0/ T4N0M0 (75%)
Stage III: anyT/N1M0/ anyTN2–3M0 (50%)
Stage IV: anyT anyN **M1** (5%)

　4. Loss of DCC gene
　5. Loss of p53 gene

SIGNS AND SYMPTOMS

- Typically asymptomatic for a long period of time; symptoms, if present, depend on location and size.
- Right-sided cancers: Occult bleeding with melena, anemia, and weakness.
- Left-sided cancers: Rectal bleeding, obstructive symptoms, change in bowel habits and/or stool caliber.
- Both: Weight loss, anorexia.

DIAGNOSIS

- Colon cancer: Flexible sigmoidoscopy or colonoscopy (need to evaluate entire colon and rectum to look for synchronous lesions).
- Rectal cancer: Digital rectal exam, proctoscopy/colonoscopy, barium enema, also consider transrectal ultrasound (TRUS), CT, or magnetic resonance imaging (MRI) to assess depth of local tumor invasion and local lymph node status.

SCREENING MEASURE/CONDITION	RECOMMENDED CANCER SCREENING MEASURE(S)/TREATMENT
Fecal occult blood test (FOBT)	Every year after 50
Flexible sigmoidoscopy	Every 5 years after 50, with FOBT
Colonoscopy	Every 10 years
Persons at high risk for colon cancer (FAP, HNPCC, UC, high-risk adenomatous polyps)	Regular endoscopic screening by a specialist
Follow-up after resection of colorectal carcinoma (CRC)	▪ Perioperative colonoscopy to remove any synchronous cancer ▪ Colonoscopy 1 year postop and yearly thereafter to look for metachronous lesions ▪ Colonoscopy 3 years after one negative test ▪ Colonoscopy every 5 years once a 3-year test is negative

STAGING AND PROGNOSIS

Dukes System (old system)
A: Limited to wall
B: Through wall of bowel but not to lymph nodes
C: Metastatic to regional lymph nodes
D: Distant mets

TNM System (more current system)
T1: Invasion of submucosa
T2: Invasion of muscularis propria
T3: Invasion of subserosa, or nonperitonealized pericolic or perirectal tissues
T4: Invasion of visceral peritoneum/direct invasion of other organs
N0: No nodal disease
N1: 1–3 pericolic or perirectal lymph nodes
N2: 4 or more lymph nodes
M0: No evidence of distant mets
M1: Distant mets

TREATMENT

- Surgical resection (see Table 10-6 and Figure 10-5):
  - Goal is to remove primary tumor along with lymphatics draining involved bowel.
  - In rectal cancer, the circumferential radial margin (CRM) is crucial to local recurrence. Total mesorectal excision (TME) reduces the rates of local recurrence.
- Adjuvant treatment:
  - Stage III: 5-fluorouracil (5-FU)-based chemotherapy.

Typical scenario: A 65-year-old male presents complaining of rectal bleeding and increasing constipation with thinning of stool caliber. A barium enema is performed (see Figure 10-4). What is the most likely diagnosis? *Think:* This elderly individual is at risk for colon cancer, and his obstructive symptoms likely indicate that it is left-sided. The "apple core" filling defect in the descending colon on barium enema is classic for left-sided colon cancer.

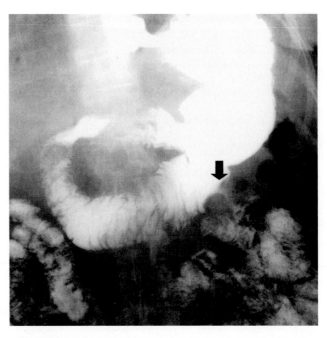

FIGURE 10-4. "Apple core" constricting adenocarcinoma of the proximal jejunum causing proximal partial bowel obstruction.

(Reproduced, with permission, from Turner D, Bass BL. Tumors of the small intestine. In Zinner MJ, Ashley SW, eds. *Maingot's Abdominal Operations*, 11th ed. New York: McGraw-Hill; 2007: 618.)

- Rectal cancer: Preop radiation using 5-FU as a radiosensitizer (this sequence is called "neoadjuvant" therapy because it occurs prior to the definitive surgical treatment.

▶ **PERIANAL AND ANAL PROBLEMS**

Hemorrhoids

See Table 10-7.

- Prolapse of the submucosal veins located in the left lateral, right anterior, and right posterior quadrants of the anal canal.
- Classified by type of epithelium: Internal if covered by columnar mucosa (above dentate line), external if covered by anoderm (below dentate line), and mixed if both types of epithelia are involved.
- **Incidence:** Male = female.
- **Risk factors:** Constipation, pregnancy, increased pelvic pressure (ascites, tumors), portal hypertension.
- **Diagnosis:** Clinical history, physical exam, visualize with anoscope.

Anal Fissure

DEFINITION

Painful linear tears in the anal mucosa below the dentate line; induced by constipation or excessive diarrhea.

There is no classification system for external hemorrhoids. They are either present or absent.

Typical scenario: A 24-year-old male with chronic constipation complains of intense anal pain. He has a tender, swollen, bluish lump at the anal orifice. What is the treatment? *Think:* This young man's history of constipation and physical exam findings are classic for a thrombosed external hemorrhoid. The treatment is surgical excision if the pain has been present for < 48 hours or is persistent. Pain typically subsides after 48 hours, and treatment is symptomatic.

TABLE 10-6. Operative Management of CRC Based on Tumor Location

TUMOR LOCATION	OPERATION
Cecum	Right hemicolectomy: ■ Resection of terminal ileum, cecum, ascending and proximal transverse colon
Right colon	Right hemicolectomy
Proximal/mid-transverse colon	Extended right hemicolectomy: ■ Resection as above plus remainder of transverse colon and splenic flexure
Splenic flexure and left colon	Left hemicolectomy: ■ Resection through descending colon
Sigmoid or rectosigmoid colon	Sigmoid colectomy
Proximal rectum	**Low anterior resection (LAR):** ■ Tumors > 4 cm from anal verge (with distal intramural spread < 2 cm) ■ Must be able to get 2-cm margin ■ Includes total mesorectum excision ■ Involves complete mobilization of rectum, with division of lateral ligaments, posterior mobilization through Waldeyer's fascia to tip of coccyx, dissection between rectum and vagina or prostate ■ Complications: Incontinence, urinary dysfunction, sexual dysfunction, anastomotic leak (5–10%), stricture (5–20%)
Distal rectum	**Abdominal-perineal resection (APR):** ■ Tumors not fitting criteria for LAR ■ Involves creation of end ostomy, with resection of rectum, total mesorectal excision (TME), and closure of anus ■ Complications: Stenosis, retraction or prolapse of ostomy, perineal wound infection
Other situations	■ Obstructing cancer: Attempt to decompress ■ Perforated cancer: Remove disease and perforated segments ■ Synchronous or metachronous lesions, or proximal perforation with distal cancer: Subtotal colectomy with ileosigmoid or ileorectal anastomosis ■ Very distal rectal tumor and/or patient not stable for big operation: Transanal excision of tumor, endoscopic microsurgery, or endocavitary radiation ■ En-bloc resection for malignant fistulas

SIGNS AND SYMPTOMS

■ Pain with defecation.
■ Bright red blood on toilet tissue.
■ Markedly increased sphincter tone and extreme pain on digital examination.
■ Visible tear upon gentle lateral retraction of anal tissue.

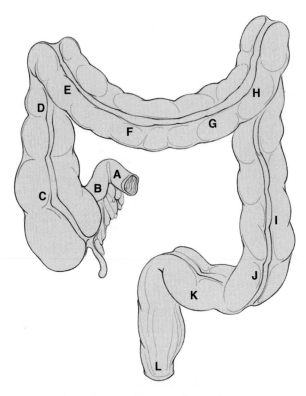

FIGURE 10-5. **Terminology of types of colorectal resections.**

A to C, ileocecectomy; + A + B to D, ascending colectomy; + A + B to F, right hemicolectomy; + A + B to G, extended right hemicolectomy; + E + F to G + H, transverse colectomy; G to I, left hemicolectomy; F to I , extended left hemicolectomy; J + K, sigmoid colectomy; + A + B to J, subtotal colectomy; + A + B to K, total colectomy; + A + B to L, total proctocolectomy.

TABLE 10-7. **Grade Description, Symptoms, and Treatments of Internal Hemorrhoids**

	GRADE DESCRIPTION	SYMPTOMS	TREATMENT
I	Protrudes into lumen, no prolapse	Bleeding	Nonresectional measures[a]
II	Prolapse with straining, spontaneous return	Bleeding, perception of prolapse	Nonresectional measures
III	Prolapse, requires manual reduction	Bleeding, prolapse, mucous soilage, pruritus	Consider trial of nonresectional measures; many require excision
IV	Prolapse cannot be reduced	Bleeding, prolapse, mucous soilage, pruritus, pain[b]	Excision

[a] Nonresectional methods (rubber-band ligation, infrared coagulation, or injection sclerotherapy) can be used in insensate tissue only (above the dentate line).

[b] Pain if thrombosed or ischemic.

Reproduced, with permission, from Niederhuber JE. *Fundamentals of Surgery.* Stamford, CT: Appleton & Lange, 1998: 317.

DIAGNOSIS

History and physical exam.

TREATMENT

- Sitz baths.
- Fiber supplements, bulking agents.
- Increased fluid intake.
- If nonsurgical therapy fails, options include lateral internal sphincterotomy or forceful anal dilation.

Anorectal Abscess

DEFINITION

Obstruction of anal crypts with resultant bacterial overgrowth and abscess formation within the intersphincteric space.

RISK FACTORS

- Constipation/diarrhea/IBD.
- Immunocompromise.
- History of recent surgery or trauma.
- History of colorectal carcinoma.
- History of previous anorectal abscess.

SIGNS AND SYMPTOMS

Rectal pain, often of sudden onset, with associated fever, chills, malaise, leukocytosis, and a tender perianal swelling with erythema and warmth of overlying skin.

TREATMENT

Surgical drainage.

Anorectal Fistulas

DEFINITION

Tissue tracts (abnormal connections between two areas) originating in the glands of the anal canal at the dentate line that are usually the chronic sequelae of anorectal infections, particularly abscesses.

CLASSIFICATION OF ANORECTAL FISTULAS

1. **Intersphincteric (most common):** Fistula tract stays within intersphincteric plane.
2. **Transsphincteric:** Fistula connects the intersphincteric plane with the ischiorectal fossa by perforating the external sphincter.
3. **Suprasphincteric:** Similar to transsphincteric, but the fistula loops above the external sphincter to penetrate the levator ani muscles.
4. **Extrasphincteric:** Fistula passes from rectum to perineal skin without penetrating sphincteric complex.

Goodsall's rule (Figure 10-6) can be used to clinically predict the course of an anorectal fistula tract. Imagine a line that bisects the anus in the coronal plane. Any fistula that originates anterior to the line will course anteriorly in a direct route. Fistulae that originate posterior to the line will have a curved path. Fistula tracts that diverge from this rule should increase one's suspicion for IBD.

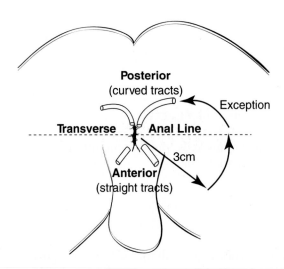

Posterior
(curved tracts)

Exception

Transverse ----- **Anal Line**

3cm

Anterior
(straight tracts)

FIGURE 10-6. Goodsall's rule to identify the internal opening of fistulas in ano.

(Reproduced, with permission, from Brunicardi FC, Andersen DK, Billiar TR, et al., eds. *Schwartz's Principles of Surgery*, 8th ed. New York: McGraw-Hill, 2005: 1108.)

SIGNS AND SYMPTOMS

Recurrent or persistent perianal drainage that becomes painful when one of the tracts becomes occluded.

DIAGNOSIS

- Bidigital rectal exam.
- Anoscopy.
- If the internal opening cannot be identified by direct probing, it should be identified by probing the external opening or by injecting a mixture of methylene blue and peroxide into the tract.

TREATMENT

Intraoperative unroofing of the entire fistula tract with or without placement of setons (heavy suture looped through the tract to keep it patent for drainage and to stimulate fibrosis).

Pilonidal Disease

- **Definition:** A cystic inflammatory process generally occurring at or near the cranial edge of the gluteal cleft.
- **Incidence:** Most commonly seen in young men in their late teens to the third decade.

SIGNS AND SYMPTOMS

Can present acutely as an abscess (fluctuant mass) or chronically as a draining sinus with pain at the top of the gluteal cleft.

TREATMENT

Incision and drainage under local anesthesia with removal of involved hairs.

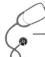

The terms *pilo* and *nidus* are Latin terms for "hair" and "origin," respectively, indicating that the lesion is associated with hair follicles. Pilonidal disease results from trauma to hair follicles in the gluteal region with resultant infection.

178

DEFINITION

Neoplasms of the anorectal region that are classified into tumors of the perianal skin (anal margin carcinomas) and tumors of the anal canal.

INCIDENCE

Rare (1–2% of all colon cancers).

RISK FACTORS

- Human papillomavirus (HPV)
- Human immunodeficiency virus (HIV)
- Cigarette smoking
- Multiple sexual partners
- Anal intercourse
- Immunosuppressed state

SIGNS AND SYMPTOMS

Often asymptomatic; can present with anal bleeding, a lump, or itching; an irregular nodule that is palpable or visible externally (anal margin tumor) or a hard, ulcerating mass that occupies a portion of the anal canal (anal canal tumor).

DIAGNOSIS

- Surgical biopsy with histopathologic evaluation.
- **Histology:** Anal margin tumors include squamous and basal cell carcinomas, Paget's disease, and Bowen's disease. Anal canal tumors are usually epidermoid (squamous cell carcinoma or transitional cell/cloacogenic carcinoma) or malignant melanoma.
- **Clinical staging:** Involves history, physical exam, proctocolonoscopy, abdominal or pelvic CT or MRI, CXR, and liver function tests.

TREATMENT

- Epidermoid carcinoma of anal canal: Chemoradiation is mainstay— 5-FU, mitomycin C, and 3,000 cGy external beam radiation (Nigro protocol) surgery is reserved for recurrence.
- Other anal margin tumors: Wide local excision alone or in combination with radiation and/or chemotherapy is successful in 80% of cases without abdominal-perineal resection (APR) if tumor is small and not deeply invasive.
- Anal canal tumors: Local excision not an option; combined chemotherapy (5-FU and mitomycin C) with radiation often successful; APR only if follow-up biopsy indicates residual tumor.

PROGNOSIS

- Anal margin tumors: 80% overall 5-year survival.
- Anal canal tumors:
  - Epidermoid carcinoma: 50% overall 5-year survival.
  - Malignant melanoma: 10–15% 5-year survival.

Two unique in situ tumors of the perianal skin are Paget's disease and Bowen's disease. Paget's disease of the anus is adenocarcinoma in situ, and anal Bowen's disease is squamous carcinoma in situ.

HIGH-YIELD FACTS

Colon, Rectum, & Anal Canal

HIGH-YIELD FACTS

Colon, Rectum, & Anal Canal

The Appendix

- The appendix begins to bud off from the cecum at around the **sixth week** of embryological development.
- The base of the appendix remains in a fixed position with respect to the cecum, whereas the tip can end up in various positions (Figure 11-1).

After you locate the cecum, you can easily find the appendix by following the three taeniae coli until they converge at the base of the appendix.

- **Mesoappendix** is the mesentery that suspends the appendix from the terminal ileum. It contains the **appendicular artery,** the blood supply to the appendix.
  - The appendicular artery is a branch of the ileocolic artery.
  - The ileocolic artery is a branch of the superior mesenteric artery.
- The appendix is composed of the same layers as the colon wall.
  - Mucosa, submucosa, inner circular muscle, outer longitudinal muscle, serosa.
  - The three distinct bands of outer longitudinal muscle, the **taeniae coli,** converge on the appendix.

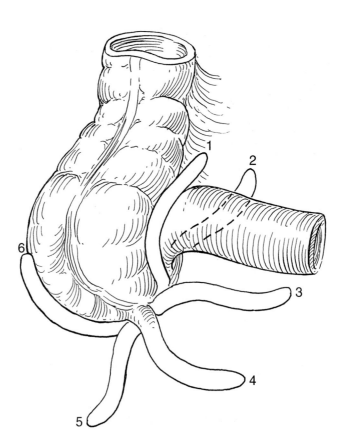

FIGURE 11-1. Anatomic variation in the position of the appendix.

(1) Preileal; (2) postileal; (3) promontoric; (4) pelvic; (5) subcecal; (6) paracolic or prececal. (Reproduced from: Smink DS, Soybel DI. Appendix and appendectomy. In Zinner MJ, Ashley SW, eds. *Maingot's Abdominal Operations,* 11th ed. New York: McGraw-Hill, 2007: 590.)

- Although many have claimed that the appendix is merely a vestigial organ, it is actually an immunological organ and **secretes IgA.** However, it is not an essential organ and can be removed without immunological compromise.
- The length can range from 2 to 20 cm but averages **6–9 cm.**
- Luminal capacity is < 1 mL.

The lifetime incidence of acute appendicitis in the United States is about 7%.

▶ ACUTE APPENDICITIS

INCIDENCE

One of the most common acute surgical diseases.

- Highest in early adulthood, at the peak of lymphoid tissue growth.
- Second peak in the incidence of appendicitis occurs in the elderly.
- There is a higher incidence of appendicitis in males than females (1.3:1), although females are more commonly misdiagnosed with acute appendicitis than males.

PATHOPHYSIOLOGY

The probable sequence of events in acute appendicitis is:

1. Luminal **obstruction.**
   - In young patients, more commonly by **lymphoid tissue hyperplasia.**
   - In older patients, **fecalith** is an increasingly common cause of obstruction.
2. **Distention** and increased intraluminal pressure.
   - The appendiceal mucosa continues to secrete normally despite being obstructed.
   - The resident bacteria multiply rapidly, further increasing intraluminal pressure.
3. Venous congestion.
   - The intraluminal pressure eventually exceeds capillary and venule pressures.
   - Arteriolar blood continues to flow in, causing vascular congestion and engorgement.
4. Impaired blood supply renders the mucosa ischemic and susceptible to **bacterial invasion.**
5. **Inflammation** and **ischemia** progress to involve the serosal surface of the appendix.

The *initial dull, diffuse (visceral) pain* that occurs at the onset of acute appendicitis is a result of the stimulation of *visceral afferent stretch fibers.* These nerve endings fire as a result of the sudden-onset distention, and the pain is commonly felt around the umbilicus (T10 distribution).

SYMPTOMS

- Right lower quadrant (RLQ) pain.
- **Migration** of pain from the periumbilical region to localize in the RLQ.
- Nausea/vomiting.
- Fever.

The shift from dull, diffuse (visceral) pain to *sharp, localized (somatic) RLQ pain* occurs when the inflamed serosa contacts the parietal peritoneum, causing *peritoneal irritation.* This pain is felt in the area directly overlying the appendix.

SIGNS

- Direct rebound tenderness, which is maximal at (or around) McBurney's point.
- Leukocytosis.
- *Rovsing's sign:* Palpation pressure exerted over left lower quadrant (LLQ) causes pain in RLQ.

McBurney's point: One third the distance along a line drawn a from the right anterior superior iliac spine to the umbilicus.

- *Iliopsoas sign:* Pain on extension at the right hip.
  - The patient will get relief by flexing the right thigh at the hip, which relaxes the psoas muscle.
  - This sign signifies retrocecal appendicitis.
- *Obturator sign* (signifies pelvic appendicitis): Pelvic pain on internal rotation of the right thigh.

DIFFERENTIAL DIAGNOSIS

Gastrointestinal Conditions
- Gastroenteritis
- Mesenteric adenitis
- Meckel's diverticulum
- Intussusception
- Typhoid fever
- Primary peritonitis

Genitourinary Conditions
- Ectopic pregnancy
- Pelvic inflammatory disease
- Ovarian torsion/cyst/tumor
- Urinary tract infection/pyelonephritis
- Ureteral stone

DIAGNOSIS

Labs
- **Complete blood count:**
  - Leukocytosis (> 10,000 in 90% of cases), usually with concomitant left shift (polymorphonuclear neutrophil [PMN] predominance).
  - Consider perforation or abscess if WBC > 18,000.
- **Urinalysis:**
  - Helpful in ruling out genitourinary causes of symptoms.
  - RBCs and WBCs may be present secondary to extension of appendiceal inflammation to the ureter.
  - Significant hematuria or pyuria, and bacteriuria from a catheterized specimen should suggest underlying urinary tract pathology.

Diagnostic Imaging
- **Abdominal x-ray:**
  - Not particularly useful in most cases.
  - May reveal appendicolith/fecalith (< 15% of cases).
- **Abdominal CT with contrast:**
  - Very sensitive (95–98%) and somewhat specific (83–90%).
  - Useful in identifying several other inflammatory processes that may present similarly to appendicitis.
  - Positive findings include:
    - Dilatation of appendix to > 6 mm in diameter.
    - Thickening of appendiceal wall (representing edema).
    - Periappendiceal streaking (densities within perimesenteric fat).
    - Presence of appendicolith (see Figure 11-2).
- **Graded compression ultrasonography:**
  - Sensitivity of 85% and specificity of 92% for diagnosing appendicitis.
  - Positive finding: Enlarged (> 6 mm), noncompressible appendix.
  - Especially useful in ruling out gynecologic pathology.

> *Yersinia enterolytica* can cause mesenteric adenitis and is a great mimicker of appendicitis.

> The appendix will become compressible after perforation is a source of false negative

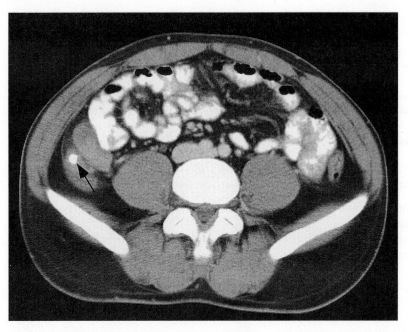

FIGURE 11-2. Abdominal CT scan demonstrating appendicolith and acute appendicitis.

TREATMENT

- Preoperative: IV fluids plus antibiotics.
- Prompt appendectomy is essential.
- For perforation: Peritoneal washout and parenteral antibiotics.

▶ APPENDICITIS IN SPECIAL POPULATIONS

Pregnant Patients

- Appendicitis is the most common surgical emergency in pregnant patients.
- Fetal mortality increases 3–8% with appendicitis and 30% with perforation.
- **Surgery** is the standard treatment, though 10–15% of women will experience premature labor.

Elderly Patients

- Tend to present atypically, leading to delayed diagnosis.
  - Present later in the course and with less pain, may present as a small bowel obstruction.
  - Delayed leukocytosis.
- Higher risk of perforation and higher mortality than in younger patients.

Immunocompromised Patients (e.g., AIDS patients, recipients of high-dose chemotherapy)

- Although they may not have absolute leukocytosis, compared to baseline WBC count, they will demonstrate relative leukocytosis.

The enlarged uterus may push the appendix up, explaining why pregnant patients may present with RUQ pain.

185

Patients will not typically have carcinoid syndrome unless the tumor has metastasized to the liver.

- The differential diagnosis is expanded to include opportunistic infections such as cytomegalovirus (CMV)-related bowel perforation and neutropenic colitis.

▶ APPENDICEAL NEOPLASMS

Carcinoid

A relatively low-grade neuroendocrine tumor (it secretes enzymes aberrantly; the enzymes typically cause nausea, diarrhea, and flushing).

- The appendix is the most common site of carcinoid tumors in the GI tract.
- Carcinoid is the second most common type of appendiceal tumor (commonest being mucinous adenocarcinoma).

DIAGNOSIS

Increased urinary 5-hydroxyindoleacetic acid (5-HIAA) and increased serum serotonin.

TREATMENT

Size is the major determinant of treatment and malignant potential:

- Tumors < 2 cm are treated with appendectomy.
- Tumors > 2 cm are treated with right hemicolectomy.
- Serotonin antagonists (e.g., cyproheptadine) or somatostatin analogues (e.g., octreotide) can be used for symptoms of carcinoid syndrome.

Mucinous Tumors

- Can rupture, causing **pseudomyxoma peritonei** with mucin implants on peritoneal surfaces and the omentum.
  - More common in women (ratio of 3:2).
  - Complications include bowel obstruction and perforation.
- Have been associated with migratory thrombophlebitis.

Adenocarcinoma

- Colon cancer that arises from the appendix; very rare and almost never diagnosed preoperatively.
- Rapid spread to regional lymph nodes, ovaries, and peritoneal surfaces.
- If confined to appendix and local lymph nodes, right hemicolectomy is the treatment of choice.

Think of an abscess in a patient who presents with the clinical picture of **appendicitis and RLQ mass.**

▶ APPENDICEAL ABSCESS

- **Signs and symptoms:** Similar to acute appendicitis.
  - Increasing RLQ pain.
  - Tender, fluctuant RLQ mass that is palpable on rectal examination.
  - Anorexia.

- Fever.
- Localizing peritonitis.
- Leukocytosis.
- **Diagnosis:** Confirmed by CT scan.
- **Treatment:** Percutateous or operative drainage.

▶ **RECENT ADVANCES**

Natural orifice transluminal endoscopic surgery (NOTES): Still experimental; in this procedure the appendix is removed via upper gastrointestinal endoscopy with the surgeon operating through the gastric wall and ultimately removing the appendix through the mouth without any external scar. The gastrotomy is closed from within the stomach.

HIGH-YIELD FACTS

The Appendix

Hernia and Abdominal Wall Problems

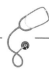

Groin hernias usually present with the complaint of a bulge in the inguinal region. The patient may describe minor pain or vague discomfort.

Hernia Calendar

- 0–2 years—indirect inguinal hernia
- 2–20 years—hernia is uncommon
- 20–50 years—indirect inguinal hernia
- > 50 years—direct inguinal hernia

▶ OVERVIEW

- Hernias are a common surgical problem.
- It is estimated that 10% of the population develops some type of hernia during life and that they are present in 3–4% of the male population.
- Fifty percent are indirect inguinal hernias, 25% are direct inguinal, and 15% are femoral.
- The male-to-female ratio is 7:1.
- Abdominal wall hernias are the most common condition requiring major surgery.

▶ DEFINITIONS

- **Hernia:** A protrusion of a viscus through an abnormal opening in the wall of a cavity in which it is contained.

▶ CLASSIFICATION OF HERNIAS

- **External hernia:** The sac protrudes completely through the abdominal wall. Examples: Inguinal (indirect and direct), femoral, umbilical, and epigastric.
- **Intraparietal hernia:** The sac is contained within the abdominal wall. Example: Spigelian hernia.
- **Internal hernia:** The sac is within the visceral cavity. Examples: Diaphragmatic hernias (congenital or acquired) and the small intestine herniating in the paraduodenal pouch.
- **Reducible hernia:** The protruding viscus can be returned to the abdomen.
- **Irreducible (incarcerated) hernia:** The protruding viscus cannot be returned to the abdomen.
- **Strangulated hernia:** The vascularity of the viscus is compromised— **surgical emergency.**

▶ GENERAL GROIN ANATOMY

See Figure 12-1.

Layers of the Abdominal Wall

Skin, subcutaneous fat, Scarpa's fascia, external oblique muscle, internal oblique muscle, transversus abdominis muscle, transversalis fascia, peritoneal fat, and peritoneum.

Internal Structures

- Inguinal canal: Length, 4 cm; boundaries:
  - Anterior wall: External oblique aponeurosis.

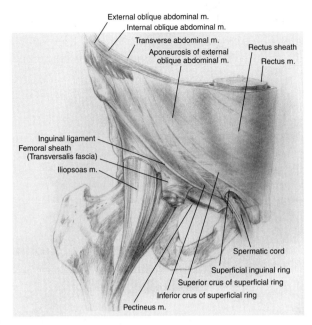
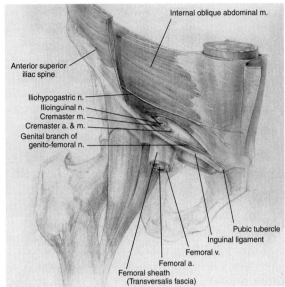

FIGURE 12-1. Groin anatomy.

- Posterior wall: Transverse abdominal muscle aponeurosis and transversalis fascia.
- Spermatic cord: Begins at the deep ring and contains the vas deferens and its artery (descend to the seminiferous tubules), one testicular artery and two to three veins, lymphatics (incline superiorly to the kidney region), autonomic nerves, and fat.

Nerves

- Genital:
  - Location: Travels along with the cremaster vessels to form a neurovascular bundle.
  - Originates: From L1 and L2.
  - Motor and sensory: Innervates the cremaster muscle, skin of the side of the scrotum and labia.
  - May substitute for the ilioinguinal nerve if it's deficient.
- Iliohypogastric, ilioinguinal nerves, and the genital branch of the genitofemoral nerve:
  - Iliohypogastric and ilioinguinal intertwine.
  - Originates: From T12 and L1.
  - Sensory: To skin of groin, base of penis, and medial upper thigh.
- Genital branch of genitofemoral nerve: Located on top of the spermatic cord in 60% of people but can be found behind or within the cremaster muscle. Often cannot be found or is too small to be seen.

Femoral Canal Structures

From lateral to medial: **N**erve, **A**rtery, **V**ein, **E**mpty space, **L**ymph nodes.

The inguinal area is examined with the patient standing and facing the physician. Presence of a discrete bulge in the inguinal area reveals the hernia. Valsalva's maneuver and cough may accentuate the bulge, making it clearly visible.

Memory aid for the femoral canal structures: **NAVEL.**

Anatomical Triangles

- **Hesselbach's triangle:** The triangular area in the lower abdominal wall. It is the site of direct inguinal hernia. The boundaries of Hesselbach's triangle are:
  - Inferior border: Inguinal ligament.
  - Medial border: Rectus abdominis.
  - Lateral border: Inferior epigastric vessels (lateral umbilical fold).
- **Triangle of Grynfeltt** (superior lumbar) bounded by the 12th rib superiorly and the internal oblique muscle anteriorly, with the floor composed of fibers of the quadratus lumborum muscle.
- **Triangle of Petit** (inferior lumbar triangle) bounded by:
  - Posteriorly: Latissimus dorsi muscle.
  - Anteriorly: External oblique muscle.
  - Inferiorly: Iliac crest.
  - The floor is composed of fibers from the internal oblique and transversus abdominis muscle.

▶ INGUINAL HERNIA

- Hernias arising above the abdominocrural crease.
- Most common site for abdominal hernias.
- Male-to-female ratio: 25:1.
- Males: Indirect > direct (2:1).
- Female: Direct is rare.
- Incidence, strangulation, and hospitalization all increase with age.
- Cause 15–20% of intestinal obstructions.

RISK FACTORS

- Abdominal wall hernias occur in areas where aponeurosis and fascia are devoid of protecting support of striated muscle.
- They can be congenital or acquired by surgery or muscular atrophy.
- Female predisposition to femoral hernias: Increased diameter of the true pelvis as compared to men, proportionally widens the femoral canal.
- Muscle deficiency of the internal oblique muscles in the groin exposes the deep ring and floor of the inguinal canal, which are further weakened by intra-abdominal pressure.
- Connective tissue destruction (transverse aponeurosis and fascia): Caused by physical stress secondary to intra-abdominal pressure; smoking; aging; connective tissue disease; systemic illnesses; fracture of elastic fibers; alterations in structure, quantity, and metabolism of collagen.
- Other factors: Abdominal distention, ascites with chronic increase in intra-abdominal pressure, and peritoneal dialysis.

SYMPTOMS

- Asymptomatic: Some patients have no symptoms.
- Symptomatic: Wide variety of nonspecific discomforts related to the contents of the sac and the pressure by the sac on adjacent tissue.
- Pain: Worse at the end of the day and relieved at night when patient lies down (because the hernia reduces).

- Groin hernias do not usually cause testicular pain. Likewise, testicular pain doesn't usually indicate the onset of a hernia.

DIAGNOSIS

Physical exam: In the standing position, have patient strain or cough. The hernia sac with its contents will enlarge and transmit a palpable impulse.

DIFFERENTIAL DIAGNOSIS

- Abdominal wall mass
- Desmoids
- Neoplasm
- Adenopathy
- Rectus sheath hematoma

RADIOLOGY

Hernia is a clinical diagnosis, and radiological tests (ultrasound/CT scan) are done only in special circumstances (e.g., morbid obesity, where clinical examination is not reliable).

MANAGEMENT

Principles of Treatment
- Tension-free repair of the hernia defect.
- Repair using fascia, aponeurosis, or mesh.
- Suture material used should hold until fibrous tissue is formed over it.
- Resuscitation in case of strangulated hernia with gangrene with shock or with intestinal obstruction.

Nonsurgical
- No role of medical management in a patient who can tolerate surgery.
- Can be considered in moribund patients.
- Hernia truss is a device to keep a reducible hernia contained by external pressure. Its use is very limited in modern practice.

Surgical
- Treatment modality of choice.
- Herniotomy is the operation where hernia sac is identified, freed, its neck ligated, and the sac reduced. This may be sufficient in young, muscular individuals and in children.
- Herniorrhaphy and hernioplasty are herniotomy along with repair of the posterior wall of the inguinal canal and the internal ring.

Hydroceles can resemble an irreducible groin hernia. To distinguish, transilluminate (hernias will not light up).

▶ TYPES OF GROIN HERNIA SURGERY

Open

- **Tissue repair:** Uses the patient's tissue for reinforcement.
  - Bassini's repair: Suturing of conjoint tendon to the incurved part of inguinal ligament. Bassini's repair is still widely practiced as it is simple to perform with good results.

- Shouldice repair: Double breasting of transversalis fascia. Technically challenging with excellent results.
- McVay's repair/Cooper's repair (used for Femoral hernias): Conjoint tendon sutured to Cooper's ligament.
- **Mesh repair:** Uses prosthetic mesh and/or plug for tension-free repair (preferred).
  - Anterior approach: For example, Lichtenstein's repair (most common).
  - Posterior approach: For example, Kugel's method, Stoppa's repair.

Laparoscopic

- Requires a very experienced and highly skilled surgeon, has decreased postop pain, requires general or regional anesthesia, and more expensive. Wound infection has been shown to decrease with laparoscopic repair.
  - Transabdominal pre-peritoneal procedure (TAPP).
  - Totally extraperitoneal procedure (TEP)—preferred.
- The choice of hernia surgery depends on the surgeon's expertise. TEP is being performed in larger numbers as surgical proficiency in laparoscopy increases, and the results are promising (see Figure 12-2).

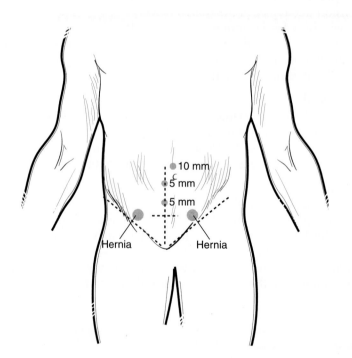

FIGURE 12-2. Laparoscopic cannula placement for a totally extraperitoneal (TEP) herniorrhaphy.

(Reproduced, with permission, from Brunicardi FC, Andersen DK, Billiar TR, et al., eds. *Schwartz's Principles of Surgery*, 8th ed. New York: McGraw-Hill, 2005: 1383.)

Indications for Surgery

Generally, all hernias should be repaired unless the risks of surgery outweigh the benefits of the repair.

Complications of Surgery

- Ischemic orchitis with testicular atrophy.
- Residual neuralgia.
- Both: More common with anterior groin hernioplasty because of the nerves and spermatic cord dissection and mobilization.

A reducible hernia in a patient with ascites should not be corrected until the ascites is controlled.

Prognosis

Recurrence:

- Expert surgeons 1–3% in 10-year follow-up.
- Caused by excessive tension on repair, deficient tissue, inadequate hernioplasty, or overlooked hernias
- Decreased with relaxing incisions.
- More common with direct hernias.

▶ CLASSIFICATION OF INGUINAL HERNIAS

- Direct
- Indirect

Direct Inguinal Hernia

A direct inguinal hernia enters the inguinal canal through its weakened posterior wall. The hernia does not pass through the internal ring.

- Lies posterior to the spermatic cord.
- Practically never enters the scrotum.
- Wide neck (strangulation uncommon).
- Occurs almost exclusively in males.
- Common in older age groups.
- Common in smokers due to weakened connective tissue.
- Predisposing factors: Hard labor, cough, straining, and so on.
- Can lead to damage to the ilioinguinal nerve.

SYMPTOMS

- Bulge in groin.
- Dull dragging pain in the inguinal region referred to testis.
- Pain increases with hard work and straining.

Indirect Inguinal Hernia

Herniation through the internal inguinal ring traveling to the external ring. If complete, can enter the scrotum while exiting the external ring.

- If congenital, associated with a patent processus vaginalis.
- Bilateral in one third of cases.
- Most common hernia in both males and females.
- Occurs at all ages.
- More common in males than in females.
- In the first decade of life, the right-sided hernia is more common than left (because of late descent of right testis).

▶ FEMORAL HERNIA

A form of indirect hernia arising out of the femoral canal beneath the inguinal ligament (medial to the femoral vessels).

- Female-to-male ratio of 2:1.
- Males affected are in a younger age group.
- Rare in children.
- Uncommon—around 2.5% of all groin hernias.
- Left side 1:2 right side: Secondary to the sigmoid colon tamponading the left femoral canal.
- Common in elderly patients.
- High incidence of incarceration due to narrow neck.
- Twenty-two percent strangulate after 3 months, and 45% after 21 months.

ANATOMY

- The femoral canal is 1.25 cm long and arises from the femoral ring to the saphenous opening.
- Femoral sac originates from the femoral canal through a defect on the medial side (common) or the anterior (uncommon) side of the femoral sheath.

SYMPTOMS

- Dull dragging pain in the groin, with swelling.
- If obstructed, can cause vomiting and constipation.
- If strangulated, can lead to severe pain and shock.
- Swelling arises from below the inguinal ligament.

DIFFERENTIAL DIAGNOSIS

- Inguinal hernia
- Saphenous varix
- Enlarged femoral lymph node
- Lipoma
- Femoral artery aneurysm
- Psoas abscess

▶ ACQUIRED UMBILICAL HERNIA

- Abdominal contents herniate through a defect in the umbilicus.
- Common site of herniation, especially in females.

ASSOCIATED FACTORS

Ascites, obesity, and repeated pregnancies.

COMPLICATIONS

- Strangulation of the colon and omentum is common.
- Rupture occurs in chronic ascitic cirrhosis. Emergency portal decompression is needed.

TREATMENT

- Surgical repair:
  - Small partial defect: Closed by loosely placed polypropylene suture.
  - Large partial defect: Managed with a prosthesis repair.
  - Mayo hemioplasty is the classical repair (not used often).

▶ PEDIATRIC UMBILICAL HERNIA

- Secondary to a fascial defect in the linea alba with protruding abdominal contents, covered by umbilical skin and subcutaneous tissue.
- Caused by a failure of timely closure of the umbilical ring, and leaves a central defect in the linea alba.
- Common in infants.
- Incarceration is rare and reduction is contraindicated.

MANAGEMENT

Usually close spontaneously within 3 years if the defect is < 1.0 cm. Surgical repair indicated if:
- The defect > 2 cm.
- Child is > 3–5 years of age.
- Protrusion is disfiguring and disturbing to the child or parents.

▶ PEDIATRIC WALL DEFECTS

See Pediatric Surgery chapter.

▶ ESOPHAGEAL HIATAL HERNIA

- A hernia in which an anatomical part (such as the stomach) protrudes through the esophageal hiatus of the diaphragm.
- Three types of esophageal hiatal hernia are identified:
  1. The sliding hernia, type I, characterized by an upward dislocation of the cardia in the posterior mediastinum.
  2. The rolling or paraesophageal hernia, type II, characterized by an upward dislocation of the gastric fundus alongside a normally positioned cardia.
  3. The combined sliding-rolling or mixed hernia, type III, characterized by an upward dislocation of both the cardia and the gastric fundus.

The end stage of type I and type II hernias occurs when the whole stomach migrates up into the chest by rotating 180° around its longitudinal axis, with the cardia and pylorus as fixed points. In this situation, the abnormality is usually referred to as an intrathoracic stomach.

Sliding Esophageal Hernia (Type I)

- The gastroesophageal junction and the stomach herniate into the thoracic cavity.
- These account for more than 90% of all hiatal hernias.
- Can lead to reflux and esophagitis that can predispose to Barrett's esophagus.
- Management can be done medically with antacids and head elevation.
- Only 15% require surgery, consisting of wrapping of the stomach fundus around the lower esophageal sphincter (Nissen fundoplication).
- See diagram in GERD section of Esophagus chapter.

Paraesophageal Hiatal Hernia (Type II)

- Herniation of the stomach into the thorax by way of the esophageal hiatus, without disruption of the gastroesophageal junction.
- Rare (< 5%).
- High frequency of complications (i.e., obstruction, strangulation, and hemorrhage).
  - **Warrants prompt surgical correction** via transthoracic or transabdominal approach.
  - Both laparoscopic and open approaches can be used.
  - Reduction, repair with or without fundoplication is done.

▶ OTHER HERNIAS

- **Richter's hernia:** Only part of the intestine wall circumference is in the hernia. May strangulate without obstruction. Seen commonly in femoral and obturator hernias.
- **Littre's hernia:** The hernial sac contains Meckel's diverticulum. It may become inflamed.
- **Garengoff's hernia:** The hernial sac has the appendix. Importance is that it may form an inflamed hernia.
- **Pantaloon hernia:** A combination of a direct and an indirect inguinal hernia.
- **Maydl's hernia:** W type of intestinal loop herniates; may strangulate with the gangrenous part being inside the abdomen, or may be reduced into the abdomen without noticing the gangrenous part.
- **Spigelian hernia:** The sac passes through the spigelian or semilunaris fascia.
- **Sliding inguinal hernia:** Any hernia in which part of the sac is the wall of a viscus. On the right, the cecum, ascending colon, or appendix is commonly involved; on the left, the sigmoid colon is involved.
- **Cooper's hernia:** Hernia that involves the femoral canal and tracts to the labia majora in females and to the scrotum in males.

- **Lumbar hernia:** Divided into congenital, spontaneous, traumatic, and incisional. Can pass through the triangle of Grynfeltt, through the inferior lumbar triangle of Petit, or previous incision.
- **Perineal hernia:** Located through pelvic diaphragm, anterior (passes through labia majora—females only) or posterior (male: enters the ischiorectal fossa; female: close to the vagina) to the superficial transverse perineal muscle.
- **Incisional hernia:** Resulting as a surgical complication. These could enlarge beyond repair. Associated with obesity, diabetes, and infection.
- **Eventration:** Loss of integrity of the abdominal wall, reducing the intra-abdominal pressure and resulting in external herniation of bowel.

The hernias associated with obesity are: Direct inguinal, paraumbilical, and hiatal hernias.

See Figure 13-1.
- Arterial supply:
  - Celiac trunk comes off the aorta, giving off the left gastric, splenic, and common hepatic arteries.

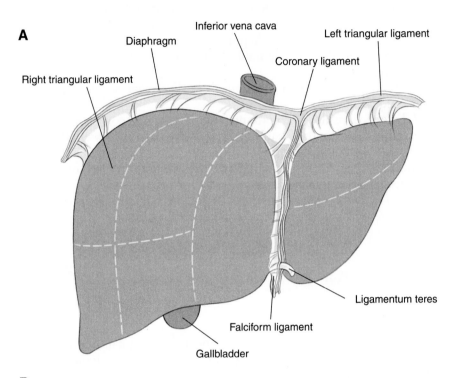

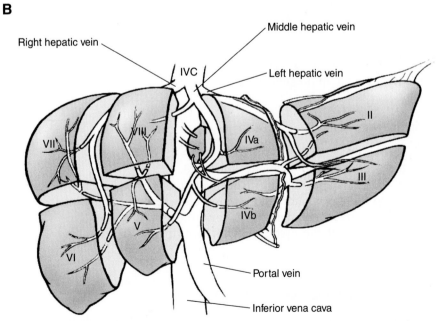

FIGURE 13-1. **Hepatic anatomy.**

Part B adapted from www.ahpba.org, the website of The American Hepato-Pancreato-Billary Association.

- Common hepatic artery divides into the hepatic artery proper and the gastroduodenal artery.
- Hepatic artery divides into the right and left hepatic arteries.
- Venous drainage: The left, middle, and right hepatic veins drain into the inferior vena cava (IVC).
- Ligaments of the liver:
  - *Falciform ligament:* Connects the anterior abdominal wall to the liver; contains the ligamentum teres (obliterated umbilical vein).
  - *Coronary ligament:* Peritoneal reflection on the cranial aspect of the liver that attaches it to the diaphragm.
  - *Triangular ligaments:* The right and left lateral extensions of the coronary ligament.
  - *Bare area:* The posterior section of the liver against the diaphragm; has no peritoneal covering.
  - **Glisson's capsule:** The peritoneal membrane that covers the liver.
  - *Cantlie's line* (portal fissure): A line that passes from the left side of the gallbladder to the left side of the IVC, dividing the liver into right and left lobes. It is based on blood supply and is the basis of the four classic types of hepatic resection.
- Liver enzymes: Aspartate transaminase (AST) and alanine transaminase (ALT) are made by hepatocytes; alkaline phosphatase (alk phos) is made by ductal epithelium.

Liver Blood Supply
The right and left hepatic arteries supply 50% of the liver's oxygen. The portal vein supplies the remaining 50%. However, the liver receives 75% of its blood supply from the portal vein and only 25% from the hepatic arteries. The different degrees of oxygen saturation within the arterial and venous systems account for this fact.

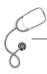

Hepatoduodenal Ligament
The hepatoduodenal ligament contains the common bile duct (CBD), portal vein, and proper hepatic artery. It forms the anterior boundary of the epipolic foramen of Winslow and connects the greater and the lesser peritoneal cavities.

► **DIAGNOSTIC IMAGING**

Ultrasonography

- Ultrasound remains the cornerstone for diagnosing gallstones and is a great tool as it is noninvasive, fast, inexpensive and very reliable for diagnosing gallstones.
- Its drawback is that it is user dependent.
- It should be the first test to be performed in all patients with a suspicion of gallstones.
- Can also detect masses and cysts.
- Test of choice in pregnancy.

Cholangiogram

- Provides image of the biliary tree.
- Oral and IV cholangiography—obsolete.
- T-tube cholangiogram: Performed after open exploration of the bile duct to rule out retained stones just before removal of the tube.
- Intraoperative cholangiogram: Performed on the operating table via cannulation of the cystic duct to confirm the anatomy and diagnose CBD stones.

Hepatobiliary Iminodiacetic Acid (HIDA) Scan

- A radionucleotide scan in which technetium-99m labeled iminodiacetic acid is injected intravenously into hepatocytes.
- A normal gallbladder would be visualized within 1 hour. Most sensitive for acute cholecystitis.
- Drawback is that it is time consuming and stones are not visualized.

Computed Tomographic (CT) Scan

- Useful for hepatic lesions and for visualizing lymph nodes.
- Not very useful for the biliary tree.
- Expensive.
- Contraindicated in pregnancy (radiation exposure).

Endoscopic Retrograde Cholangiopancreatography (ERCP)

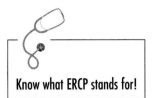

Know what ERCP stands for!

- Involves passage of an endoscope into the duodenum, introduction of a catheter into the ampulla of Vater, and injection of contrast medium into the CBD and/or pancreatic duct; conscious sedation is necessary.
- Can be diagnostic (biopsy and show pancreatic cancer or cholangiocarcinoma) and therapeutic (remove stones, or stent an obstruction).
- One percent risk of pancreatitis from procedure.

ERCP with Sphincterotomy (Papillotomy)

- A cut through the sphincter of Oddi to allow the passage of stones from the CBD into the duodenum.
- Often performed during ERCP but can also be performed as part of open surgery (sphincteroplasty).

Percutaneous Transhepatic Cholangiography (PTCA)

- Involves passing a needle through the skin and subcutaneous tissues into the hepatic parenchyma and advancement into a peripheral bile duct. When bile is aspirated, a catheter is introduced through the needle and radiopaque contrast medium is injected.
- It is very useful in cases with distal obstruction where ERCP is not possible or has failed.

▶ BILE

- Constituents: Cholesterol, lecithin, bile acids, and bilirubin.
- Function: Emulsifies fats.
- Enterohepatic circulation: Bile acids are released from the liver into the duodenum, reabsorbed at the terminal ileum, and transported back to the liver via the portal vein.
- Cholecystokinin:
  - Released by duodenal mucosal cells.
  - Stimulates gallbladder contraction and release of bile (along with vagal stimulation).
  - Causes opening of the ampulla of Vater and slows gastric emptying.
  - Is stimulated by fat, protein, amino acids, and hydrochloride (HCl).
  - Trypsin and chymotrypsin inhibit its release.

▶ JAUNDICE

DEFINITION

Yellowing of the skin and sclera due to an elevation in total bilirubin > 2.5. Categorized into prehepatic, hepatic, or posthepatic causes (see Table 13-1).

TABLE 13-1. Causes of Increased Bilirubin

CLASSIFICATION	CAUSES	DIRECT BILIRUBIN	INDIRECT BILIRUBIN
Prehepatic	Hemolysis, Gilbert's disease, Crigler-Najjar syndrome	Normal	High
Hepatic	Alcoholic cirrhosis, acute hepatitis, primary biliary cirrhosis	High	High
Posthepatic	Gallstones, tumor	High	Normal

In obstructive jaundice, the alkaline phosphatase (ALP) level rises more quickly than the bilirubin level. Also, when the obstruction is relieved, the ALP level falls more quickly than the bilirubin level.

SIGNS AND SYMPTOMS

- Yellow skin and sclera.
- Pruritus.
- Can have hepatomegaly, tenderness of the right upper quadrant (RUQ), or signs of cirrhosis.
- Dark urine, clay-colored stools, anorexia, and nausea indicate obstructive jaundice.

DIAGNOSIS

See Table 13-1.

TREATMENT

Treat the underlying disorder.

▶ LIVER INJURY

See Table 13-2.

INITIAL TREATMENT

- Airway, breathing, circulation (ABCs).
- Ascertain details about mechanism of injury.
- CT: Will detect blood and solid organ damage; is useful for grading injury. CT is contraindicated in the unstable or marginal patient.
- Ultrasound, if accessible, should be performed initially as focused abdominal sonography for trauma (FAST), and may then be used for serial examinations following delineation of injury on CT.

Though the liver has been found to be protective against other organ injuries, for the same reasons (size, position), it is very vulnerable to injury itself.

NONOPERATIVE MANAGEMENT

- Approximately one half of patients are eligible.
- For penetrating trauma: Operative management remains standard of care.
- For blunt trauma: May attempt trial of observation if:
  - Patient is stable or stabilizes after fluid resuscitation.
  - There are no peritoneal signs.
  - The injury can be precisely delineated and graded by CT scan.
  - There are no associated injuries requiring laparotomy.
  - There is no need for excessive hepatic-related blood transfusions.

GRADE[a]	TYPE OF INJURY	DESCRIPTION OF INJURY
I	Hematoma	Subcapsular, < 10% surface area
	Laceration	Capsular tear, < 1 cm parenchymal depth
II	Hematoma	Subcapsular, 10–50% surface area; intraparenchymal < 10 cm in diameter
	Laceration	Capsular tear, 1–3 parenchymal depth, < 10 cm in length
III	Hematoma	Subcapsular, > 50% surface area of ruptured subcapsular or parenchymal hematoma; intraparenchymal hematoma > 10 cm or expanding 3-cm parenchymal depth
	Laceration	Parenchymal disruption involving 25–75% hepatic lobe or 1–3 Couinaud's segments
IV	Laceration	Parenchymal disruption involving > 75% of hepatic lobe or > 3 Couinaud's segments within a single lobe
V	Vascular	Juxtahepatic venous injuries (i.e., retrohepatic vena cava/central major hepatic veins)
	Vascular	Hepatic avulsion

[a]Advance one grade for bilateral injuries up to grade III

Reproduced, with permission, from the American Association for Surgery of Trauma, www.aast.org/injury/injury.html.

- Repeat CT scan in 2–3 days to look for expansion or resolution of injury.
- Patients may resume normal activities after 2 months.

OPERATIVE MANAGEMENT

- As a rule, any hemodynamically unstable patient due to a liver injury should be explored.
  - Generally needed for 20% of patients with grade III or higher injuries who present with hemodynamic instability due to hemorrhage.
- Laparotomy is undertaken through a long midline incision.
- The primary goal is the control of bleeding with direct pressure and packing.
- Patient should then be resuscitated as needed, with attention to temperature control, volume status, and acid-base balance.
- Specifics of trauma liver surgery include:
  - Pringle maneuver: Occlusion of the portal triad manually or with an atraumatic vascular clamp.
  - Finger fracture of liver to expose damaged vessels and bile ducts.
  - Debridement of nonviable tissue.
  - Placement of an omental pedicle (with its blood supply) at the site (using omentum to plug up bleeding site).
  - Closed suction drainage.
  - Major hepatic resection is indicated when the parenchyma was totally destroyed by the trauma, the extent of injury is too great for

Use stability as the deciding factor in choosing operative or nonoperative management.

Imaging of the liver: If contrast pool or blush is noted on CT and patient remains stable, consider an **angiogram.**

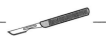

Pringle maneuver: Occlusion of the portal triad manually or with an atraumatic vascular clamp. Occlusion should not exceed 20 minutes if feasible.

If the Pringle maneuver fails to stop hemorrhage, consider an injury to the retrohepatic IVC.

Watch for increasing abdominal distention with decreasing hematocrit as potential indicators of postop bleeding.

In the United States, most hepatic abscesses (80%) are of bacterial origin.

The most common organisms isolated from pyogenic abscesses are *Escherichia coli*, *Klebsiella*, and *Proteus*. Amebic abscesses are classically described as "anchovy paste" in appearance and are caused by *Entamoeba histolytica*, which gains access to the liver via the portal vein from intestinal amebiasis.

packing, the injury itself caused a near-resection, or resection is the only way to control life-threatening hemorrhage.

- Damage control surgery: Packing the perihepatic space with a planned reoperation in 24–36 hours is indicated when the patient is severely coagulopathic, there is bilobar bleeding that cannot be controlled, there is a large expanding hematoma, other methods to control bleeding have failed, or the patient requires transfer to a level I trauma center.
- Complications:
  - Hemorrhage (5%).
  - Hemobilia (1%): Signs and symptoms—upper gastrointestinal (GI) bleed, RUQ pain, positive fecal occult blood, and jaundice.
  - Abscess.
  - Biliary fistula (7–10%): Definition—> 50 mL/d drainage for > 14 days.

▶ **NONTRAUMATIC LIVER CONDITIONS**

Hepatic Abscesses

DEFINITION

A collection of pus in the liver of bacterial, fungal, or parasitic origin that most commonly involves the right lobe. The two main subtypes are pyogenic (bacterial) and amebic.

INCIDENCE

- Pyogenic: 8–15/100,000
- Amebic: 1.3/100,000

RISK FACTORS

- Pyogenic: Usually secondary to bacterial sepsis or biliary or portal vein infection; can also occur from a perforated infected gallbladder, cholangitis, diverticulitis, liver cancer, or liver metastases.
- Amebic: Patients from Central America, homosexual men, institutionalized patients, and alcoholics.

SIGNS AND SYMPTOMS

Fever, chills, RUQ pain, jaundice, sepsis, and weight loss; amebic abscesses tend to have a more protracted course.

DIAGNOSIS

- Leukocytosis.
- Elevated liver function tests (LFTs).
- Ultrasound or CT of the liver.
- Serology for amebic abscesses.

TREATMENT

- Pyogenic: Ultrasound or CT-guided percutaneous drainage with IV antibiotics; operative drainage indicated if percutaneous attempts fail or cysts are multiple or loculated.

- Amebic: Operative drainage not indicated unless abscesses do not resolve with IV metronidazole or are superinfected with bacteria.

PROGNOSIS

Mortality is low for uncomplicated abscesses, but complicated abscesses carry a 40% mortality risk.

Hepatic Cysts

HYDATID CYST

DEFINITION

A hepatic cyst caused by *Echinococcus multilocularis* or *Echinococcus granulosus* that is usually solitary and involves the right lobe of the liver.

RISK FACTORS

Exposure to dogs, sheep, cattle, foxes, wolves, domestic cats, or foreign travel.

SIGNS AND SYMPTOMS

Most commonly asymptomatic; can cause hepatomegaly.

DIAGNOSIS

Often picked up incidentally on ultrasound, CT, or abdominal films, which may show calcifications outlining the cyst; eosinophilia, serology.

TREATMENT

Never aspirate these cysts or they will spill their contents. Treat with albendazole or mebendazole followed by resection.

NONPARASITIC CYSTS

DEFINITION

Benign cysts within the liver parenchyma that most commonly involve the right lobe; are thought to be of congenital origin.

INCIDENCE

Rare; 4:1 female-to-male ratio.

SIGNS AND SYMPTOMS

Most cysts are small and asymptomatic; large cysts (rare) can present with increasing abdominal pain and girth and can bleed or become infected.

DIAGNOSIS

Usually incidental; ultrasound or CT.

TREATMENT

Small asymptomatic cysts require no treatment; large, symptomatic cysts should be surgically excised.

Nonparasitic cysts of the liver are associated with polycystic kidney disease.

Benign Liver Tumors

CAVERNOUS HEMANGIOMA

DEFINITION

A benign vascular tumor resulting from abnormal differentiation of angioblastic tissue during fetal life; usually located in the right posterior segment of the liver.

INCIDENCE

Most common tumor of the liver; occurs at all ages.

SIGNS AND SYMPTOMS

Usually asymptomatic; rarely presents with pain, a mass, or hepatomegaly.

DIAGNOSIS

Usually discovered incidentally; can be detected by ultrasound, CT, magnetic resonance imaging (MRI), radionuclide scan, or arteriography; **do not** biopsy, as hemorrhage can occur.

TREATMENT

Surgical resection if symptomatic or in danger of rupture; otherwise, observe.

HAMARTOMA

DEFINITION

- A benign focal lesion of the liver that consists of normal tissue that has differentiated in an abnormal fashion.
- Multiple subtypes, depending on the types of cells involved (e.g., bile duct hamartoma, mesenchymal hamartoma, etc.).

INCIDENCE

Rare.

SIGNS AND SYMPTOMS

Typically asymptomatic; can present with RUQ pain or fullness.

DIAGNOSIS

Usually discovered incidentally during radiologic imaging; may require histopathologic evaluation.

TREATMENT

Surgical excision.

HEPATOCELLULAR ADENOMAS

DEFINITION

A mass lesion of the liver characterized by a benign proliferation of hepatocytes.

INCIDENCE

Ninety-five percent occur in women of childbearing years.

Hepatocellular adenomas present with abdominal pain secondary to tumor rupture or bleeding in approximately one third of patients.

Typical scenario: A 27-year-old female presents to her obstetrician with a history of a hepatocellular adenoma that resolved after discontinuing oral contraceptives (OCPs). She now wants to get pregnant. Does she have any specific health risks? *Think:* Hepatocellular adenomas treated by cessation of OCPs rather than by resection are at risk for rupture and hemorrhage during future pregnancies.

RISK FACTORS

OCP use, long-term anabolic steroid therapy, glycogen storage disease.

SIGNS AND SYMPTOMS

- Abdominal pain.
- Abdominal mass.
- Bleeding (from spontaneous rupture of large tumors).
- Can also be asymptomatic.

DIAGNOSIS

Ultrasound with needle biopsy.

TREATMENT

- Cessation of OCPs
- Surgical excision

FOCAL NODULAR HYPERPLASIA (FNH)

DEFINITION

A benign hepatic tumor, thought to arise from hepatocytes and bile ducts, that has a characteristic "central scar" on pathologic evaluation.

INCIDENCE

Most common in premenopausal females.

Like hepatic adenomas, FNH is associated with long-term OCP use.

SIGNS AND SYMPTOMS

Usually asymptomatic; 10% of patients present with abdominal pain and/or an RUQ mass.

DIAGNOSIS

- Usually incidental on ultrasound or CT.
- Can be differentiated from hepatocellular adenoma by a Tc-99 study.

TREATMENT

Resect if patient is symptomatic.

Malignant Liver Tumors

HEPATOCELLULAR CARCINOMA (HEPATOMA)

DEFINITION

A malignant tumor derived from hepatocytes frequently found in association with chronic liver disease, particularly cirrhosis.

INCIDENCE

- Accounts for 80% of liver cancers, but < 2% of all cancers.
- Much more common in males (3:1).
- Usually diagnosed in the fifth or sixth decade.

Eighty to ninety percent of patients with hepatocellular carcinoma have underlying cirrhosis, with alcoholic cirrhosis being the predominant type in Western countries. In the Far East, posthepatitis cirrhosis is more common.

RISK FACTORS

- Hepatitis B
- Hepatitis C
- Cirrhosis
- Aflatoxins (found in peanuts)
- Liver flukes
- Hemochromatosis
- α_1-antitrypsin deficiency
- Anabolic steroid use

SIGNS AND SYMPTOMS

- Weight loss
- Weakness
- Dull pain in the RUQ or epigastrium
- Nausea, vomiting
- Jaundice
- Nontender hepatomegaly
- Splenomegaly (33%)
- Ascites (50%)

A bruit can commonly be heard over a hepatocellular carcinoma due to its abundant vascularity.

DIAGNOSIS

- Increased ALP, AST, ALT, γ-glutamyl transferase (GGT), α-fetoprotein (AFP), and des-γ-carboxy prothrombin (DCP).
- Contrast CT and ultrasound can visualize the tumor.
- CT or ultrasound-guided needle biopsy will give the definitive diagnosis.

TREATMENT

- Surgical resection is the only cure, consisting of either lobectomy or segmental resection. A 1-cm margin is required.
- Transplant is also a possibility, but there often is a high recurrence rate due to the continued presence of the underlying risk factor (e.g., hepatitis B, hepatitis C, etc.).
- Local chemotherapy infusion into the hepatic artery, hepatic artery embolization, and liposomal chemotherapy are the newer treatment options being explored.

Why do ascites and anasarca occur in liver disease? Because the liver makes albumin, which is necessary to generate oncotic pressure and maintain fluids in the vasculature.

PROGNOSIS

Most patients die within the first 4 months if the tumor is not resected. After resection or transplant, the 5-year survival rate is approximately 25%.

METASTATIC NEOPLASMS

SIGNS AND SYMPTOMS

- Patients are usually asymptomatic until the disease has become advanced and the liver begins to fail.
- Symptoms may include fatigue, weight loss, epigastric fullness, dull RUQ pain, ascites, jaundice, or fever.

DIAGNOSIS

- Increased ALP, GGT, lactic dehydrogenase (LDH), AST, and ALT (nonspecific).
- Metastases will enhance on contrast CT (see Figure 13-2).
- Intraoperative ultrasound with liver palpation is the most sensitive diagnostic tool.

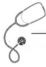

The most common hepatic malignancy is metastases. The primary is usually from colon, breast, or lung, with bronchogenic carcinoma being the most common primary cancer.

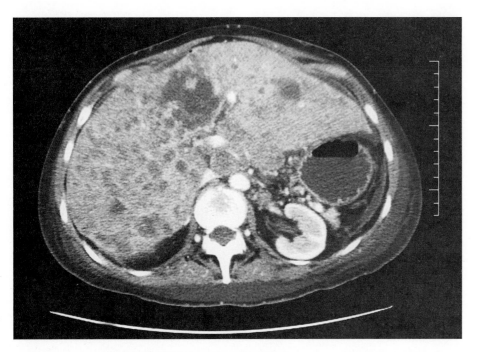

FIGURE 13-2. **Abdominal CT in hepatic metastasis.**

Note slitlike appearance of intrahepatic IVC secondary to compression by mets. Also note presence of ascites and bilateral pleural effusions, left greater than right.

TREATMENT

- Resection, if possible, is the treatment of choice.
- Radiofrequency ablation (RFA) is now extensively done even for multiple lesions, and the short-term results are promising.

► LIVER FAILURE

Child-Pugh Score

Child's classification estimates hepatic reserve in patients with liver failure (see Table 13-3).

► PORTAL HYPERTENSION

DEFINITION

Portal pressure >10 mm Hg (measure with indirect hepatic vein wedge pressure).

CAUSES

- Prehepatic: Congenital atresia, cyanosis, or portal vein thrombosis.
- Intrahepatic: Cirrhosis, hepatic fibrosis from hemochromatosis, Wilson's disease, or congenital fibrosis.
- Posthepatic: Budd-Chiari syndrome (thrombosis of the hepatic veins), hypercoagulable state, lymphoreticular malignancy.

The most common cause of portal hypertension in the United States is cirrhosis from alcoholism. The most common cause outside North America is schistosomiasis.

TABLE 13-3. Child-Pugh Score for Liver Failure

	NUMBER OF POINTS ACCORDED		
VARIABLE	1	2	3
Bilirubin (mg/dL)	< 2.0	2.0–3.0	> 3.0
Albumin (mg/dL)	> 3.5	2.8–3.5	< 2.8
Ascites (clinical evaluation)	None	Easily controlled	Poorly
Neurologic disorder	None	Minimal	Advanced
Prothrombin time (sec < control)	< 4.0	4.0–6.0	> 6.0

Correlation with Child's class: 5–6 points, Class A; 7–9 points, Class B; 10–15 points, Class C.

Rule of two thirds for portal hypertension: Two thirds of patients with cirrhosis develop portal hypertension. Two thirds of patients with portal hypertension develop esophageal varices. Two thirds of patients with esophageal varices will bleed from them. *Note:* Only 10–15% of alcoholics develop cirrhosis.

SIGNS AND SYMPTOMS

- Jaundice
- Splenomegaly
- Palmar erythema
- Spider angiomata
- Ascites
- Truncal obesity with wasting of the extremities
- Asterixis (a flapping hand tremor)
- Hepatic encephalopathy

Portosystemic Collaterals and Their Clinical Manifestations

- Left gastric vein to the esophageal veins—esophageal varices.
- Umbilical vein (via the falciform ligament) to the epigastric veins—caput medusa.
- Superior hemorrhoidal vein to the middle and inferior hemorrhoidal veins—hemorrhoids.
- Veins of Retzius (posterior abdominal wall veins) to the retroperitoneal lumbar veins—retroperitoneal varices.

DIAGNOSIS

- Suggestive history and physical examination.
- Duplex Doppler ultrasound: Initial procedure of choice.
- Venous phase of visceral angiography: Defines portal anatomy more precisely.

TREATMENT

- Aimed at reducing portal pressure.
- Shunts (see Figure 13-3):
    - **Splenorenal (Warren shunt):** Connects the splenic vein to the left renal vein. Used for patients with esophageal varices and a history of bleeding.
    - **End to side:** Connects the end of the portal vein to the side of the IVC. This is considered a total shunt.
    - **Side to side:** Connects the side of the portal vein to the side of the IVC. This is considered a partial shunt.

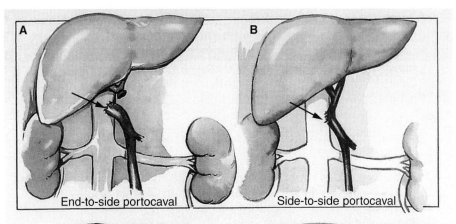

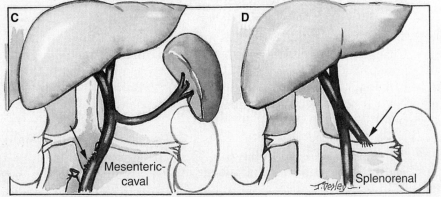

A. End-to-side portocaval B. Side-to-side portocaval

C. Mesenteric-caval D. Splenorenal

FIGURE 13-3. **Types of portocaval shunts.**

(Copyright © 2003 Mayo Foundation.)

- **Portacaval H graft:** A synthetic graft is attached from the portal vein to the IVC. This is considered a partial graft.
- **Mesocaval H graft:** A synthetic graft is attached from the superior mesenteric vein (SMV) to the IVC.
- **Complications:** Increased incidence of hepatic encephalopathy because more toxins are diverted to the systemic circulation (except for the Warren shunt), and death from hepatic failure due to decreased blood flow to the liver.
- **Liver transplant:** Ideal candidate is a young patient with cirrhosis and an episode of bleeding from esophageal varices.

Splenomegaly is the most common clinical finding in portal hypertension. Removal is almost never warranted.

► **MORBIDITIES RESULTING FROM LIVER FAILURE**

Hepatic Encephalopathy

DEFINITION

- Altered mental status due to hepatic insufficiency.
- Toxins that are normally cleared by the liver are retained in the circulation.
- The exact toxin that causes the central nervous system (CNS) changes is unknown but has been theorized to be ammonia, γ-aminobutyric acid (GABA), mercaptens, or short-chain fatty acids.

EPIDEMIOLOGY

- Occurs in all cases of fulminant hepatic failure.
- Occurs in one half of patients with end-stage liver disease requiring transplantation.
- Occurs in one third of patients with cirrhosis.

CAUSE

Precipitating factors include:

- Infection (watch for spontaneous bacterial peritonitis [SBP]).
- Potassium, magnesium, or other electrolyte depletion.
- Use of opiates, sedatives, or other hepatically cleared drugs.
- GI bleed.
- Excess dietary protein.

SIGNS AND SYMPTOMS

- Change in level of consciousness, mood disturbance, decreased attention span.
- Lethargy, coma.
- Normal electroencephalogram (EEG).
- Asterixis flapping tremor of hand.

DIAGNOSIS

An elevated serum ammonia level along with signs of altered mental status and altered LFT is diagnostic.

TREATMENT

Lactulose and neomycin (PO or PR) to reduce intestinal formation and absorption of ammonia.

In hepatic encephalopathy, the serum ammonia level **does not** correlate with the degree of encephalopathy.

Ascites

DEFINITION

- Excess fluid in the peritoneal cavity.
- Sodium and fluid retention by the kidney, low plasma oncotic pressure due to low albumin production by the failing liver, and elevated hydrostatic pressure in the hepatic sinusoids or portal veins cause fluid to be lost into the peritoneal cavity.
- Ascitic fluid is frequently the site of spontaneous bacterial peritonitis (SPB) in patients with liver disease.

SIGNS AND SYMPTOMS

Distended abdomen, fluid wave, shifting dullness.

A **LeVeen shunt** is a peritoneal-jugular shunt used to decrease ascites. One drawback is that it may increase hepatic encephalopathy.

TREATMENT

- Reduce sodium intake.
- Potassium-sparing diuretic (e.g., spironolactone).
- Abdominal paracentesis.
- Removing too much ascitic fluid or removing the fluid too quickly will cause intravascular fluid to be drawn into the peritoneal cavity. This leads to a loss of intravascular volume and can cause hypovolemic shock.

Esophageal Varices

DEFINITION

Engorged esophageal or gastric veins, usually resulting from increase portal pressure from liver disease.

SIGNS AND SYMPTOMS

- Asymptomatic unless rupture occurs.
- With rupture: Upper GI bleeding with hematemesis, melena, and/or hematochezia.

DIAGNOSIS

Esophagogastroduodenostomy (EGD).

TREATMENT OF RUPTURED VARICES

Options include:

- Endoscopic sclerotherapy.
- Vasopressin or somatostatin injection.
- Balloon tamponade (Sengstaken-Blakemore tube).
- Transjugular intrahepatic portacaval shunt (TIPS): This is used more for long-term management, rather than during an acute bleed; it shunts pressure away from the esophageal vessels.
- Intraoperative placement of a portacaval shunt.
- Liver transplant.
- β-blockers can be used to decrease portal pressure and reduce the incidence of rupture.

PROGNOSIS

Poor, even with treatment. Ruptured esophageal varices have a 50% death rate.

Caput Medusa

DEFINITION

Engorged abdominal wall veins—a sign of increased portal pressure.

SIGNS AND SYMPTOMS

Mass of veins extending from around the umbilicus, periumbilical bruit (Cruveilhier-Baumgarten bruit).

▶ THE BILIARY SYSTEM

Anatomy of the Biliary Tree

See Figure 13-4.

- Intrahepatic ducts converge to become the right and left hepatic ducts.
- Right and left hepatic ducts converge, forming the common hepatic duct.
- Cystic duct comes off the gallbladder and joins the common hepatic duct to become the common bile duct.
- CBD empties into the duodenum via the ampulla of Vater.

Calot's triangle: Inferior border of the liver, common hepatic duct, and cystic duct. The cystic artery runs through it, and the associated lymph node is called Calot's node. The right hepatic artery is adjacent to the cystic duct in Calot's triangle and, as such, is susceptible to injury during cholecystectomy.

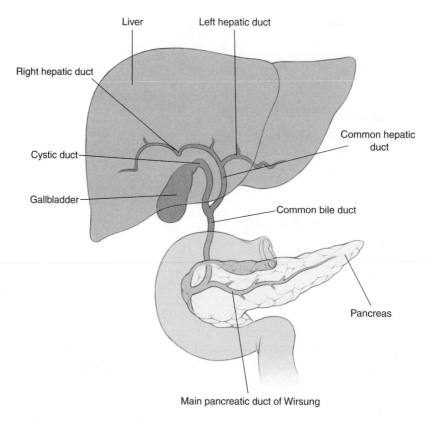

FIGURE 13-4. **Anatomy of the biliary tree.**

Anatomy of the Gallbladder

The infundibulum of the gallbladder is also called **Hartman's pouch.**

- The proximal end of the gallbladder near the cystic duct is called the *infundibulum,* and the larger distal end of the gallbladder is called the *fundus.*
- The valves within the cystic duct are called the *spiral valves of Heister.*
- The gallbladder collects bile directly from the liver via small bile ducts called *ducts of Luschka.*

► CONDITIONS OF THE GALLBLADDER AND THE BILIARY TREE

Cholelithiasis

DEFINITION

Only 15% of gallstones have enough calcium to be radiopaque. The majority of kidney stones, however, have sufficient calcium to be radiopaque on plain films.

Stones in the gallbladder. Eighty-five percent of stones are composed primarily of cholesterol, while the remaining 15% are pigmented.

INCIDENCE

Approximately 10% of the U.S. population has gallstones.

RISK FACTORS

- The typical ones are: Female, fat, fertile, and forty.
- Other risk factors include Native American race, pregnancy, oral contraceptives, Western diet, inflammatory bowel disease (IBD), hyperlipi-

demia, ileal resection (due to loss of enterohepatic circulation), and total parenteral nutrition (TPN).

SIGNS AND SYMPTOMS

- Most patients are asymptomatic.
- Symptomatic patients classically complain of severe RUQ pain that radiates to the back, epigastrium, or left upper quadrant (LUQ) that tends to be worse after eating (especially after fatty foods) and may be associated with nausea and vomiting.
- The symptom complex is called *biliary colic* and typically resolves over a few hours.

DIAGNOSIS

- Often incidental, as most patients are asymptomatic.
- Abdominal plain films pick up 15% of gallstones.
- Ultrasound: Procedure of choice; classic findings include an acoustic shadow ("headlight") and gravity-dependent movement of gallstones with patient repositioning (see Figure 13-5).

TREATMENT

Asymptomatic cholelithiasis does not require cholecystectomy unless the patient:

- Has a porcelain gallbladder (which has an increased incidence of carcinoma).
- Has sickle cell anemia.
- Has a stone > 2–3 cm.

Risk factors for cholelithiasis:
- **Female**
- **Fat**
- **Fertile**
- **Forty**
- **Flatulent**
- **Familial**
- **Fibrosis, cystic**
- **F-Hgb (sickle cell disease)**

Mirizzi's syndrome is external compression of the common hepatic duct by a gallstone impacted in the cystic duct.

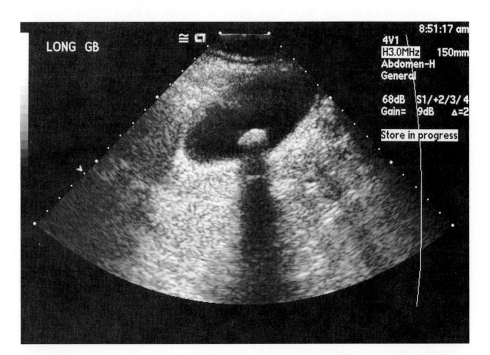

FIGURE 13-5. Sonogram demonstrating classic "headlight" appearance of cholelithiasis.

Hydrops of the gallbladder: Complete obstruction of the cystic duct by a gallstone, causing the gallbladder to fill with fluid from the gallbladder mucosa. The fluid is often milky white.

In acute cholecystitis, the pain is similar in character to cholelithiasis but typically lasts longer (> 3 hours).

- Is a pediatric patient.
- Is immunocompromised.

Symptomatic cholelithiasis requires cholecystectomy. A laparoscopic cholecystectomy can be performed on 95% of patients. Medical treatment of cholelithiasis involves chenodeoxycholic acid or ursodeoxycholic acid, drugs.

Cholecystitis

ACUTE CHOLECYSTITIS

DEFINITION

Inflammation of the gallbladder wall, usually due to obstruction of the cystic duct by gallstones.

SIGNS AND SYMPTOMS

- RUQ tenderness and guarding are present, usually for > 3 hours.
- Fever, nausea, vomiting, and anorexia are nonspecific and variable.
- Murphy's sign: Pain on deep inspiration resulting in inspiratory arrest (positive in about one third of patients).
- Sonographic Murphy's: Pain over RUQ when palpated with ultrasound probe (87% sensitivity).
- One third of patients develop exquisitely tender RUQ mass late in course.

DIAGNOSIS

- Labs: Leukocytosis with or without increased ALP, LFTs, amylase, and total bilirubin.
- Ultrasound: Reveals inflammation of the gallbladder wall (> 4 mm), pericholecystic fluid and stones in the gallbladder. Positive predictive value of all three is 90%. Will also see dilation of the CBD if the stone has passed.
- HIDA scan (most sensitive): Nonfilling of the gallbladder even when the small bowel is visualized is characteristic of acute cholecystitis (see Figures 13-6 and 13-7).

TREATMENT

- NPO.
- IV fluids.
- IV antibiotic.
- IV analgesia.
- Cholecystectomy within 24–48 hours.
- Often done laparoscopically; if inflammation prevents adequate visualization of important structures, convert to open cholecystectomy.

EMPHYSEMATOUS CHOLECYSTITIS

See Figures 13-8 and 13-9.

- Severe variant of cholecystitis caused by gas-forming bacteria.
- Relatively rare.
- Often results in perforation of the gallbladder, high mortality and morbidity.
- Typically affects elderly diabetic men.

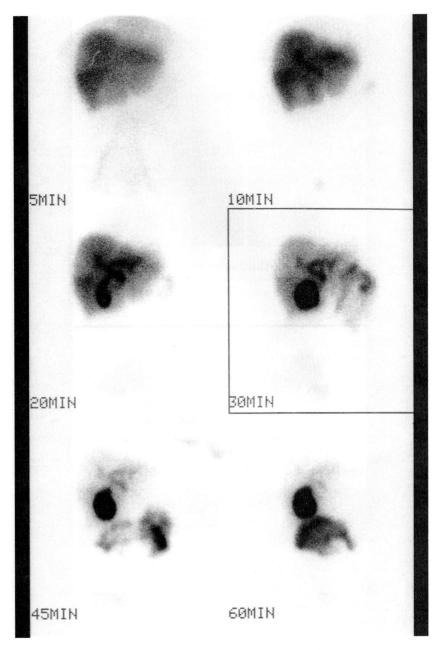

FIGURE 13-6. Normal HIDA scan, demonstrating uptake of contrast in intrahepatic bile ducts and gallbladder at 20 minutes and excretion into small bowel at 30 minutes.

ACALCULOUS CHOLECYSTITIS

DEFINITION

Acute cholecystitis without evidence of gallstones; thought to be due to biliary stasis.

INCIDENCE

Ten percent of cases of acute cholecystitis.

- Laparoscopic is by 4-port technique (umbilical 10-mm, subxiphoid 10-mm and two 5-mm ports).
- Safe dissection of the Calot's triangle is key.
- If the whole GB cannot be safely removed partial cholecystectomy should be done.

Choledocholithiasis

DEFINITION

Stones in the CBD. This can, but does not necessarily, cause cholecystitis.

INCIDENCE

Found in 6–15% of acute calculous cholecystitis and 1–2% of acalculous cholecystitis at surgery.

SIGNS AND SYMPTOMS

Epigastric or RUQ pain and tenderness, jaundice, cholangitis, or recurrent attacks of acute pancreatitis without other known risk factors.

DIAGNOSIS

- Labs: Increased ALP, LFTs, and total and direct bilirubin.
- ERCP: Gold standard for diagnosis of CBD stones; also provides a therapeutic option (see below).
- Endoscopic ultrasound: Less sensitive than ERCP but also less invasive; more sensitive than transabdominal ultrasound.
- Transabdominal ultrasound: Highly specific but not very sensitive for CBD stones.

TREATMENT

- ERCP: Involves endoscopic sphincterotomy with retrieval of the CBD stone(s) with a basket (85–90% successful).
- If ERCP fails, the CBD can be opened surgically and the stones removed. A T-tube is placed so bile can drain externally. It is removed 2–3 weeks later on an outpatient basis.

Cholangitis

ACUTE (ASCENDING) CHOLANGITIS

DEFINITION

Bacterial infection of the bile ducts usually associated with obstruction of the CBD by a gallstone.

SIGNS AND SYMPTOMS

- Fever, chills.
- Nausea, vomiting.
- Abdominal pain with or without altered mental status and septic shock.

DIAGNOSIS

- Labs: Leukocytosis with increased bilirubin, ALP, and LFTs.
- Ultrasound: Should be the initial study; dilation of common and intrahepatic bile ducts along with gallstones, and a thickened, edematous gallbladder wall.

Ascending cholangitis is a life-threatening emergency. It can be precipitated by any irritation or obstruction of the biliary tree.

Charcot's triad:
- RUQ pain
- Fever
- Jaundice

Reynolds' pentad:
- Charcot's triad plus
- Central nervous system (CNS) symptoms
- Septic shock

Common causes of CBD obstruction: **SINGE**
Stricture
Iatrogenic causes (ERCP/ PTC or biliary stent placement)
Neoplasm
Gallstones
Extrinsic compression (e.g., pancreatic pseudocyst/ pancreatitis)

- ERCP/percutaneous transhepatic cholangiography (PTCA): Provides a definitive diagnosis; can also be therapeutic.
- Bile cultures: Obtain to facilitate proper antibiotic treatment; offending organisms are usually enteric gram negatives and enterococci.

TREATMENT

- NPO, IV fluids, and IV antibiotics.
- If patient is in shock, decompress bile duct and remove obstruction immediately by ERCP/PTC. If unsuccessful, intraoperative decompression with T-tube placement is indicated.
- If the patient is stable, continue conservative management with definitive treatment later.

SCLEROSING CHOLANGITIS

DEFINITION

A chronic, progressive inflammatory process of the biliary tree of unknown etiology that results in strictures and, in most cases, leads to cirrhosis and liver failure. Associated with autoimmune phenomena, particularly ulcerative colitis.

INCIDENCE

Two-to-one male predominance with median age of onset at 40 years.

RISK FACTORS

Inflammatory bowel disease (ulcerative colitis), pancreatitis, diabetes, trauma to the common hepatic duct.

SIGNS AND SYMPTOMS

Many patients are asymptomatic at the time of diagnosis, but symptoms can include fever, weight loss, fatigue, pruritus, jaundice, hepatomegaly, splenomegaly, and hyperpigmentation.

Seventy percent of patients with sclerosing cholangitis have IBD, whereas 3–7.5% of patients with IBD have sclerosing cholangitis.

DIAGNOSIS

ERCP/PTC reveal a "beads on a string" appearance of the bile ducts (see Figure 13-10). ALP is almost always elevated.

TREATMENT

- Balloon dilation with stent placement can be performed for palliative purposes, but definitive treatment varies depending on the location of the strictures.
- Extrahepatic strictures: Hepatoenteric anastomosis with removal of the extrahepatic ducts and T-tube placement for external drainage of bile.
- Intrahepatic strictures: Liver transplant.

PROGNOSIS

- Ten percent of patients develop cholangiocarcinoma.
- Ten-year survival is 75%.

Complications of sclerosing cholangitis:
- Cirrhosis
- Cholangitis
- Obstructive jaundice
- Cholangiocarcinoma

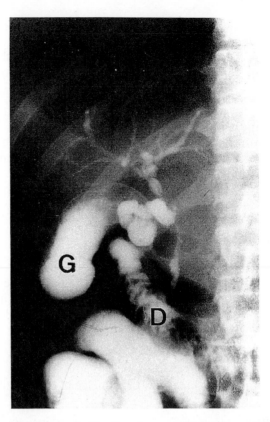

FIGURE 13-10. ERCP demonstrating "beads on a string" appearance of bile ducts in sclerosing cholangitis.

G, gallbladder; D, duodenum. (Reproduced, with permission, from Nakanuma Y et al. Definition and pathology of primary sclerosing cholangitis. *J Hepatobiliary Pancreat Surg* 1999; 6: 333–342.)

Typical scenario: A 75-year-old female with a past history of cholelithiasis presents complaining of RUQ pain that radiates to her back, with nausea, vomiting, and abdominal distention. Abdominal plain films show air in the biliary tree and a "stepladder" appearance of the small bowel. *Think:* The history is consistent with both cholelithiasis and small bowel obstruction, and findings on abdominal radiograph are suggestive of gallstone ileus.

Gallstone Ileus

DEFINITION

- Small bowel obstruction caused by a gallstone; the ileocecal valve is the most common site of obstruction.
- Most often, a large stone has eroded a hole through the gallbladder wall to the duodenum, causing a cholecystenteric fistula. A gallstone escapes through this hole into the GI tract and eventually gets stuck in the ileum, causing small bowel obstruction.

INCIDENCE

Most common in women over 70.

SIGNS AND SYMPTOMS

Symptoms of acute cholecystitis followed by signs of small bowel obstruction (nausea, vomiting, abdominal distention, RUQ pain).

DIAGNOSIS

- Abdominal plain films: May show the pathognomonic features of pneumobilia, dilated small bowel, and a large gallstone in the right lower quadrant (RLQ).

- Ultrasound: Useful to confirm cholelithiasis; may also identify the fistula.
- Upper and lower GI series: Other diagnostic options that are usually unnecessary.

TREATMENT

Exploratory laparotomy, removal of the gallstone, and possible small bowel resection with or without cholecystectomy and fistula repair.

Carcinoma of the Gallbladder

DEFINITION

Malignant neoplasm of the gallbladder, the majority of which are adenocarcinomas.

INCIDENCE

Extremely rare (< 1% of patients with cholelithiasis); incidence increases with age with a peak at 75 years; female-to-male ratio 3:1.

RISK FACTORS

Include porcelain gallbladder, gallstones, choledochal cysts, gallbladder polyps, and typhoid carriers with chronic inflammation.

SIGNS AND SYMPTOMS

Most patients are asymptomatic until late in the course when findings may include abdominal pain, nausea, vomiting, weight loss, RUQ mass, hepatomegaly, or jaundice.

DIAGNOSIS

Ultrasound, CT, MRI, or ERCP/PTC.

Courvoisier's sign: A palpable, nontender gallbladder often associated with cancer in the head of the pancreas or the gallbladder.

TREATMENT

- Varies depending on the extent of tumor involvement.
- Tumor confined to gallbladder mucosa: Cholecystectomy.
- Tumor involving muscularis or serosa: Radical cholecystectomy, wedge resection of overlying liver, and lymph node dissection.
- Tumor involving liver: Consider palliative measures such as decompression of the proximal biliary tree or a bypass procedure of the obstructed duodenum.

Benign Tumors of the Bile Ducts

DEFINITION

Tumors that arise from ductal glandular epithelium most commonly found at the ampulla of Vater; most are adenomas, of polypoid morphology, and < 2 cm in size.

SIGNS AND SYMPTOMS

Intermittent jaundice and RUQ pain.

DIAGNOSIS

Intraoperative cholangiogram, ultrasound, ERCP/PTC.

TREATMENT

Resection of the tumor with a margin of duct wall either intraoperatively or endoscopically.

Cholangiocarcinoma

DEFINITION

An uncommon tumor that may occur anywhere along the intrahepatic or extrahepatic biliary tree but is most commonly located at the bifurcation of the right and left hepatic ducts (60–80% of cases). Nearly all are adenocarcinomas.

INCIDENCE

- Increases with age with peak at 55–65 years; 1/100,000 people per year.
- No sex predilection.

RISK FACTORS

Choledochal cyst, ulcerative colitis, sclerosing cholangitis, liver flukes, toxins, contrast dye.

SIGNS AND SYMPTOMS

- Jaundice
- Clay-colored stools
- Dark urine
- Pruritus
- Pain
- Malaise
- Weight loss

DIAGNOSIS

- Ultrasound: Shows bile duct dilation.
- CT: Identifies tumors located near the hilum of the liver.
- Biopsy via ERCP/PTC under ultrasound guidance.

TREATMENT

- Varies depending on location of the tumor.
- Proximal tumors: Resect with a Roux-en-Y hepaticojejunostomy.
- Distal tumors: Whipple procedure.
- If both hepatic ducts or the main trunk of the portal vein are extensively involved, the tumor may be unresectable.

PROGNOSIS

Five-year survival rate is 15–20%.

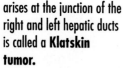

A cholangiocarcinoma that arises at the junction of the right and left hepatic ducts is called a **Klatskin tumor.**

The Pancreas

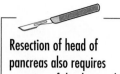

Resection of head of pancreas also requires resection of duodenum due to their shared blood supply (gastroduodenal artery).

▶ EMBRYOLOGY

- During the fourth week of gestation, the pancreas begins development from the duodenal endoderm.
- Two buds form, which rotate and fuse by eighth week.
  - Ventral pancreatic bud: Uncinate process and part of the head.
  - Dorsal pancreatic bud: remaining part of the head, neck, body, and tail.
- **Heterotopic pancreas:** Pancreatic tissue in an abnormal location such as the stomach, duodenum, or Meckel's diverticulum.
- **Pancreas divisum:** Due to a failure of the ventral and dorsal ducts to fuse, the majority of pancreatic drainage is accomplished via the accessory papilla and duct of Santorini. This is the most common congenital anomaly of the pancreas (5% of population) but is usually asymptomatic. Rarely, however, chronic pain and recurrent pancreatitis may result from inadequate drainage.
- **Annular pancreas:** Usually presents in infancy with duodenal obstruction (postprandial vomiting). Caused by malrotation of the ventral pancreas leading to a ring of pancreatic tissue around the second portion of the duodenum. Pancreatitis and peptic ulcers may also result.
- **Treatment:** Duodenojejunostomy.

▶ ANATOMY

- Location: Retroperitoneal (posterior to stomach, transverse mesocolon, and lesser omentum) at the level of the body of L2.
- Head: Includes uncinate process and abuts the second part of the duodenum.
- Neck: Portion anterior to superior mesenteric vein.
- Body: Lies to the left of the neck, forms posterior floor of lesser sac (omental bursa).
- Tail: Enters splenorenal ligament, adjacent to splenic hilum; susceptible to injury during splenectomy.
- Ducts: The duct of Wirsung is the main duct; runs entire length of pancreas. It joins the common bile duct and empties into the second part of the duodenum at the ampulla of Vater. The duct of Santorini (small duct) is an accessory duct often joining the duodenum more proximally than the ampulla of Vater.
- Sphincter of Oddi: Smooth muscle around the ampulla of Vater.

▶ BLOOD SUPPLY AND INNERVATION

See Figure 14-1.
- Head:
  - **Anterior and posterior superior pancreaticoduodenal arteries**—branches of the gastroduodenal artery.
  - **Anterior and posterior inferior pancreaticoduodenal arteries**—branches of the superior mesenteric artery.
- Neck, body, and tail:
  - **Splenic artery and branches (dorsal pancreatic artery).**

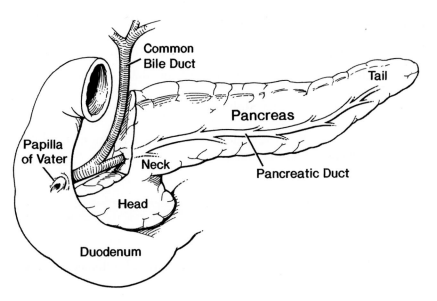

FIGURE 14-1. The pancreas and its relationships.

- Sympathetics: Pain sensation is provided by the celiac plexus (via the splanchnic nerves).
- Parasympathetics: Islets, acini, and ducts are innervated by branches of the vagus nerve.

Celiac plexus block can be done for pain control in pancreatic disease.

▶ PHYSIOLOGY

Exocrine

Secretion of 1–2 L/day of clear, isosmotic, alkaline (pH 7.0–8.3) fluid containing digestive enzymes.

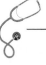

Secretin is the most potent endogenous stimulant of bicarbonate secretion.

- **Acinar cells:** Secrete enzymes (e.g., chymotrypsin, trypsin, carboxypeptidase, amylase, lipase). These enzymes are secreted as inactive zymogen granules until they are activated intraluminally by enterokinase in the duodenum.
- **Centroacinar and ductal cells:** Secrete water and electrolytes (e.g., Na^+, K^+, HCO_3^-, Cl^-) in response to secretin stimulation.
- Phases:
  1. Cephalic phase: Sight and smell of food activates vagal fibers. Gastric acid production → duodenal acidification → secretin release → pancreatic HCO_3^- release.
  2. Gastric phase: Antral distention and ingested protein cause release of gastrin → gastric acid secretion → duodenal acidification → secretin release → pancreatic HCO_3^- release.
  3. Intestinal phase: Duododenal acid and bile stimulate secretin. Ingested fat and protein in the duodenum stimulate release of CCK → acinar cells release pancreatic enzymes.

The exocrine pancreas makes up 85% of pancreatic volume; the endocrine pancreas accounts for only 2%, with the rest composed of extracellular matrix and vessels or ducts.

Somatostatin may be used clinically to:

- Treat symptoms of neuroendocrine tumors (islet cell, carcinoid, gastrinoma, VIPoma, and acromegaly).
- Convert high-output fistulae to low-output fistulae (because of its antimotility and antisecretory effects).

Causes of pancreatitis:
Posterior perforation of peptic ulcer
Alcohol
Neoplasm
Cholelithiasis (biliary disease)
Renal disease (end stage)
ERCP
Anorexia (malnutrition)
Trauma
Infections
Toxins (drugs)
Incineration (burns)
Surgery/**S**corpion bite

Endocrine

Islets of Langerhans make up 2% of pancreas by weight:

- Insulin: From **beta** cells in islets of Langerhans (glucose absorption and storage).
- Glucagon: From islet **alpha** cells (glycogenolysis and release of glucose).
- Somatostatin: From islet **delta** cells (generally causes inhibitory functions of gastrointestinal tract).

▶ ACUTE PANCREATITIS

DEFINITION

Inflammation of the pancreas due to parenchymal autodigestion by proteolytic enzymes.

ETIOLOGY

Most common etiologies in the United States:

1. Alcohol abuse (40–50%)
2. Gallstones (40%)
3. Idiopathic (10%)

Other causes of acute pancreatitis:

- Hyperlipidemia
- Hypercalcemia: Secondary to hyperparathyroidism
- Trauma
- Postop and post-ERCP (endoscopic retrograde cholangiopancreatography)
- Pancreatic duct obstruction (e.g., tumor, pancreatic divisum)
- Vasculitis
- Scorpion venom
- Viral infection (e.g., mumps, coxsackie B, cytomegalovirus)
- Drugs (e.g., isoniazid, glucocorticoids, cimetidine)

SIGNS AND SYMPTOMS

- Severe, constant epigastric pain **radiating to the back.** Pain may be improved by sitting forward or standing.
- Nausea, vomiting.
- Physical exam:
  - Low-grade fever, tachypnea, tachycardia, upper abdominal tenderness with guarding but no rebound. Bowel sounds may be absent due to adynamic ileus. Signs of hypovolemic shock may also be present due to massive retroperitoneal fluid sequestration and dehydration.
  - Cullen's sign (bluish discoloration of periumbilicus), Grey-Turner's sign (bluish discoloration of flank), and Fox's sign (bluish discoloration of inguinal ligament) are indicative of severe, hemorrhagic pancreatitis.

Laboratory Studies
- Elevated lipase: Only found in gastric and intestinal mucosa and liver, in addition to the pancreas, so is more specific for pancreatitis than amylase.
- Elevated amylase:
  - Also found in salivary glands, small bowel, ovaries, testes, and skeletal muscle, so is not a specific marker for pancreatitis.
  - Although amylase may be persistently elevated in renal insufficiency, a level three times the upper limit of normal is suggestive of pancreatitis.
  - Neither amylase nor lipase is a part of Ranson's criteria.
  - Ranson's criteria listed in Table 14-1.

Abdominal Imaging
- Abdominal x-ray: Sentinel loop sign and colon cutoff sign.
- Ultrasound: May demonstrate pseudocysts, phlegmon, abscesses or cholelithiasis.
- Computed tomographic (CT) scan: Diagnostic test of choice (90% sensitive and 100% specific). Demonstrates pseudocysts, phlegmon, abscesses or pancreatic necrosis (see Figure 14-2).

DIFFERENTIAL DIAGNOSIS
- Acute cholecystitis
- Gastritis/peptic ulcer disease

Beware of **MEDVIPS**, which may cause drug-induced pancreatitis.
Methyldopa/ Metronidazole
Estrogen
Didanosine
Valproate
Isoniazid
Pentamidine
Sulfonamides

Cullen's sign: Think of c**UL**len and Umbi**L**icus.
Grey-Turner's sign: Think of **TURN**ing on your side/flank).

HIGH-YIELD FACTS

The Pancreas

TABLE 14-1. Ranson's Criteria (Predicts Risk of Mortality in Pancreatitis)

ON ADMISSION	AFTER 48 HOURS
Age > 55	Base deficit > 4
Blood sugar > 200	Increase in blood urea nitrogen (BUN) > 5
Serum aspartate aminotransferase (AST) < 250	Fluid deficit > 6 L
Lactic dehydrogenase (LDH) > 350	Calcium < 8
White blood count (WBC) > 16,000	Drop in hematocrit > 10%
	PO_2 < 60 mmHg

NUMBER OF RISK FACTORS	MORTALITY
< 3	1%
3 or 4	16%
5 or 6	40%
> 6	70–100%

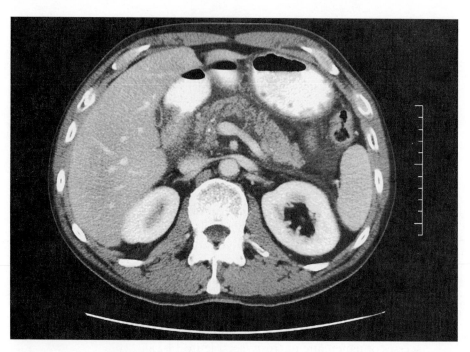

FIGURE 14-2. Abdominal CT demonstrating stranding in the peripancreatic region, consistent with acute pancreatitis.

High amylase levels are also seen in intestinal disease, perforated ulcer, ruptured ectopic pregnancy, salpingitis, salivary gland disorders, renal failure, and diabetic ketoacidosis.

A sentinel loop is distention and/or air-fluid levels near a site of inflammation. In pancreatitis, it is secondary to pancreatitis-associated ileus.

- Perforated esophagus/peptic ulcer
- Myocardial infarction
- Ruptured abdominal aortic aneurysm
- Acute mesenteric ischemia
- Pneumonia

TREATMENT

- Aggressive hydration with electrolyte monitoring to maintain adequate intravascular volume.
- Nasogastric tube: For severe disease with vomiting.
- Antibiotics: If infection identified.
- NPO with nutritional support via post pyloric feeding or total parenteral nutrition (TPN).
- Avoid use of morphine due to possible spasm of sphincter of Oddi. Use meperidine (Demerol) instead for pain management.
- Surgery indicated for:
  - Infected necrosis of pancreas.
  - Correction of associated biliary tract disease: Gallstone pancreatitis should be treated with early interval cholecystectomy only *after* acute pancreatic inflammation has resolved. Acutely, ERCP with endoscopic sphincterotomy may be used to relieve biliary obstruction.

PROGNOSIS

See Table 14-1 for Ranson's criteria.

DEFINITION

Chronic inflammation or recurrent acute pancreatitis causes irreversible parenchymal fibrosis, destruction, and calcification, leading to loss of endocrine and exocrine function.

ETIOLOGY

- Most commonly alcohol abuse (70%).
- Idiopathic (20%).
- Other (10%): Hyperparathyroidism, hypertriglyceridemia, congenital pancreatic anomalies, hereditary, obstruction.

SIGNS AND SYMPTOMS

- Recurrent or constant epigastric and/or back pain.
- Malabsorption/malnutrition (exocrine dysfunction).
- Steatorrhea (exocrine dysfunction)—fat-soluble vitamin deficiency.
- Type 1 diabetes mellitus (endocrine dysfunction).
- Polyuria.

DIAGNOSIS

- History.
- Fecal fat analysis.
- X-ray (kidneys, ureters, bladder): **Pancreatic calcifications.**
- ERCP: **Chain-of-lakes** pattern—ductal irregularities with dilation and stenosis.
- CT: **Pseudocysts** (see Figure 14-3) (use ultrasound for follow-up of pseudocysts). **Gland enlargement/atrophy, calcifications, masses** also seen on CT.

Gallstones are not a common cause of chronic pancreatitis.

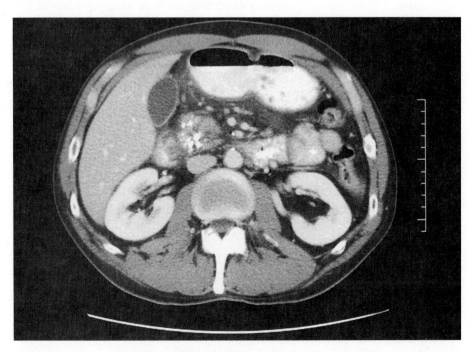

FIGURE 14-3. Abdominal CT demonstrating calcification involving the entire head of the pancreas, consistent with chronic pancreatitis.

DIFFERENTIAL DIAGNOSIS

- Peptic ulcer disease.
- Pancreatic cancer.
- Biliary tract disease (cholecystitis).

INDICATIONS FOR SURGERY

- Persistent pain
- Gastrointestinal or biliary obstruction
- Pseudocyst infection, hemorrhage, or rupture
- Enlarging pseudocysts

TREATMENT

- **Nonoperative management:** Includes control of abdominal pain, endocrine and exocrine insufficiency (insulin and pancreatic enzyme therapy).
- **Operative management** (must do preop ERCP to evaluate anatomy):
  - Pain relief: Celiac plexus block.
  - Ampullary procedures: ERCP with endoscopic sphincterotomy.
  - Ductal decompression procedures:
    - Puestow procedure (longitudinal pancreaticojejunostomy) for segmental ductal dilation.
    - Duval procedure (retrograde drainage with distal resection and end-to-end pancreaticojejunostomy).
  - Ablative procedures (resection of portions of pancreas):
    - Frey procedure (longitudinal pancreaticojejunostomy with partial resection of the pancreatic head).
    - Whipple procedure (pancreaticoduodenectomy with choledochojejunostomy, pancreaticojejunostomy, and gastrojejunostomy).
    - Near-total pancreatectomy.
- Pseudocysts: Nonepithelialized, encapsulated pancreatic fluid collections. Up to 30% of pseudocysts resolve on their own with bowel rest (TPN and NPO). If after 6 weeks they have not resolved and are > 6 cm in size, internal drainage of the mature cyst is indicated via cyst gastrostomy or Roux-en-Y cyst jejunostomy.

Pancreatic calcifications and stones are associated with chronic pancreatitis.

▶ OTHER COMPLICATIONS OF PANCREATITIS

- Pancreatic abscess
- Pancreatic fistulae

▶ PANCREATIC ADENOCARCINOMA

ETIOLOGY

- Originates in the exocrine pancreas (ductal cells).
- Two thirds occur in the head of the pancreas.

RISK FACTORS

- Male gender (2:1 male-to-female).
- African-American heritage (2:1 Black-to-White).
- Tobacco use (2× increased risk).

Tumors of the pancreatic tail are usually unresectable because they are asymptomatic during growth and thus present at a late stage. Tumors in the head of the pancreas, however, often present earlier because they cause **biliary obstruction.**

- Diabetes, alcohol abuse, chronic pancreatitis, and increased age are also associated with increased risk.

SIGNS AND SYMPTOMS

- Weight loss.
- Jaundice (due to obstruction in head).
- Posterior epigastric pain radiating to the back.
- Migratory thrombophlebitis: Trousseau's syndrome is seen especially in tumors of the body or tail.

DIAGNOSIS

- Elevated carcinoembryonic antigen (CEA) or CA 19-9 (tumor markers).
- CT scan is study of choice.
- Percutaneous transhepatic cholangiography (PTC) and ERCP (double duct sign) useful in periampullary lesions.
- Angiography may also be useful.

TREATMENT

- Tumors of the head: The only chance for a cure is the Whipple procedure (pancreaticoduodenectomy), and most tumors are **not** resectable at the time of diagnosis.
- Tumors of the body/tail: Distal "near-total" pancreatectomy.
- If unresectable (due to liver/peritoneal metastases, nodal metastases beyond the zone of resection, or tumor invasion of the superior mesenteric artery), palliative procedure considered:
  - **Relieve biliary obstruction.**
  - **Relieve duodenal obstruction.**
  - **Splanchnic nerve block (pain control).**
- Postoperative chemoradiation therapy controversial, but typically includes 5-fluorouracil (5-FU) and external-beam radiation.

PROGNOSIS

- The mean survival for patients with unresectable disease is 4–6 months, with a 5-year survival rate of < 3%.
- The median survival for patients who undergo successful resection is approximately 12–19 months, with a 5-year survival rate of 15–20%.

▶ CYSTADENOCARCINOMA

- Commonly females age 40–60 years.
- In body and tail.
- Less than 2% of all pancreatic exocrine tumors.
- Prognosis better than adenocarcinoma.
- **Treatment:** Surgical resection—distal/total pancreatectomy.

▶ CYSTADENOMA

- Older and middle-aged women
- Two types:

Courvoisier's sign:
Jaundice with a palpable nontender gallbladder.

Whipple procedure:
Removal of gallbladder, common bile duct (CBD), antrum of stomach, duodenum, proximal jejunum and head of pancreas (en bloc); Reconstruction with pancreaticojejunostomy, choledochojejunostomy, and gastrojejunostomy.

HIGH-YIELD FACTS

The Pancreas

237

Pancreatic cystadenoma:
Mucinous = **M**alignant
potential

- Serous: Benign
  - Mucinous: Generally benign but has potential to be malignant
- **Treatment:** Surgical resection

▶ ENDOCRINE TUMORS (ISLET CELL TUMORS)

Insulinoma

DEFINITION

Beta cell neoplasm with overproduction of insulin.

EPIDEMIOLOGY

- Most common islet cell tumor.
- Ninety percent are benign.
- Most are solitary lesions with even distribution in the head, body, and tail of the pancreas.
- If associated with multiple endocrine neoplasia (MEN) I syndrome (< 10% of cases), then multiple insulinomas may be present.

SIGNS AND SYMPTOMS

Most symptoms related to hypoglycemia triggered catecholamine release.

DIFFERENTIAL DIAGNOSIS

Surreptitious insulin administration.

DIAGNOSIS

- Fasting serum insulin level > 10 uU/mL (normal: < 6 uU/mL).
- Fasting insulin-to-glucose ratio > 0.3.
- Proinsulin or C-peptide levels should be measured to rule out surreptitious exogenous insulin administration.

TREATMENT

- Surgical enucleation or resection is usually curative (90% of patients).
- Diazoxide can improve hypoglycemic symptoms by inhibiting pancreatic insulin release.

Typical scenario: A
30-year-old male complains
of feeling faint and
confused most notably after
he exercises. His symptoms
improve after he has a soft
drink. *Think:* Insulinoma—
check fasting serum insulin
level.

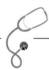

Insulinoma is characterized
by **Whipple's triad:**
1. Symptoms of
   hypoglycemia with
   fasting
2. Fasting glucose < 50
   mg/dL
3. Relief of symptoms after
   eating

Twenty-five percent of
gastrinomas are associated
with MEN-1.

Gastrinoma

DEFINITION

- Neoplasm associated with overproduction of gastrin.
- Also known as Zollinger-Ellison syndrome.

EPIDEMIOLOGY

- Second most frequent islet cell tumor.
- Ninety percent are located in the "gastrinoma triangle" (Figure 14-4) bordered by:
  - Junction of second and third part of the duodenum.
  - The cystic duct.

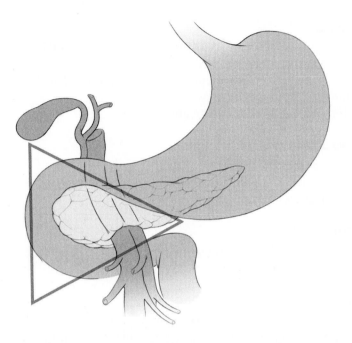

FIGURE 14-4. Gastrinoma triangle—the anatomic triangle in which approximately 90% of gastrinomas are found.

- The superior mesenteric artery under the neck of the pancreas.
- Small, slow-growing, multiple, 60% malignant.

SIGNS AND SYMPTOMS

- Signs of peptic ulcer disease (especially in patients with recurrent or unusually located ulcers).
- Epigastric pain most prominent after eating.
- Profuse watery diarrhea.

DIAGNOSIS

- Fasting serum gastrin level > 500 pg/mL (normal: < 100 pg/mL).
- Secretin stimulation test will cause a paradoxical increase in gastrin in patients with Zollinger-Ellison syndrome (double fasting level or increase of 200 pg/dL over the fasting level).
- Ulcers in unusual locations (e.g., third part of duodenum or jejunum) is highly suggestive.
- Octreotide scan to localize tumor.

Typical scenario: A 40-year-old male complains of chronic epigastric pain shortly following meals and notices needing increasing doses of his anti-ulcer medication. *Think:* Gastrinoma.

TREATMENT

- Proton pump inhibitor to alleviate symptoms.
- Surgical resection (curative or debulking).
- Chemotherapy.

VIPoma

DEFINITION

Overproduction of vasoactive intestinal peptide (VIP).

EPIDEMIOLOGY

- Also known as Verner-Morrison syndrome or **WDHA** syndrome (**Wa**tery **D**iarrhea, **H**ypokalemia, **A**chlorhydria).
- Most are malignant; majority have metastasized to lymph nodes and the liver at time of diagnosis.
- Ten percent are extrapancreatic.

SIGNS AND SYMPTOMS

- Severe watery diarrhea.
- Signs of hypokalemia—palpitations/arrhythmias, muscle fasiculations/tetany, paresthesias.

DIAGNOSIS

Fasting serum VIP level > 800 pg/mL (normal: < 200 pg/mL) with exclusion of other causes of diarrhea.

TREATMENT

- Surgical resection, chemotherapy.
- Octreotide (somatostatin analogue)—diarrhea control.

Glucagonoma

DEFINITION

Rare alpha cell neoplasm resulting in overproduction of glucagon.

EPIDEMIOLOGY

Most are malignant, large primary tumors that have usually metastasized to lymph nodes and liver at the time of diagnosis.

SIGNS AND SYMPTOMS

- Mild diabetes (hyperglycemia).
- Anemia.
- Mucositis.
- Weight loss due to low amino acid levels.
- Severe dermatitis—often a red psoriatic-like rash with serpiginous borders over trunk and lower limbs.

DIAGNOSIS

- Fasting serum glucagon level > 1000 pg/mL (normal: < 200 pg/mL).
- Skin biopsy to confirm presence of necrolytic migratory erythema.

TREATMENT

- Surgery and chemotherapy.
- Octreotide to inhibit the release of glucagon.

Somatostatinoma

- Very rare tumor.
- Malignant.
- Treated by surgery and chemotherapy.

PANCREATIC TRAUMA

See Trauma chapter.

PANCREAS TRANSPLANTATION

See Transplant chapter.

HIGH-YIELD FACTS IN

The Endocrine System

DEFINITION

A chemical substance secreted into the bloodstream by cells in one part of the body that acts on distant organs or tissues.

CLASSES

- Steroid:
  - Adrenal cortical: Cortisol, aldosterone.
  - Ovarian, testicular, and placental hormones (not discussed here).
- Tyrosine-derived:
  - Thyroid: Triiodothyronine (T_3), thyroxine (T_4).
  - Adrenal medulla: Epinephrine, norepinephrine.
- Protein/peptide:
  - Pituitary:
    - Anterior: Growth hormone (GH), adrenocorticotropic hormone (ACTH), thyroxine-stimulating hormone (TSH), follicle-stimulating hormone (FSH), luteinizing hormone (LH), prolactin (PRL).
    - Posterior: Antidiuretic hormone (ADH), oxytocin.
  - Parathyroid: Parathyroid hormone.
  - Pancreas: Insulin, glucagon, somatostatin.

MECHANISMS OF ACTION

See Table 15-1.

All **protein** hormones are produced in locations starting with **P:**
Pituitary
Parathyroid
Pancreas

General

Autosomal dominant genetic disorder.

MEN I (Wermer's Syndrome)

- Chromosomal deletion: 11q12–13.
- Parathyroid hyperplasia (90%).
- Pancreatic (and duodenal) islet cell tumors (50%).
- Pituitary adenomas (25%) (prolactinoma is most common).

MEN I tumors are the
3 P's:
Pituitary
Parathyroid
Pancreas

MEN IIA (Sipple's Syndrome)

- RET oncogene mutation on chromosome 10q11.2; missense mutations on chromosome 1.
- Medullary thyroid carcinoma (100%)—20% of all medullary cancers are due to MEN.
- Pheochromocytoma (33%)—majority are bilateral.
- Parathyroid hyperplasia (50%).

MEN IIB

- Mucosal neuroma may be earliest sign present (100%)—hypertrophied lips, thickened eyelids.

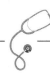

MEN IIA and IIB both consist of medullary thyroid carcinoma and pheochromocytoma. The additional components differ: Another **P** in MEN IIA (think **P**arathyroid), and **M** in MEN IIB (think **M**ucosal neuromas and **M**arfanoid habitus).

TABLE 15-1. Summary of Endocrine Hormones and Their Functions

ENDOCRINE ORGAN	HORMONE	FUNCTIONS	STIMULATED BY	INHIBITED BY
Anterior pituitary	Growth hormone (GH)	▪ Opposes insulin ▪ Stimulates amino acid uptake ▪ Stimulates release of fatty acid from storage sites ▪ Mediates immunoglobulin F (IGF) synthesis ▪ Stimulates growth of nearly all tissues	▪ Growth hormone–releasing hormone (GHRH) ▪ Hypoglycemia ▪ Arginine ▪ Exercise ▪ L-dopa ▪ Clonidine ▪ Propranolol	Somatostatin
	Adrenocorticotropic hormone (ACTH)	▪ Stimulates secretion of adrenocortical hormones	▪ Corticotropin-releasing hormone (CRH) ▪ Stress	Cortisol (negative feedback)
	Thyroid-stimulating hormone (TSH)	▪ Regulates secretion of triiodothyronine (T_3) and thyronine (T_4)	▪ Thyrotropin-releasing hormone (TRH)	Negative feedback
	Follicle-stimulating hormone (FSH)	▪ Stimulates ovarian follicular growth (female) ▪ Stimulates spermatogenesis and testicular growth (male)	▪ Gonadotropin-releasing hormone (GnRH)	Negative feedback
	Luteinizing hormone (LH)	▪ Ovulation (female) ▪ Luteinization of follicle (female) ▪ Stimulates production of estrogen and progesterone (female) ▪ Promotes production of testosterone (male)	▪ GnRH	Negative feedback
	Prolactin (PRL)	▪ Facilitates breast development in preparation for milk production	▪ TRH ▪ Estrogen ▪ Stress ▪ Exercise	Bromocriptine
Posterior pituitary	Antidiuretic hormone (ADH, vasopressin)	▪ Promotes water absorption in collecting ducts of kidney ▪ Vasoconstriction of peripheral arterioles, increasing blood pressure	▪ Increased plasma osmolality ▪ Decreased plasma volume	
	Oxytocin	▪ Increases frequency and strength of uterine contractions ▪ Stimulates breast milk ejection	▪ Suckling ▪ Vaginal stimulation	

ENDOCRINE ORGAN	HORMONE	FUNCTIONS	STIMULATED BY	INHIBITED BY
Thyroid	T_3, T_4	■ Increase basal metabolic rate (BMR), oxygen consumption ■ Increase protein synthesis, lipolysis, glycogenolysis, gluconeogenesis ■ Increase heart rate and contractility ■ Increase catecholamine sensitivity ■ Stimulate release of steroid hormones ■ Stimulate erythropoiesis and 2,3-diphosphoglycerate (DPG) production ■ Increase bone turnover	TSH	Negative feedback
	Calcitonin	■ Increases serum calcium (by inhibiting osteoclasts) ■ Increases phosphate excretion	High serum calcium	Low serum calcium
Parathyroid	Parathyroid hormone (PTH)	■ Kidney: Increases calcium resorption in proximal convoluted tubule ■ Rapid ■ Also increased excretion of sodium, potassium, phosphate, and bicarbonate ■ Bone: Increases calcium mobilization ■ Rapid phase: Equilibration with extracellular fluid (ECF) ■ Slow phase: Enzyme activation (promoting bone resorption) ■ GI tract (indirect): Increases absorption via vitamin D	Low serum calcium	High serum calcium
Pancreas	Insulin (B cell)	Effects on liver: ■ Glycogenesis, glycolysis, synthesis of protein, triglycerides, cholesterol, very low-density lipoprotein (VLDL) ■ Inhibits glycogenolysis, ketogenesis, gluconeogenesis Effects on muscle: ■ Protein synthesis, glycogen synthesis Effects on fat: ■ Promotes triglyceride storage	Hyperglycemia	Hypoglycemia

HIGH-YIELD FACTS

The Endocrine System

ENDOCRINE ORGAN	HORMONE	FUNCTIONS	STIMULATED BY	INHIBITED BY
Pancreas (continued)	Glucagon (A cell)	Metabolic effects: ■ Glycogenolysis, gluconeogenesis, ketogenesis (liver); lipolysis (adipose tissue); insulin secretion Effects on gastrointestinal (GI) secretion: ■ Inhibition of gastric acid and pancreatic exocrine secretion Effects on GI motility: ■ Inhibition of peristalsis Cardiovascular effects: ■ Increase in HR and force of contraction	Hypoglycemia	Hyperglycemia
	Somatostatin (D cell)	■ Inhibition of gastric acid, pepsin, pancreatic exocrine secretion ■ Inhibition of ion secretion ■ Inhibition of motility ■ Reduction of splanchnic blood flow ■ Inhibition of insulin, glucagons, pancreatic polypeptide secretion		
	Pancreatic polypeptide (F cell)	■ Function not known, but level rises after a meal (possible inhibition of pancreatic exocrine secretion)		
Adrenal cortex	Cortisol (zona fasciculata and reticularis)	■ Stimulation of hepatic gluconeogenesis, inhibition of protein synthesis, increased protein catabolism, lipolysis, inhibition of peripheral glucose uptake ■ Inhibition of fibroblast activity, inhibition of bone formation, reduction of GI calcium absorption ■ Inhibition of leukocytes, decreased migration of inflammatory cells to site of injury, decreased production of mediators of inflammation	■ ACTH circadian rhythm ■ Stress	Negative feedback
	Androgens (zona fasciculata and reticularis)	■ Dehydroepiandrosterone (DHEA), DHEA sulfate are converted to testosterone and dihydrotestosterone in the periphery ■ Adrenal androgens make up < 5% of total testosterone production in the normal male		

Endocrine Organ	Hormone	Functions	Stimulated By	Inhibited By
	Aldosterone (zona glomerulosa)	▪ Stimulates renal tubular sodium absorption in exchange for potassium and hydrogen ▪ Net effect: Fluid reabsorption and intravascular volume expansion		
Adrenal medulla	Epinephrine and norepinephrine	▪ Increased oxygen consumption ▪ Increased heat production ▪ Stimulation of glycogenolysis, lipolysis, inhibition of insulin secretion	Stress Receptors α: Vasoconstriction β₁: Cardiac inotropic and chronotropic stimulation β₂: Noncardiac smooth muscle relaxation (vessels, uterus, bronchi)	

- Medullary thyroid carcinoma (85%).
- Pheochromocytoma (50%).
- Marfanoid habitus—skeletal abnormalities of spine (e.g., kyphosis), pectus excavatum.

TREATMENT

- Perform subtotal or total parathyroidectomy with autotransplantation for parathyroid hyperplasia (MEN I and MEN IIA).
- Perform total thyroidectomy for medullary thyroid cancer (MEN II). May require nodal dissection if palpable nodes present.

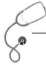

Persistence of the thyroid-pharynx connection may occur via a sinus or cyst, called a thyroglossal duct cyst. These cysts present as midline neck masses that move with swallowing and are usually seen in children or adolescents. They should be surgically excised because of the risk of infection.

▶ THYROID

General

The thyroid gland is responsible for the metabolic activity of the body. Dysfunction of the thyroid can result in hyper or hypo states of hormone production. Several different types of cancer can also form in the thyroid gland. These conditions may ultimately require surgical correction.

Development

- The thyroid develops at the base of the tongue between the first pair of pharyngeal pouches, in an area called the foramen cecum.
- The thyroid gland then descends down the midline to its final location overlying the thyroid cartilage, and develops into a bilobed organ with an isthmus between the two lobes.

- It remains connected to the floor of the pharynx via the thyroglossal duct, which subsequently obliterates around the second month of gestation. However, the thyroglossal duct may fail to obliterate and form a thyroglossal cyst or fistula instead. These are most commonly seen in children and should be surgically excised.
- A pyramidal lobe can be seen in 50–80% of the population and represents a remnant of the distal thyroglossal tract. The pyramidal lobe extends superiorly from the median isthmus.

Anatomy

See Figure 15-1.

Gross Anatomy

- Two lobes, isthmus, pyramidal lobe (pyramidal lobe present in 50–80%).
- Suspended from larynx, attached to trachea (cricoid cartilage and tracheal rings).
- Weighs 20–25 g in adults.
- Relationships:
  - Anterior: Strap muscles (sternohyoid, sternothyroid, thyrohyoid, omohyoid).
  - Posterior: Trachea.
  - Posterolateral: Common carotid arteries, internal jugular veins, vagus nerves.
- Parathyoid glands on posterior surface of thyroid, and may be within capsule.

Lymphatics ultimately drain to internal jugular nodes. Intraglandular lymphatics connect both lobes, explaining the relatively high frequency of multifocal tumors in the thyroid.

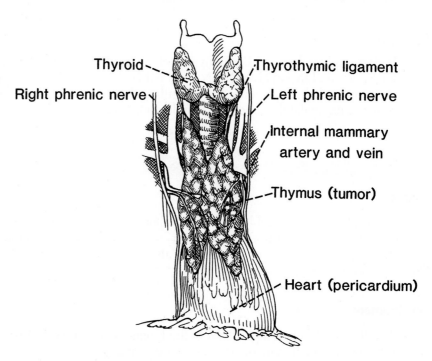

FIGURE 15-1. Thyroid anatomy.

Vasculature

See Figure 15-2.

Arterial
- Superior thyroid arteries (on each side).
  - First branch of external carotid artery at the level of the carotid bifurcation.
- Inferior thyroid artery (on each side).
  - From thyrocervical trunk of subclavian artery.
- Ima (sometimes present).
  - From aortic arch or innominate artery.

Venous
- Superior thyroid vein (on each side).
  - Drains to internal jugular (IJ).
- Middle thyroid vein (on each side).
  - Drains to IJ.
- Inferior thyroid vein (on each side).
  - Drains to brachiocephalic vein.

Innervation

- The right recurrent laryngeal nerve (RLN) branches from the right vagus nerve, loops under the right subclavian artery, and ascends to the larynx (posterior to the thyroid) between the trachea and esophagus. It may be anterior or posterior to the inferior thyroid artery. The left RLN branches from the left vagus nerve, loops under the aortic arch, and then ascends along the tracheoesophageal groove to the larynx. Both recurrent laryngeal nerves innervate the muscles of the true vocal cords.
- Sympathetic: Superior and middle cervical sympathetic ganglia (vasomotor).
- Parasympathetic: From vagus nerves, via branches of laryngeal nerves.

> The RLN innervates all the intrinsic muscles of the larynx, except the cricothyroid (supplied by the superior laryngeal nerve), and provides sensory innervation to the mucous membranes below the vocal cord. It can be damaged during a thyroid operation, so the surgeon must know its course well. Damage produces ipsilateral vocal cord paralysis and results in hoarseness or sometimes shortness of breath due to the narrowed airway.

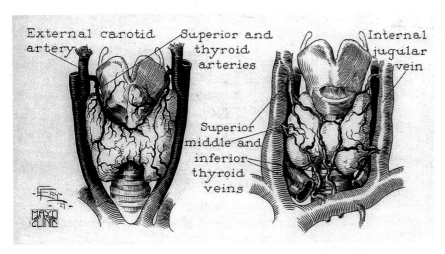

FIGURE 15-2. Thyroid blood supply.

(Copyright © 2003 MAYO Foundation.)

Hormones

The thyroid gland produces thyroid hormone (TH) using iodide and tyrosine.

HORMONE REGULATION

- TSH causes:
  - Increased formation of TH.
  - The release of TH into circulation within 30 minutes.
- The increased TH level in blood then feeds back to the pituitary and results in decreased TSH secretion, by an incompletely understood mechanism.

EFFECTS OF THYROID HORMONE

- Cardiovascular system: Increased heart rate (HR), cardiac output (CO), blood flow, blood volume, pulse pressure (no change in mean arterial pressure [MAP]).
- Respiratory system: Increased respiratory rate (RR), depth of respiration.
- Gastrointestinal (GI) system: Increased motility.
- Central nervous system (CNS): Nervousness, anxiety.
- Musculoskeletal system: Increased reactivity up to a point, then response is weakened; fine motor tremor.
- Sleep: Constant fatigue but decreased ability to sleep.
- Nutrition: Increased basal metabolic rate (BMR), need for vitamins, metabolism of carbohydrate, lipid, and protein; decreased weight.

Assessment of Function

- If T_4 production is increased, both total T_4 (tT_4) and free T_4 (fT_4) increase.
- If production decreases, both tT_4 and fT_4 decrease.
- If amount of thyroid-binding globulin (TBG) changes, only tT_4 changes, not fT_4.

Congenital Anomalies

- Persistent sinus tract remnant of developing gland: **Thyroglossal duct cyst**—may occur anywhere along course as a midline structure with thyroid epithelium, usually between the isthmus and the hyoid bone:
  - Most common congenital anomaly.
  - Few symptoms but may become infected.
  - Easier to see when tongue is sticking out.
  - Surgical treatment: Excision of duct remnant and central portion of hyoid bone (Sistrunk's operation).
- Complete failure to develop.
- Incomplete descent: Lingual or subhyoid position (if gland enlarges, patient will have earlier respiratory symptoms).
- Excessive descent: Substernal thyroid.
- Malformation of branchial pouch.

Hyperthyroidism

CAUSES

- Graves' disease.
- Toxic nodular goiter.
- Toxic thyroid adenoma.
- Subacute thyroiditis.
- Functional metastatic thyroid cancer.
- Struma ovarii (abnormal thyroid tissue in ovary).

GRAVES' DISEASE

- Most common cause of hyperthyroidism (in the United States).
- **Mechanism:** Autoimmune disorder that causes an excess of TH to be produced due to the presence of thyroid-stimulating immunoglobulins that stimulates production of TSH.
- Affects nearly 2% of American women; six times more common in women.
- Onset age 20–40.
- Families with Graves' disease have increased risk of other autoimmune disorders (e.g., diabetes, Addison's) and other thyroid disorders as well.

SIGNS AND SYMPTOMS

- Nervousness, increased sweating, tachycardia, goiter, pretibial myxedema, tremor (90%).
- Heat intolerance, palpitations, fatigue, weight loss, dyspnea, weakness, increased appetite, exophthalmos, thyroid bruit (50–90%).
- Other: Amenorrhea, decreased libido and fertility.

DIAGNOSIS

- Labs: Thyroid function tests (TFTs)—increased T_3 and/or T_4 and decreased TSH (negative feedback of ↑ hormone levels).
- Radioactive iodide uptake test (RAIU): Scan shows diffusely increased uptake.

TREATMENT

- Antithyroid drugs.
- Radioiodide ablation with ^{131}I.
- Subtotal or total thyroidectomy.
- Choosing a treatment:
  - Consider: Age, severity, size of gland, surgical risk, treatment side effects, comorbidities.
  - Radioablation is the most common choice in the United States:
    - Indicated for small or medium-sized goiters, if medical therapy has failed, or if other options are contraindicated.
    - Most patients become euthyroid within 2 months.
    - Most patients ultimately require thyroid hormone replacement (e.g., levothyroxine).
    - Complications include exacerbation of thyroid storm initially.
    - Contraindicated in pregnant patients, women of childbearing age and newborns.
  - Surgical treatment:
    - Indicated when radioablation is contraindicated (e.g., young or pregnant patients) or if medical management cannot be used.

Ten percent of patients will have atrial fibrillation that may be refractory to medical treatment until hyperthyroidism is controlled.

Typical scenario: A 28-year-old female presents with a recent unintentional 10-lb weight loss, and complaining of insomnia despite extreme fatigue. She also complains of amenorrhea and decreased sexual desire. She appears anxious and fidgety during your assessment. On exam, she is tachycardic and with an enlarged thyroid. Laboratory studies reveal TSH of 0.08 and T_4 of 250 nmol/L. *Think:* Graves' disease. You can control her tachycardia with β-blockers and optimize her for surgery.

Risks of thyroid surgery include recurrent laryngeal nerve injury, hypoparathyroidism, and persistent hyperthyroidism (with subtotal thyroidectomy).

- Patients should be euthyroid prior to excision.
- Advantage over radioablation is immediate cure.
- Medical therapy:
  - β-blockers provide symptomatic relief.
  - Antithyroid drugs (propylthiouracil [PTU], methimazole) inhibit hormone production and peripheral conversion of $T_4 \rightarrow T_3$.
  - Potassium iodide reduces hormone production (via Wolff-Chaikoff effect), used to shrink gland prior to surgical excision.
  - High recurrence rate with medical therapy.
  - May cause side effects such as rash, fever, or peripheral neuritis.
  - Patients relapse if meds are discontinued.
  - Check TFTs after any treatment to determine if patient is successfully euthyroid or requires hormone replacement.

TOXIC NODULAR GOITER (PLUMMER'S DISEASE)

- Causes hyperthyroidism, but without the extrathyroidal symptoms.
- Treatment is surgical since medical therapy and radioablation has a high failure rate.
- Solitary nodule: Lobectomy.
- Multinodular goiter: Subtotal thyroidectomy.

THYROID STORM (THYROTOXICOSIS)

- Life-threatening extreme exacerbation of hyperthyroidism precipitated by surgery on an inadequately prepared patient (i.e., incomplete β-blockade and noneuthyroid patients), infection, labor, iodide administration, or recent radioablation.
- Patient presents with fever, tachycardia, muscle stiffness or tremor, disorientation/altered mental status.
- Fifty percent of patients with thyroid storm develop congestive heart failure (CHF).
- Has a 20–40% mortality rate.
- Best way to treat this is by avoiding it. Prophylaxis includes achieving euthyroid state preop.
- **Treatment:** Fluids, antithyroid medication (thionamide, PTU, methimazole), β-blockers (propanolol, metoprolol), corticosteroids (hydrocortisone), sodium iodide (NaI) or Lugol's solution (KI), and a cooling blanket.

Hypothyroidism

CAUSES

- Autoimmune thyroiditis.
- Iatrogenic: s/p thyroidectomy, s/p radioablation, secondary to antithyroid medications.
- Iodine deficiency.

SIGNS AND SYMPTOMS

Differ, depending on age of diagnosis:

- Infants/peds: Characteristic Down's-like facies, failure to thrive, mental retardation.
- Adolescents/adults (particularly when due to autoimmune thyroiditis):
  - Eighty percent female.
  - Physiologic effects: Bradycardia, decreased CO, hypotension, shortness of breath secondary to effusions.

- Presentation includes: Fatigue, weight gain, cold intolerance, constipation, menorrhagia, decreased libido and fertility.
- Less common complaints: Yellow-tinged skin, hair loss, tongue enlargement.

DIAGNOSIS

- History and physical exam findings.
- Labs:
  - Decreased T_4, T_3.
  - TSH:
    - Increased in primary hypothyroidism.
  - Decreased in secondary hypothyroidism.
  - Confirm with TRH challenge: TSH will not respond in secondary hypothyroidism.
  - Thyroid autoantibodies present in autoimmune thyroiditis.
  - Low hematocrit (Hct).
- Electrocardiogram (ECG): Decreased voltage and flat or inverted T waves.

Immediate treatment (of infants) with thyroid hormone will help minimize the neurologic and intellectual deficits.

TREATMENT

Thyroxine PO or IV emergently if patient presents in myxedema coma.

Thyroiditis

ACUTE

- **Infectious etiology:** *Streptococcus pyogenes, Staphylococcus aureus, Pneumococcus pneumoniae.*
- **Risk factors:** Female sex, goiter, thyroglossal duct.
- **Signs and symptoms:** Unilateral neck pain and fever, euthyroid state, dysphagia.
- **Treatment:** IV antibiotics and surgical drainage.

The bacteria that cause acute suppurative thyroiditis usually spread through lymphatics from a nearby locus of infection.

SUBACUTE (DE QUERVAIN'S)

- **Etiology:** Post–viral upper respiratory infection (URI).
- **Risk factors:** Female sex.
- **Signs and symptoms:** Fatigue, depression, neck pain, fever, unilateral swelling of thyroid with overlying erythema, firm and tender thyroid, transient hyperthyroidism usually preceding hypothyroid phase.
- **Diagnosis:** Made by history and exam.
- **Treatment:**
  - Usually self-limited disease (within 6 weeks).
  - Manage pain with nonsteroidal anti-inflammatory drugs (NSAIDs).

Ten percent of patients with subacute thyroiditis become permanently hypothyroid.

CHRONIC (HASHIMOTO'S THYROIDITIS)

- **Etiology:** Autoimmune.
- **Risk factors:** Down's syndrome, Turner syndrome, familial Alzheimer's disease, history of radiation therapy as child.
- **Signs and symptoms:** Painless enlargement of thyroid, neck tightness, presence of other autoimmune diseases.
- **Diagnosis:** Made by history, physical, and labs.
  - Labs: Circulating antibodies against microsomal thyroid cell, thyroid hormone, T_3, T_4, or TSH receptor.

Typical scenario: A 35-year-old female who emigrated from Russia in 1990 is referred to you for a solitary right thyroid mass. On exam, you find a solitary mass, 2×1 cm, that is firm and fixed. There are no palpable lymph nodes. What is a likely diagnosis? *Think:* Papillary thyroid cancer, which is the most common variety. Fine-needle aspiration in 85–90% of patients shows cuboidal cells with abundant cytoplasm and psammoma bodies. Computed tomography (CT) shows no other foci of disease. What's your next step? *Think:* Near-total thyroidectomy.

FNA of thyroid nodule has 1% false-positive rate and 5% false-negative rate.

- **Pathology:** Firm, symmetrical, enlargement; follicular and Hürthle cell hyperplasia; lymphocytic and plasma cell infiltrates.
- **Treatment:**
  - Thyroid hormone (usually results in regression of goiter).
  - With failure of medical therapy, partial thyroidectomy is indicated.

RIEDEL'S FIBROSING THYROIDITIS

- Rare.
- Fibrosis replaces both lobes and isthmus.
- **Risk factors:** Associated with other fibrosing conditions, like retroperitoneal fibrosis, sclerosing cholangitis.
- **Signs and symptoms:** Usually remain euthyroid; neck pain, possible airway compromise; firm, nontender, enlarged thyroid.
- **Diagnosis:** Open biopsy required to rule out carcinoma or lymphoma.
- **Pathology:** Dense, invasive fibrosis of both lobes and isthmus. May also involve adjacent structures.
- **Treatment:**
  - With airway compromise: Isthmectomy.
  - Without airway compromise: Medical treatment with steroids.

Workup of a Mass

- Fifteen percent of solitary thyroid nodules are malignant.
- If multinodular thyroid gland, risk of malignancy is only 5%.
- Ninety to ninety-five percent present as well-differentiated cancer.
- Lateral aberrant thyroid: Usually well-differentiated papillary cancer metastatic to cervical lymph nodes.
- **Risk factors:** History of radiation, family history of thyroid cancer, age, gender.
- **Signs and symptoms:**
  - Voice and/or airway symptoms, sudden enlargement of nodule.
  - History of head and neck radiation therapy leads to 40% risk of developing thyroid cancer, so if patient presents with this history, proceed directly to surgery.
  - Exam: Check size, mobility, quality, adherence of mass, and presence of lymphadenopathy. Concerning findings include hard, fixed gland or palpable cervical lymph nodes.

DIAGNOSIS

Fine-needle aspiration (FNA) is the standard of care for thyroid nodule workup.

- *Benign* (65%):
  - Ultrasound (US) for sizing and to differentiate nodules and cysts.
  - Obtain thyroglobulin level and follow over time. No need for surgery.
- *Suspicious or nondiagnostic* (15%): Usually follicular (20% will be malignant).
- Obtain ^{123}I scan:
  - Eighty-five percent are "cold" nodules with a 10–25% chance of malignancy.
  - Five percent are "hot" nodules with only a 1% chance of malignancy.
  - Surgery is indicated if serial T_4 levels fail to regress and future biopsies are worrisome.
- *Malignant* (15%): Surgery.

■ Cyst: Drain completely (curative in 75% of cases). If cyst is > 4 cm, complex, or recurring even after three aspirations, send to OR for removal.

Thyroid Cancer

See Table 15-2.

▶ PARATHYROID

Development

■ Superior parathyroid glands (2) develop from fourth pharyngeal pouch.
■ Inferior parathyroid glands (2) develop from third pharyngeal pouch.

FNA is less reliable if patient has history of irradiation, and initial OR biopsy may be appropriate.

TABLE 15-2. Thyroid Cancer

	PAPILLARY	FOLLICULAR	MEDULLARY	ANAPLASTIC
	Most common type of thyroid cancer	Not common in populations that do not have iodine deficiency		Rarest but worst prognosis
Percent	80–85 (75% of pediatric thyroid cancer)	5–20%	5–10%	1–5%
Risk factors	Radiation	Dyshormonogenesis	MEN II in 30–40%	■ Prior diagnosis of well-differentiated thyroid cancer ■ Iodine deficiency
Age group	30–40	40–50	50–60	60–70
Sex (F/M)	2/1	3/1	1.5/1	1.5/1
Signs and symptoms	■ Painless mass ■ Dysphagia ■ Dyspnea ■ Hoarseness ■ Euthyroid	■ Painless mass ■ Rarely hyperfunctional	■ Painful mass ■ Palpable lymph node (LN) (15–20%) ■ Dysphonia ■ Dyspnea ■ Hoarseness	■ Rapidly enlarging neck mass (large mass at presentation) ■ Neck pain ■ Dysphagia ■ Hard, fixed LN (50%)
Diagnosis	■ FNA ■ CT or MRI (to assess local invasion)	■ FNA ■ CT or MRI (to assess local invasion)	■ FNA ■ Presence of amyloid is diagnostic ■ Check for calcitonin	■ FNA

TABLE 15-2. **Thyroid Cancer (continued)**

	PAPILLARY	**FOLLICULAR**	**MEDULLARY**	**ANAPLASTIC**
Metastases	Lymphatic (5% at time of presentation)	Hematogenous	■ Lymphatic (local neck and mediastinal nodes) ■ Local (into trachea and esophagus)	■ Aggressive local disease ■ 30–50% have synchronous pulmonary mets at time of diagnosis
Treatment	■ Minimal cancer (< 1.5 cm): Limited lobectomy and isthmectomy ■ Other: Total or near-total thyroidectomy for cancers > 1.5 cm ■ For + LN, modified radical neck dissection ■ ^{131}I ablation or thyroid suppression (with thyroid hormone) for patients with residual thyroid tissue or LN mets	■ Minimal cancer (< 4 cm): Lobectomy and isthmectomy ■ Other: Total or near-total thyroidectomy for cancers > 4 cm ■ For + LN, modified radical neck dissection ■ ^{131}I ablation for patients with residual thyroid tissue or LN mets	■ Sporadic (80%): Total thyroidectomy ■ Familial (20%): Total thyroidectomy and central neck node dissection ■ No value for ^{131}I ablation ■ Follow patients with calcitonin levels	■ Debulking resection of thyroid gland and adjacent structures ■ External radiation therapy (XRT) ■ Doxorubicin-based chemotherapy
Prognosis	■ Worse for older patients and those with distant mets ■ Presence of + LN not strongly correlated with overall survival	■ Worse for older patients, those with distant mets, tumor size > 4 cm, high tumor grade ■ Presence of + LN not strongly correlated with overall survival		Poor prognosis
Survival	10-year survival: 74–93%	10-year survival: 60–80%	10-year survival: 70–80%	Median survival: 4–5 months

Anatomy

- Weight < 50 mg/gland.
- $3 \times 3 \times 3$ mm.
- Adult position of superior gland constant and next to the superior lobes of thyroid.
- Inferior glands have more variable position (posterior/lateral to thyroid and below inferior thyroid artery).

- Not uncommon for one of the inferior glands to be "missing."
- Most common location in thymus. Other sites include intravagal, groove in carotid sheath.
- Yellow-brown tissue similar to surrounding fatty tissue.
- Histology: Normal gland contains mainly chief cells (produce parathyroid hormone [PTH]), with occasional oxyphils.
- Vasculature: Inferior thyroid arteries; superior, middle, and inferior thyroid veins.

Physiology/Calcium Homeostasis

- **Primary function:** Regulation of calcium and phosphate metabolism by PTH, vitamin D, and calcitonin.
- Primary organ systems involved: Gastrointestinal (GI) tract, bone, kidney.

PTH

- Synthesized by the parathyroid glands (see Figure 15-3).
- Serum calcium levels regulate secretion of cleaved PTH by negative feedback mechanism.
- Bone:
  - Stimulates osteoclasts (increased bone resorption).
  - Inhibits osteoblasts (stops bone production).
  - This causes release of calcium and phosphate.
- Kidney:
  - Increases reabsorption of calcium.
  - Increases phosphate excretion.
- GI tract:
  - Stimulates hydroxylation of 25-OH D → 1,25 OH D.
  - 1,25 OH D (vitamin D) increases the intestinal absorption of dietary calcium (primarily in duodenum) and phosphate.
  - Promotes mineralization.
  - Enhances PTH's effect on bone (synergistic effect).

Of the half of serum calcium in an ionized, active form, 80% is bound to albumin, and 20% is found in a citrate complex.

Hypercalcemic crisis (calcium > 13 mg/dL and symptomatic): Treat with saline, furosemide, bisphosphonates, and, if needed, antiarrhythmic agents.

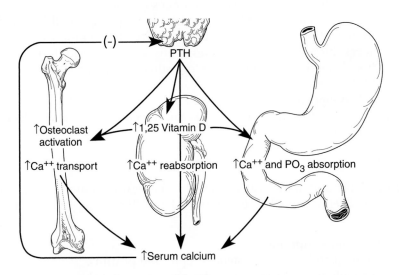

FIGURE 15-3. Actions of parathyroid hormone.

Hyperparathyroidism = ↑ Ca²⁺. *Think:* Stones, bones, groans, and moans.

Calcitonin

- Secreted by thyroid C cells.
- Inhibits bone resorption (inhibits calcium release).
- Increases urinary excretion of calcium and phosphate.
- Works as a counterregulatory hormone to PTH.

Hyperparathyroidism

PRIMARY

Due to overproduction of PTH, causing increased absorption of calcium from intestines, increased vitamin D_3 production, and decreased renal calcium excretion, thereby raising the overall serum level of calcium and lowering the amount of phosphorus.

- **Incidence:** 1/4000 in the United States.
- **Risk factors:** MEN I, MEN IIA, history of radiation.
- **Signs and symptoms:**
  - "Stones": Kidney stones.
  - "Bones": Bone pain, pathologic fractures, subperiosteal resorption.
  - "Groans": Nausea, vomiting, muscle pain, constipation, pancreatitis, peptic ulcer disease.
  - "Moans": Lethargy, confusion, depression, paranoia.
- **Etiology:**
  - Solitary adenoma: 85–90%
  - Four-gland hyperplasia: 10%
  - Cancer: < 1%
- **Preop imaging:** Ultrasound, Sestamibi scan, CT/magnetic resonance imaging (MRI), operative exploration.
- **Diagnosis:** Elevation of plasma PTH, with inappropriately high serum calcium. Check urine for calcium to rule out diagnosis of familial hypocalciuric hypercalcemia (will be low if familial disease, and high if primary hyperparathyroidism).
- **Treatment:**
  - Solitary adenoma: Solitary parathyroidectomy with neck exploration to identify +/– biopsy 3 remaining glands. If preop sestamibi scan is done to localize area, no need for neck exploration.
  - Multiple gland hyperplasia: Remove three glands, or all four with reimplantation of at least 30 g of parathyroid tissue in forearm or other accessible site to retain function (this makes it easier to resect additional parathyroid gland if hyperparathyroid state persists).
  - Outcome:
    - First operation has 98% success rate.
    - Reoperation has 90% success rate if remaining gland is localized preop.

SECONDARY

Increased PTH due to hypocalcemia that is the result of chronic renal failure (phosphate retention → low calcium), GI malabsorption, osteomalacia, or rickets.

- **Signs and symptoms:**
  - Bone pain from renal osteodystrophy and pruritus.
  - Patients are often asymptomatic.

Not all patients with hypercalcemia have hyperparathyroidism. Hypercalcemia of malignancy (due to tumor-secreted PTH-related protein) must be ruled out. Malignancies commonly implicated include colon, lung, breast, prostate, head, neck, and multiple myeloma.

- **Diagnosis:** Made by labs in asymptomatic patient; usually due to four-gland hyperplasia.
- **Treatment:**
  - Nonsurgical: In renal failure patients, correct calcium and phosphate.
    - Restrict phosphorus intake, treat with phosphorus-binding agents and calcium/vitamin D supplementation. Adjust dialysate to maximize calcium and minimize aluminum.
  - Surgical: Indicated for intractable bone pain or pruritus, or pathologic fractures, with failure of medical therapy. No role for parathyroid surgery in secondary HPTH.
    - Perform renal transplant if necessary.

TERTIARY

Due to persistent hyperparathyroidism after treatment for secondary hyperparathyroidism. Due to autonomously functioning parathyroid glands that are resistant to negative feedback from high calcium levels. Usually s/p renal transplant.

- Usually a short-lived phenomenon.
- If persistent, surgery is indicated (3½-gland parathyroidectomy).

Hypoparathyroidism

- Uncommon.

ETIOLOGY

- Surgically induced: Following total thyroidectomy; usually transient and treated if symptoms develop.
- Congenital absence of all four glands.
- DiGeorge syndrome: Absence of parathyroid and thymus.
- Functional: Chronic hypomagnesemia.

SIGNS AND SYMPTOMS

- Numbness and tingling of circumoral area, fingers, toes.
- Anxiety, confusion.
- May progress to tetany, hyperventilation, seizures, heart block.

TREATMENT

- Supplementation with PO calcium and vitamin D (to help GI absorption).
- Pseudohypoparathyroidism: Familial disease causing resistance of PTH at target tissue. Patients remain hypocalcemic and hyperphosphatemic despite bone resorption from elevated PTH. Treatment consists of calcium and vitamin D supplementation.

Parathyroid Cancer

SIGNS AND SYMPTOMS

- Forty to fifty percent present with firm, fixed mass that is palpable.
- Extremely high calcium and PTH levels. Usually has high levels of human chorionic gonadotropin (hCG—tumor marker).
- Neck pain, voice change (due to lesion in recurrent laryngeal nerve).

Patients with familial hyperparathyroidism (i.e., MEN I/IIa) have a high recurrence rate; total parathyroidectomy with forearm reimplantation is indicated to facilitate potential reoperation if HPTH persists. Patients with sporadic four-gland hyperplasia may undergo total parathyroidectomy with reimplantation or three-gland excision.

Typical scenario: A patient complains of tingling around her lips on postoperative day 1 s/p total thyroidectomy. *Think:* Iatrogenic hypoparathyroidism causing hypocalcemia. Supplement calcium and vitamin D. Continue to follow calcium levels.

Hypocalcemia
Chvostek: Contraction of facial muscles when tapping on facial nerve.
Trousseau: Development of carpal spasm by occluding blood flow to forearm.

TREATMENT

- En bloc surgical resection of mass and surrounding structures, along with ipsilateral thyroid lobectomy, and ipsilateral lymph node dissection.
- Postop external radiation therapy (XRT) and chemotherapy are not usually beneficial.
- Postop complications: Recurrent laryngeal nerve damage, severe hypocalcemia (hungry bone syndrome).
- Five-year survival: 70%.

▶ ADRENAL GLAND

Anatomy

- Bilateral retroperitoneal organs, anterior and medial to superior pole of kidneys.
- At level of T11.
- Size: 3–6 g, 5 × 2.5 cm.
- Vasculature: Branches of aorta, inferior phrenic, and renal arteries.
- Venous drainage: Right side drains to inferior vena cava (IVC), and left side drains to the left renal vein.

HISTOLOGY

- Cortex.
- Glomerulosa: 15%; aldosterone synthesis.
- Fasciculata: 75%; steroids and cortisol synthesis.
- Reticularis: 10%; cortisol, androgen, and estrogen secretion.

Physiology

See section on endocrine organs and Figure 15-4.

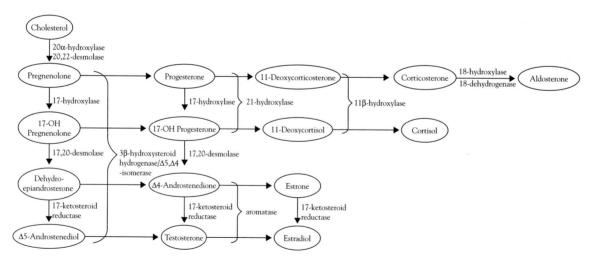

FIGURE 15-4. **Pathways of adrenal steroid synthesis.**

Hyperplasia

Area of cortex expands and becomes hyperfunctioning.

Adenoma

- Most are unilateral.
- If adrenal gland < 6 cm, usually observe unless hormonally active (↑ cortisol, ↑ ACTH) or increasing in size.
- If adrenal gland > 6 cm, surgically resect due to increased risk of adrenocortical carcinoma.

Adrenal Cortical Carcinoma

DEFINITION

Very rare adrenal tumor.

EPIDEMIOLOGY

Affects women more than men, peak < 5 years old or 30–40 years old.

SIGNS AND SYMPTOMS

- Vague abdominal complaints (due to enlarging retroperitoneal mass).
- Symptoms related to overproduction of a steroid hormone (most tumors are functional).

DIAGNOSIS

- Twenty-four-hour urine collection for cortisol, aldosterone, catecholamines, metanephrine, vanillylmandelic acid, 17-OH corticosteroids, 17-ketosteroids.
- CT (lesions > 7 mm) or magnetic resonance imaging (MRI) (especially for assessing IVC invasion).
- Chest x-ray (CXR) to rule out pulmonary metastases.

TREATMENT

- Radical en bloc resection, but only 1/3 of adrenal carcinomas are operable.
- If resection cannot be completed, debulk to reduce amount of cortisol-secreting tissue.
- Bone metastases should be palliated with XRT.
- No role for chemotherapy.
- Monitor steroid hormone levels postop.
- Recurrence also warrants resection.
- Recurrence: Lungs, lymph nodes, liver, peritoneum, bone.
  - In 10% of bilateral adrenalectomies, patients may develop Nelson's syndrome—excess production of ACTH from pituitary adenoma. Pituitary adenoma often causes visual disturbances (due to mass effect on chiasm), hyperpigmentation (↑ melanocyte-stimulating hormone [MSH]), and amenorrhea as well.

Fifty percent of adrenal cortical carcinomas secrete cortisol, resulting in Cushing's syndrome.

PROGNOSIS

- Seventy percent present in stage III or IV.
- Five-year survival 40% for complete resection.
- If local invasion, median survival time is 2–3 years.

Cushing's Syndrome

DEFINITION

Excessive cortisol production.

CAUSES

- Iatrogenic administration of corticosteroids most common cause!
- Pituitary tumor that secretes ACTH (i.e., Cushing's disease).
- Ectopic ACTH secretion by tumor elsewhere stimulates adrenal cortisol production.
- Adrenal tumor that secretes cortisol.

SIGNS AND SYMPTOMS

Appearance
- Weight gain
- Truncal obesity
- Extremity wasting
- Buffalo hump
- Moon facies
- Acne
- Purple striae
- Hirsutism

Physiologic
- Mild glucose intolerance
- Amenorrhea
- Decreased libido
- Depression
- Impaired memory
- Muscle weakness

Typical scenario: A young male presents with weight gain, especially in the trunk; loss of muscle mass; and a buffalo hump. He has recently been noted to be mildly glucose intolerant. His past medical history is significant for severe asthma, for which he is chronically on steroids. *Think:* Cushing's syndrome secondary to exogenous administration of steroids.

DIAGNOSIS

See Table 15-3.

- Confirm presence of hypercortisolism:
  - Low-dose dexamethasone test.
  - Twenty-four-hour urinary cortisol looking for cortisol or its metabolites (e.g., 17-hydroxycorticosteroids).
  - Direct measurement of serum cortisol.
- Determine whether cortisol production is pituitary dependent or independent: High-dose dexamethasone test.
- CT (adrenals): Can distinguish cortical hyperplasia from tumor with sensitivity > 95%, but lacks high specificity.
- MRI (sella).
- Petrosal sinus sampling (will see elevated ACTH if pituitary tumor).
- Adrenal cortisol production: High cortisol, low plasma ACTH (due to negative feedback from cortisol production), and no suppression of cortisol with high-dose dexamethasone suppression test.

Most common cause of ectopic ACTH production is small cell lung cancer (a.k.a. oat cell carcinoma), followed by carinoid tumors.

TABLE 15-3. Assays in the Workup of Cushing's Syndrome

TEST	RESULT	INTERPRETATION
24-hour urinary free cortisol or single dose dexamethasone suppression test	Normal	Hypercortisolism can be ruled out: ▪ Low-dose dexamethasone (2 mg) normally decreases urinary cortisol levels in normal patients. Lack of suppression confirms hypercortisolism ▪ High-dose dexamethasone (8 mg) will only decrease urinary cortisol if pituitary-dependent cause of ↑ ACTH (Cushing's disease), but will not suppress cortisol at all if cause is either ectopic ACTH production or a primary adrenal tumor
Plasma ACTH	Very high	Ectopic ACTH production
	Intermediate value	Pituitary tumor
	Low or undetectable	Adrenal source: Either adenoma, hyperplasia, or, very rarely, cancer
Urinary 17-ketosteroids	< 10 mg/day	Adenoma
	> 60 mg/day	Cancer
	In between	Likely hyperplasia
Metyrapone test	Increased ACTH	Pituitary cause
Petrosal sinus sampling	Sinus/plasma ACTH ratio > 3 after corticotropin-releasing hormone (CRH) administration	Identifies Cushing's disease with 100% sensitivity

- Ectopic ACTH production: Increased plasma cortisol and ACTH, and no suppression of cortisol (because only ACTH from pituitary, and not ectopic source, is capable of negative feedback).
- Pituitary tumor (Cushing's disease): Mild elevation of ACTH and cortisol is successfully suppressed with high-dose dexamethasone (negative feedback on pituitary).

TREATMENT

- Cushing's disease: Transsphenoidal resection of pituitary adenoma.
- Adrenal adenoma: Adrenalectomy.
- Adrenal carcinoma: Adrenalectomy.
- Ectopic ACTH: Resection of primary lesion (usually in lung).
- Unresectable lesions and recurrence should be debulked for palliation.
- Medical treatment to suppress cortisol production: Metyrapone (inhibits cortisol production), amino-glutethimide, mitotane, ketoconazole.

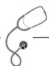

Low-dose dexamethasone suppression test: Single dose of steroid at 11 P.M., followed by measurement of serum and urinary cortisol levels at 8 A.M.
Normal: < 5 μg/dL (because evening dose suppresses further release).
Abnormal: > 5 μg/dL high-dose dexamethasone (8 mg) distinguishes pituitary cause (suppression) from adrenal or ectopic cause (no suppression).

Most common cause of secondary adrenal insufficiency is iatrogenic due to long-term glucocorticoid therapy.

The sudden cessation of long-term glucocorticoid therapy can precipitate adrenal insufficiency because it suppresses the intrinsic control by the hypothalamus and pituitary. Six months may be required for the intrinsic controls to return to normal.

Typical scenario: A patient with known Addison's disease presents with acute upper abdominal pain, with peritoneal signs and confusion. *Think:* Addisonian crisis.

Patients with Addison's disease or who have been taking exogenous steroids for 6 months or longer are likely to require stress-dose steroids perioperatively. The timing and dose may vary depending on the planned procedure and baseline doses of the patient.

Addison's Disease

DEFINITION

Adrenal insufficiency:

- Primary: Due to destruction of adrenal cortex with sparing of medulla.
- Secondary: Failure due to hypothalamic or pituitary abnormalities.

ETIOLOGY

Primary
- Post-adrenalectomy.
- Autoimmune adrenalitis.
- Tuberculosis (TB).
- Fungal infection.
- Acquired immune deficiency syndrome (AIDS).
- Metastatic cancer.
- Familial glucocorticoid deficiency.

Secondary
- Exogenous steroids.
- Craniopharyngioma.
- Pituitary surgery or irradiation.
- Empty sella syndrome.

Addisonian Crisis
- Acute situation due to some extrinsic stressor (i.e., infection, surgery).

SIGNS AND SYMPTOMS

- Nausea.
- Vomiting.
- Abdominal pain.
- Tachycardia.
- Weight loss.
- Weakness.
- Fatigue.
- Lethargy.
- Hyperpigmentation (low levels of cortisol cause ↑ pituitary production of proopiomelanocortin [POMC], which is precursor to both ACTH as well as MSH).
- Fever and hypovolemic shock in Addisonian crisis.

DIAGNOSIS

- Hyponatremia, hyperkalemia (due to ↓ adosterone, which is normally produced in adrenals).
- ACTH stimulation test: Give ACTH and measure cortisol level after 30 minutes. If adrenal failure is present, there will be no increase in cortisol.
- Baseline ACTH level is elevated in patients with primary failure due to absence of negative feedback.

TREATMENT

- Glucocorticoid therapy for primary and secondary causes.
- Additional mineralocorticoid therapy for primary cause.
- Addisonian crisis: Volume (D_5NS) and glucocorticoids IV.

Hyperaldosteronism

DEFINITION

- Hyperaldosteronism
- Primary
- Secondary

ETIOLOGY

- Primary (due to excessive aldosterone secretion): Conn's syndrome:
  - Aldosterone-secreting tumor (66%)
  - Idiopathic adrenocortical hyperplasia (30%)
- Secondary (due to elevated renin → elevated aldosterone):
  - Renal artery stenosis
  - Cirrhosis
  - CHF
  - Normal pregnancy

SIGNS AND SYMPTOMS

- Hypertension
- Muscle weakness and cramping
- Headache
- Polyuria
- Polydipsia
- Hypokalemia

DIAGNOSIS

- **Primary/Conn's syndrome:**
  - Diastolic hypertension without edema.
  - Elevated plasma aldosterone.
  - Normals or low plasma renin.
  - Hypokalemia, elevated urinary potassium (off antihypertensive medications).
  - Post-captopril plasma aldosterone:
    - Normally results in decreased aldosterone.
    - Diagnostic of hyperaldosteronism if ratio > 50.
  - Imaging:
    - CT picks up tumors > 1 cm. If there is an aldosteronoma, opposite adrenal appears atrophied.
    - Iodocholesterol scan: Picks up 90% of aldosteronomas and shows how functional they are. Hyperplasia will present as bilateral hyperfunction versus unilateral (for tumor).
    - If all imaging is nondiagnostic, then sample adrenal vein for aldosterone and cortisol pre- and post-ACTH.
    - Unilateral elevation of aldosterone or aldosterone/cortisol ratio indicates aldosterone-secreting adenoma.
    - Bilateral elevation of aldosterone is consistent with hyperplasia.

TREATMENT

- Primary:
  - Hyperplasia: Medical treatment with spironolactone, nifedipine, amiloride and/or other antihypertensive. **No surgery!**
  - Adenoma: Laparoscopic adrenalectomy.

Renin is produced in the juxtaglomerular (JG) cells of the kidney when blood pressure is low, and stimulates conversion of angiotensinogen to angiotensin I in the kidney. Angiotensin I is converted to angiotensin II in the lung. Angiotensin II causes adrenals to produce aldosterone.

In working up a patient for suspected Conn's syndrome, make sure it isn't just a patient with uncontrolled hypertension on potassium-wasting diuretics.

Sheehan's Syndrome

Postpartum infarction and necrosis of pituitary leading to hormonal failure.

ETIOLOGY

Pituitary ischemia due to hemorrhage, hypovolemic shock, pituitary portal venous thrombosis.

SIGNS AND SYMPTOMS

- Failure of lactation.
- Amenorrhea.
- Progressive decreased adrenal function and thyroid function.

Posterior Pituitary Disorders

SYNDROME OF INAPPROPRIATE ANTIDIURETIC HORMONE (SIADH)

- Occurs in 15% of hospital patients.
- Impaired water secretion.
- Hypersecretion of ADH results in increased urinary sodium with elevation of urine osmolality.
- Causes: CNS injury, cancer, trauma, drugs.

DIABETES INSIPIDUS

- Decreased ADH secretion.
- Impaired water conservation; large volumes of urine, leads to increased plasma osmolality and thirst.
- One third idiopathic; two thirds due to tumor or trauma.

The Spleen

Most common indications for splenectomy:
1. Trauma
2. Idiopathic thrombocytopenic purpura (ITP) refractory to steroids

Note: In the past it was staging for Hodgkin's disease, but now splenectomy is not required for this.

Conditions associated with rupture of the spleen:
- Mononucleosis
- Malaria
- Blunt LUQ trauma
- Splenic abscess

▶ DESCRIPTION

Immunologic organ without distinct lobes or segments that weighs about 100–175 g. The spleen is responsible for the removal of old red blood cells and bacteria from the blood circulation.

▶ ANATOMIC BOUNDARIES

Left upper quadrant (LUQ) of the abdomen, between the 8th and 11th ribs (see Figure 16-1).

- Superior: Left diaphragm leaf.
- Inferior: Colon, splenic flexure, and phrenocolic ligament.
- Medial: Pancreas (tail) and stomach.
- Lateral: Rib cage.
- Anterior: Rib cage, stomach.
- Posterior: Rib cage.

▶ SPLENECTOMY

See Table 16-1 for indications.

Types

- Laparoscopic
- Open

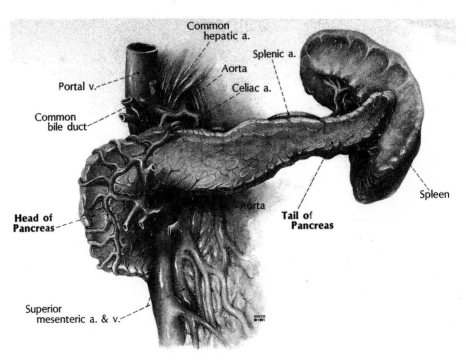

FIGURE 16-1. The spleen and its relationships.

(Copyright © 2003 Mayo Foundation.)

TABLE 16-1.   **Indications for Splenectomy**

These conditions themselves do not always require a splenectomy, but in certain situations, they do. Many of these conditions can cause splenomegaly. Splenectomy in such cases may be necessary due to sheer bulk, or problems resulting cytopenias due to splenic sequestration.

1. Red cell disorders
   a. Congenital
      i. Hereditary spherocytosis
      ii. Hemoglobinopathies
         (1) Sickle cell disease
         (2) Thalassemia
         (3) Enzyme deficiencies
   b. Acquired
      i. Autoimmune hemolytic anemia
      ii. Parasitic diseases
2. Platelet disorders
   a. Idiopathic thrombocytopenic purpura (ITP)
   b. Thrombotic thrombocytopenic purpura (TTP)
3. Lymphoid disorders
   a. Non-Hodgkin's lymphomas
   b. Portal hypertension
   c. Splenic artery aneurysm
4. Bone marrow disorders (myeloproliferative disorders)
   a. Myelofibrosis (myeloid metaplasia)
   b. Chronic myeloid leukemia (CML)
   c. Acute myeloid leukemia (AML)
   d. Chronic myelomonocytic leukemia (CMML)
   e Essential thrombocythemia
   f. Polycythemia vera
5. Miscellaneous disorders and lesions
   a. Infections/abscess
   b. Storage diseases/infiltrative disorders
      i. Gaucher's disease
      ii. Nieman-pick disease
      iii. Amyloidosis
   c. Felty syndrome's
   d. Sarcoidosis
   e Cysts and tumors
   f. Portal hypertension
   g. Splenic artery aneurysm

Reproduced, with permission, from Brunicardi FC, Andersen DK, Billiar TR, et al. *Schwartz's Principles of Surgery*, 8th ed. New York: McGraw-Hill, 2004: 1301.

Escherichia coli O157:H7 is an invasive gastroenteritis resulting in hemolytic-uremic syndrome (HUS). HUS differs from TTP in severity and lack of neurologic symptoms.

Diagnostic pentad for TTP:
FAT RN
Fever
Anemia
Thrombocytopenia
Renal dysfunction
Neurologic dysfunction

Transfusing platelets in TTP is thought to "fuel the fire" and exacerbate consumption of platelets and clotting factors, resulting in more thrombi in the microvasculature. Plasmapheresis is the treatment of choice.

The spleen is the most commonly injured organ in blunt abdominal trauma, and trauma is the most common reason for splenectomy.

Complications

- **Overwhelming postsplenectomy sepsis.**
- Atelectasis (not taking deep breaths due to pain)/pneumonia (due to atelectasis sequestering bacteria).
- Pleural effusion (usually on the left).
- Subphrenic abscess.
- Injury to pancreas (because tail of pancreas "hugs" spleen).
- Postoperative hemorrhage.
- Thrombocytosis—many of the platelets that were sequestered in the spleen are now out in the circulation.

▶ TUMORS OF THE SPLEEN

Benign
- Hemangioma/lymphangioma
- Hamartomas
- Primary cyst/echinococcal cyst

Malignant
- Either lymphomas or myeloproliferative diseases.
- Rare site for solid tumor metastatic disease.
- A common site for metastases especially in lung and breast. However, it is rarely clinically significant and usually an autopsy finding.

▶ SPLENIC INJURY

SIGNS AND SYMPTOMS

- History: Check for preexisting diseases that cause splenomegaly (these patients are more vulnerable to splenic injury), details of injury mechanism.
- Exam: Look for peritoneal irritation, Kehr's sign, left-sided lower rib fractures, external signs of injury.

TREATMENT

Initial
- Airway, breathing, circulation (ABCs).
- Patients who are stable or who stabilize with fluid resuscitation may be considered for conservative management.
- Further diagnostic tools:
    - Computed tomographic (CT) scan: Able to define injury precisely.
    - Ultrasound (US): May be used for initial assessment to detect hemoperitoneum as a part of focused abdominal sonography for trauma (FAST) exam.
    - Diagnostic peritoneal lavage (DPL): Not specific for splenic injury but will show hemoperitoneum.
    - Angiogram: May be able to use therapeutically in the stable patient (embolization of CT-identified injury).

Definitive
- Nonoperative management criteria:
    - Stable.

TABLE 16-2. AAST Spleen Injury Scale (1994 Revision)

GRADE	INJURY TYPE	DESCRIPTION OF INJURY
I	Hematoma	Subcapsular, nonexpanding, < 10% surface area
	Laceration	Capsular tear, < 1 cm parenchymal depth
II	Hematoma	Subcapsular, 10–50% surface area; intraparenchymal, nonexpanding , < 5 cm in diameter
	Laceration	Capsular tear, 1–3 cm parenchymal depth that does not involve a trabecular vessel
III	Hematoma	Subcapsular, > 50% surface area or expanding; ruptured subcapsular hematoma with active bleeding; parenchymal hematoma ≥ 5 cm or expanding
	Laceration	> 3 cm parenchymal depth or involving trabecular vessels
IV	Hematoma	Ruptured intraparenchymal hematoma with active bleeding
	Laceration	Laceration involving segmental or hilar vessels producing major devascularization (> 25% of spleen)
V	Laceration	Completely shattered spleen
	Vascular	Hilar vascular injury with devascularized spleen

Reproduced, with permission, from the American Association for Surgery of Trauma, www.aast.org/injury/injury.html.

- Injury grade I or II (see Table 16-2).
- No evidence of injury to other intra-abdominal organs.
- Consists of bed rest, nasogastric tube (NGT) decompression, monitored setting, serial exam, and hematocrits.
- Operative management indications:
  - Signs and symptoms of ongoing hemorrhage.
  - Injury ≥ grade III.
  - Failure of nonoperative management.
- Exploratory laparotomy:
  - Perform splenectomy if the spleen is the primary source of exsanguinating hemorrhage.
  - If not, pack the area and search for other, more life-threatening injuries; address those first.
  - Subsequently, return to inspection of spleen. Mobilize fully unless the only injury is a minor nonbleeding one.
- Capsular bleeding and most grade II injuries: Apply direct pressure ± topical hemostatic agent.
- Persistently bleeding grade II or III injuries: Suture lacerations.
- Multiple injuries: Consider mesh splenorrhaphy for splenic preservation (especially in children).
- Complex fractures: Perform anatomic resection if possible, based on demarcation after segmental artery ligation.
- Perform splenectomy (see indications).

Causes of splenic rupture:
- Trauma: Rib fractures on the left (especially the 9th and 10th, which make up 20% of cases).
- Spontaneous rupture (associated with mononucleosis).

Thirty percent of patients with splenic injury will present with hypotensive shock due to hemorrhage.

Radiographic signs of splenic injury:
- CT: Low-density mass or intrasplenic accumulation of contrast.
- US: Perisplenic fluid, enlarged spleen, irregular borders, abnormal position, increase in size over time.

Patients with a vascular blush on CT scan are likely to fail nonoperative management.

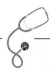

Patients who fail nonoperative management usually do so within 48–72 hours.

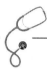

Pneumococcal vaccine will be needed for patients undergoing splenectomy. It may be given on the day of hospital discharge.

▶ **SPLENIC ABSCESS**

CAUSES

- Sepsis seeding
- Infection from adjacent structures
- Trauma
- Hematoma
- IV drug use

SIGNS AND SYMPTOMS

- Fever, chills.
- LUQ tenderness and guarding.
- Spleen may or may not be palpable.

DIAGNOSIS

- US: Enlarged spleen with areas of lucency contained within.
- CT: Abscess will show lower attenuation than surrounding spleen parenchyma. Defines abscess better than US.

TREATMENT

- Splenectomy for most cases.
- Percutaneous drainage for a large, solitary juxtacapsular abscess.

COMPLICATIONS

- Spontaneous rupture
- Peritonitis
- Sepsis

The Breast

Skin dimpling and retraction of nipple in breast cancer is due to traction on Cooper's ligaments.

The breast is a modified sebaceous gland composed of glandular, fibrous, and adipose tissue (see Figure 17-1).

- Lies within layers of superficial pectoral fascia.
- Each mammary gland consists of approximately 15–20 lobules, each of which has a lactiferous duct that opens on the areola.
- Has ligaments that extend from the deep pectoral fascia to the superficial dermal fascia that provide structural support referred to as **Cooper's ligaments.**
- Frequently extends into axilla as the **axillary tail of Spence.**
- Is partitioned into quadrants by vertical and horizontal lines across the nipple: Upper inner quadrant (UIQ), lower inner quadrant (LIQ), upper outer quadrant (UOQ), and lower outer quadrant (LOQ).

Blood Supply

- Arterial: Axillary artery via the lateral thoracic and thoracoacromial branches, internal mammary artery via its perforating branches, and adjacent intercostal arteries.

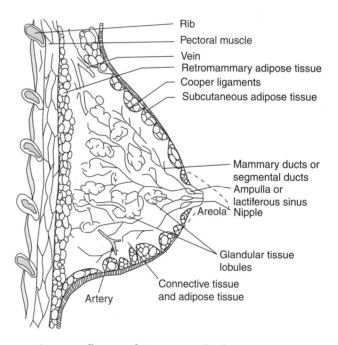

FIGURE 17-1.   Cut-away diagram of a mature resting breast.

The breast lies cushioned in fat between the overlying skin and the pectoralis major muscle. Both the skin and the retromammary space under the breast are rich with lymphatic channels. Cooper's ligaments, the suspensory ligaments of the breast, fuse with the overlying superficial fascia just under the dermis, coalesce as the interlobular fascia in the breast parenchyma, and then join with the deep fascia of breast over the pectoralis muscle. The system of ducts in the breast is configured like an inverted tree, with the largest ducts just under the nipple and successively smaller ducts in the periphery. After several branching generations, small ducts at the periphery enter the breast lobule, which is the milk-forming glandular unit of the breast. (Reproduced, with permission, from Peart O. *Lange Q&A: Mammography Examination*, 2nd ed. New York: McGraw-Hill, 2009: 124.)

■ Venous: Follows arterial supply; axillary, internal mammary, and intercostal veins; axillary vein responsible for majority of venous drainage.

Lymphatic Drainage

See Figure 17-2.

- ■ Level I: Lateral to lateral border of pectoralis minor.
- ■ Level II: Deep to pectoralis minor.
- ■ Level III: Medial to medial border of pectoralis minor.
- ■ **Rotter's nodes** lie between the pectoralis major and pectoralis minor muscles.
- ■ Lymphatic drainage from nipple, areola, and lobules all drain in a subareolar lymphatic plexus.
- ■ There is a quadrant-wise drainage:
  - ■ Lateral quadrants: Axillary nodes and supraclavicular through the pectoral, interpectoral (Rotter's) and deltopectoral.

Venous drainage is largely responsible for metastases to the spine through **paravertebral plexus of Batson.**

Lymph node involvement by tumor tends to progress from level I to III. The higher the level, the worse the prognosis.

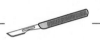

The medial pectoral nerve is actually lateral to the lateral pectoral nerve. The nerves are named according to their origin from the brachial plexus, not by their relation to one another on the chest wall.

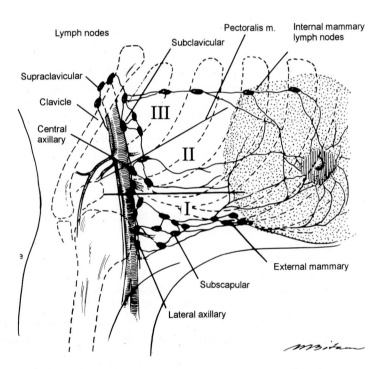

FIGURE 17-2. Contents of the axilla.

In this figure there are five named and contiguous groupings of lymph nodes in the full axilla. Complete axillary dissection, as done in the historical radical mastectomy, removes all these nodes. However, note that the subclavicular nodes in the axilla are continuous with the supraclavicular nodes in the neck and nodes between the pectoralis major and minor muscles, named the *interpectoral nodes* or *Rotter's lymph nodes*. The internal mammary nodes probably drain independently from the breast. The sentinel lymph node, located in modern sentinel biopsy, is functionally the first and lowest node in the axillary chain. Anatomically, the sentinel lymph node is usually found in the external mammary group. (Reproduced from: Zollinger RM Jr, Zollinger RM Sr. *Zollinger's Atlas of Surgical Operations*, 8th edition. New York, NY: McGraw-Hill; 2003: 397.)

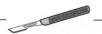

Perform breast self-examination at same time each month (one week after menstrual period is ideal).

Typical scenario: A female with one or more risk factors for breast cancer presents with a mass in the upper outer quadrant of the breast. *Think:* She's at risk for cancer, and 50% of breast cancers occur in the upper outer quadrant. Therefore, the mass is likely to be malignant.

The smallest mass palpable on physical exam is 1 cm.

- Medial quadrants: Parasternal nodes.
- Lower quadrants: Inferior phrenic (abdominal) nodes.

Nerves

See Table 17-1.

▶ **BOUNDARIES FOR AXILLARY DISSECTION**

See Figure 17-2.
- *Superior:* Axillary vein.
- *Posterior:* Long thoracic nerve.
- *Medial:* Either lateral to, underneath, or medial to the medial border of the pectoralis minor muscle, depending on the level of nodes taken.
- *Lateral:* Latissimus dorsi muscle.

▶ **INITIAL EVALUATION OF PATIENTS WITH POSSIBLE BREAST DISEASE**

- Complete medical history, including risk factors for breast cancer (see below). Be sure to inquire about any history of nipple discharge or any changes in the size, shape, symmetry, or contour of the breasts.
- Physical examination (see Figure 17-3).
- Inspection: Note color, symmetry, size, shape, and contour, and check for dimpling, erythema, edema, or thickening of skin with a porous appearance (**peau d'orange**).
- Palpation: Palpate all four quadrants and the nipple-areolar complex for any discharge.
- Axillary nodes are palpated along the lateral border of anterior and posterior axillary fold, the medial and lateral wall of the axilla and the apex of the axilla.

TABLE 17-1. Neural Structures Encountered During Major Breast Surgery

NERVES	MUSCLE(S)/AREA SUPPLIED	FUNCTIONAL DEFICIT IF INJURED
Long thoracic nerve (of Bell)	Serratus anterior	Winging of scapula
Thoracodorsal nerve	Latissimus dorsi	Cannot push oneself up from a sitting position
Medial and lateral pectoral nerves	Pectoralis major and minor	Weakness of pectoralis muscles
Intercostobrachial nerve	Crosses axilla transversely to supply inner aspect of arm	Area of anesthesia on inner aspect of arm

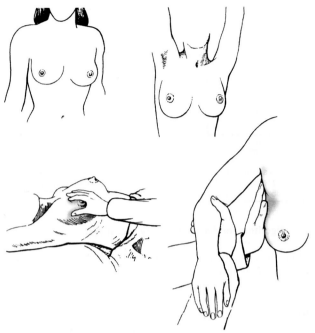

FIGURE 17-3. Examination of the breast.

A. Inspection of the breast with arms at sides. B. Inspection of the breast with arms raised. C. Palpation of the breast with the patient supine. D. Palpation of the axilla. (Reproduced, with permission, from Brunicardi FC, Andersen DK, Billiar TR, et al. *Schwartz's Principles of Surgery*, 8th ed. New York: Mc-Graw-Hill, 2004: 475.)

► **EVALUATION OF A PALPABLE BREAST MASS**

APPROACH

See Figures 17-4 and 17-5. If age < 30, serial physical examination with observation for 2–4 weeks or until next menstrual period is an option.

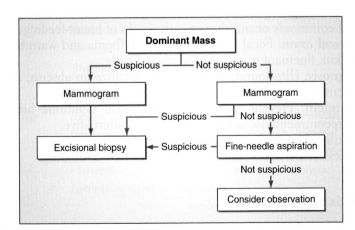

FIGURE 17-4. Algorithm for diagnosis of any breast mass (triple method—physical exam, radiology, and tissue diagnosis).

(Reproduced, with permission, from Fauci AS, Braunwald E, Kasper DL, et al. *Harrison's Principles of Internal Medicine*, 17th ed. New York: McGraw-Hill, 2008: 518.)

Fine-needle aspiration (FNA) is not sensitive enough to rule out malignancy (10% false-negative rate).

All persistent breast masses require evaluation.

Only presentations nonsuspicious of cancer:
- Lactating woman with focal erythematous warm swelling.
- Cyclical changing mass in young woman with clear aspirate.

Everything else is extensively worked up.

Typical scenario: A 42-year-old woman presents with an undiagnosed breast mass. *Think:* Evaluate without delay. Observation is not an option if age > 30.

A 14-year-old male complains of gynecomastia. Wait and watch. Perform surgery only if progressive.

Causes of gynecomastia:
- Increased estrogen (tumors, endocrine disorders, liver failure, obesity).
- Decreased testosterone (aging, primary or secondary testicular failure, Klinefelter's, renal failure).
- Drugs (e.g., spironolactone).

Tumors Running and Leaping Promptly to Bone:
- **Thyroid**
- **Renal**
- **Lung**
- **Prostate**
- **Breast**

Twenty percent of infiltrating lobular breast carcinoma have simultaneous contralateral breast cancer.

Gynecomastia

- **Definition:** Development of female-like breast tissue in males.
- May be physiologic (neonatal, adolescent, and senescent) or pathologic.
- At least 2 cm of excess subareolar breast tissue is required to make the diagnosis.
- **Treatment:** Treat underlying cause if specific cause identified; if normal physiology is responsible, only surgical excision (subareolar mastectomy) may be effective. Surgery is recommended only for progressive gynecomastia or for cosmetic reasons.

▶ PREMALIGNANT DISEASE

See Table 17-3.

▶ MALIGNANT TUMORS

Infiltrating Ductal Carcinoma

- Most common invasive breast cancer (80% of cases).
- Most common in perimenopausal and postmenopausal women.
- Ductal cells invade stroma in various histologic forms described as scirrhous, medullary, comedo, colloid, papillary, or tubular.
- Metastatic to axilla, bones, lungs, liver, brain.

Infiltrating Lobular Carcinoma

- Second most common type of invasive breast cancer (10% of cases).
- Originates from terminal duct cells and, like LCIS, has a high likelihood of being bilateral.
- Presents as an ill-defined thickening of the breast.
- Like LCIS, lacks microcalcifications and is often multicentric.
- Tends to metastasize to the axilla, meninges, and serosal surfaces.

Paget's Disease (of the Nipple)

- Two percent of all invasive breast cancers.
- Usually associated with underlying LCIS or ductal carcinoma extending within the epithelium of main excretory ducts to skin of nipple and areola.
- **Presentation:** Tender, itchy nipple with or without a bloody discharge with or without a subareolar palpable mass.
- **Treatment:** Usually requires a modified radical mastectomy.

Inflammatory Carcinoma

- Two to three percent of all invasive breast cancers.
- Most lethal breast cancer.
- Frequently presents as erythema, "peau d'orange," and nipple retraction.

- Dermal lymphatic invasion seen at pathologic evaluation.
- Inflammatory picture is due to the blockage of the efferent lymphatic ducts causing edema—"peau d'orange."
- **Treatment:** Consists of chemotherapy followed by surgery and/or radiation, depending on response to chemotherapy.

TABLE 17-3. Premalignant Disease

DISEASE	DCIS	LCIS
Cell of origin	Inner layer of epithelial cells in major ducts	Cells of terminal duct–lobular unit
Definition	Proliferation of ductal cells that spread through the ductal system but lack the ability to invade the basement membrane	A multifocal proliferation of acinar and terminal ductal cells
Age and sex	More than half of cases occur after menopause; 5% of male cancer	Vast majority of cases occur prior to menopause; Never seen in males
Palpable mass	Sometimes	Never
Diagnosis	Clustered microcalcifications on mammogram, malignant epithelial cells in breast duct on biopsy	Typically a clinically occult lesion; undetectable by mammogram and incidental on biopsy
Lymphatic invasion	< 1%	Rare
Risk of invasive	Considered the anatomic precursor of breast carcinoma. Increased risk in ipsilateral breast, usually same quadrant; infiltrating ductal carcinoma most common histologic type; comedo type has the worst prognosis	Considered as a marker of breast carcinoma. Equally increased risk in either breast, infiltrating ductal carcinoma also most common histologic type (counterintuitive); associated with simultaneous LCIS in the contralateral breast in over half of cases
Treatment	• If small (< 2 cm): Lumpectomy with either close follow-up or radiation • If large (> 2 cm): Lumpectomy with 1-cm margins and radiation • If breast diffusely involved: Simple mastectomy	None; bilateral mastectomy an option if patient is high risk

Typical scenario: A 65-year-old female presents with a pruritic, scaly rash of her nipple–areolar complex and a bloody nipple discharge. *Think:* Paget's disease. Biopsy and pathologic exam required to confirm diagnosis.

Greater than 75% of patients have axillary metastases at time of diagnosis of inflammatory breast carcinoma, and distant metastases are common.

Paget's disease of vagina is a similar disease, presenting as a scaly, pruritic rash of the vagina.

Typical scenario: A 45-year-old female presents with enlargement of her left breast with nipple retraction, erythema, warmth, and induration. *Think:* Inflammatory breast carcinoma.

HIGH-YIELD FACTS

The Breast

Fibrocystic changes of the breast alone are not a risk factor for breast cancer.

Despite all known risk factors, most women with breast cancer (75%) present without any identifiable risk factors.

Genetic syndromes associated with breast cancer:
- Autosomal dominant:
    - Li-Fraumeni
    - Muir-Torre
    - BRCA1 and BRCA2 Cowden's syndrome
    - Peutz–Jeghers syndrome
- Autosomal recessive:
    - Ataxia-telangiectasia

EPIDEMIOLOGY

- One in eight women will develop breast cancer in their lifetime.
- Second most common cause of cancer death among women overall (lung cancer is number 1).
- Incidence increases with increasing age.
- One percent of breast cancers occur in men.

RISK FACTORS

- Any change that causes increased exposure to estrogen without the protective effects of progesterone.
- Early menarche (< 12).
- Late menopause (> 55).
- Nulliparity or first pregnancy > 30 years.
- White race.
- Old age.
- History of breast cancer in mother or sister (especially if bilateral or premenopausal).
- Genetic predisposition (BRCA1 or BRCA2 positive, Li-Fraumeni syndrome).
- Prior personal history of breast cancer.
- Previous breast biopsy.
- DCIS or LCIS.
- Atypical ductal or lobular hyperplasia.
- Postmenopausal estrogen replacement (unopposed by progesterone).
- Radiation exposure.

GENETIC PREDISPOSITION

- Five to ten percent of breast cancers are associated with an inherited mutation.
- p53: A tumor suppressor gene; Li-Fraumeni syndrome results from a p53 mutation.
- Both BRCA1 and BRCA2 function as tumor-suppressor genes, and for each gene, loss of both alleles is required for the initiation of cancer.
    - BRCA1 and BRCA2 both are inherited in an autosomal dominant fashion with varying penetrance.
    - BRCA1: On 17q, also associated with ovarian cancer.
    - BRCA2: On chromosome 13q, also associated with male breast cancer.
- Somatic mutation of p53 in 50% and of Rb in 20% of breast cancers.

SCREENING RECOMMENDATIONS (FROM THE AMERICAN CANCER SOCIETY)

See Table 17-4. Screening reduces mortality by 30–40%.

DIAGNOSIS AND TREATMENT

Diagnostic Options
- **Ultrasound:**
    - (++) No ionizing radiation.
    - (+) Good for identifying cystic disease and can also assist in therapeutic aspiration.
    - (+) Results easily reproducible.

TABLE 17-4. American Cancer Society Recommendations for Breast Cancer Detection in Asymptomatic Women

AGE GROUP	EXAMINATION	FREQUENCY
20–39	Breast self-examination	Monthly
	Clinical breast examination	Every 3 years
40 and older	Breast self-examination	Monthly
	Clinical breast examination	Annually
	Mammography	Annually

Reproduced, with permission, from Chen MYM, Pope TL, Ott DJ. *Basic Radiology*. New York: McGraw-Hill, 1996: 123.

- ▪ (–) Resolution inferior to mammogram.
- ▪ (–) Will not identify lesions < 1 cm.
- ▪ **Mammography:** See Figure 17-6.
  - ▪ Identifies 5 cancers/1,000 women.
  - ▪ Sensitivity 85–90%.
  - ▪ False positive 10%, false negative 6–8%.
  - ▪ If cancer is first detected by mammogram, 80% have negative lymph nodes (versus 45% when detected clinically). Mammography picks up early disease and hence is a good screening test.
    - ▪ Suspicious finding: Stellate, speculated mass with associated microcalcifications.
- ▪ **Reporting mammogram results (Breast Imaging Reporting and Data System—BIRADS):**
  0: Assesment incomplete
  1: Negative
  2: Benign finding

Start yearly mammograms 10 years before the age at which first-degree relative was diagnosed with breast cancer.

Mammography is more useful if age > 30 because the large proportion of fibrous tissue ("dense tissue") in younger women's breasts make mammograms more difficult to interpret.

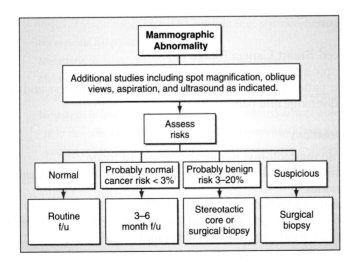

FIGURE 17-6. Approaches to abnormalities detected by mammogram.

(Reproduced, with permission, from Fauci AS, Braunwald E, Kasper DL, et al. *Harrison's Principles of Internal Medicine*, 17th ed. New York: McGraw-Hill, 2008: 518.)

TABLE 17-6. **Staging System for Breast Cancer**

Stage 0	DCIS or LCIS
Stage I	Invasive carcinoma ≤ 2 cm in size (including carcinoma in situ with micro invasion) without nodal involvement and no distant metastases
Stage II	Invasive carcinoma ≤ 5 cm in size with involved but movable axillary nodes and no distant metastases, or a tumor > 5 cm without nodal involvement or distant metastases
Stage III	Breast cancers > 5 cm in size with nodal involvement; or any breast cancer with fixed axillary nodes; or any breast cancer with involvement of the ipsilateral internal mammary lymph nodes; or any breast cancer with skin involvement, pectoral and chest wall fixation, edema, or clinical inflammatory carcinoma, if distant metastases are absent
Stage IV	Any form of breast cancer with distant metastases

- Breast conservation is considered for all patients with stage I or II cancer because of the important cosmetic advantages. Relative contraindications to breast conservation therapy include:
  - Prior radiation therapy to the breast or chest wall.
  - Involved surgical margins or unknown margin status following reexcision.
  - Multicentric disease.
  - Scleroderma or other connective-tissue disease.
- **Sentinel node biopsy:** Recently developed alternative to complete axillary node dissection:
  - Done only if there are no palpable nodes.
  - Based on the principle that metastatic tumor cells migrate in an orderly fashion to first draining lymph node(s).
  - Lymph nodes are identified on preoperative nuclear scintigraphy and blue dye is injected in the periareolar area.
  - Axilla is opened and inspected for blue and/or "hot" nodes identified by a gamma probe.
  - When sentinel node(s) is positive, an axillary dissection is completed.

TABLE 17-7. **Hormone Receptor Status Response to Therapy**

HORMONE RECEPTOR STATUS	RESPONSE TO HORMONAL THERAPY (ESTROGEN BLOCKERS OR AROMATASE INHIBITORS)
ER+/PR+	80%
ER–/PR+	45%
ER+/PR–	35%
ER/PR–	10%

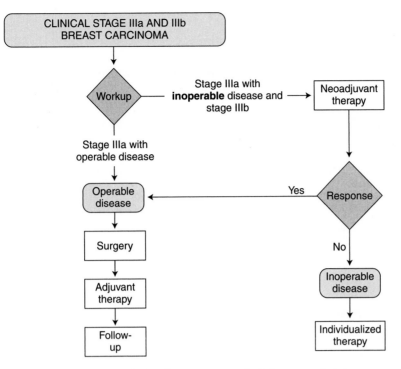

FIGURE 17-7. Treatment pathways for stage IIIa and IIIb breast carcinoma.

- When sentinel node(s) is negative, an axillary dissection is not performed unless axillary lymphadenopathy is identified.

HORMONAL THERAPY: TAMOXIFEN

- Selective estrogen receptor modulator (SERM) that blocks the uptake of estrogen by target tissues.
- Side effects will simulate menopause: Hot flashes, irregular menses; thromboembolism and increased risk for endometrial cancer due to selective hormone agonist action.
- Therapy of choice for postmenopausal women with positive receptors. Survival benefit for pre- and postmenopausal women, but benefit greater for ER-positive patients.
- May get additional benefit by combining tamoxifen with chemotherapy.

CHEMOTHERAPY

- Any number of regimens are acceptable. Adriamycin, 5-fluorouracil, methotrexate, cyclophosphamide, and paclitaxel (Taxol) are some of the agents used.
- Herceptin is used for HER2/neu-positive patients.

RECONSTRUCTION

- Done in patients after mastectomy.
- Can use either prosthetic or autologous implants. May also use an expander and implant at a later date.
- Prosthetic implant may be either saline or silicone based.
- Autologous tissue can be either rectus muscle or latissimus dorsi muscle myocutaneous flap.

Raloxifene is another SERM that has been used for breast cancer prevention. It does not increase uterine cancer risk.

RECURRENCE

- Five to ten percent local recurrence at 10 years.
- Metastases in < 10% of cases.
- Local chest wall recurrence most common within 2–3 years, if at all.

METASTASIS

- Median survival 2 years.
- Palliative therapy indicated.

PROGNOSIS

The 5-year survival rate is:

- Stage I: 94%
- Stage II: 70–85%
- Stage III: 48–52%
- Stage IV: 18%

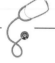

Termination of pregnancy is not part of the treatment plan for breast cancer and does not improve survival.

Breast Cancer in Pregnant and Lactating Women

- Three breast cancers are diagnosed per 10,000 pregnancies.
- A fine-needle aspiration should be performed. If it identifies a solid mass, then it should be followed by biopsy.
- Mammography is possible as long as proper shielding is used.
- Radiation is not advisable for the pregnant woman. Thus, for stage I or II cancer, a modified radical mastectomy should be done rather than a lumpectomy with axillary node dissection and postoperative radiation.
- If lymph nodes are positive, delay chemotherapy until the second trimester.
- Suppress lactation after delivery. If it is diagnosed in the third trimester, lumpectomy can be done and radiation given postpartum.

Males with breast cancer often have direct extension to the chest wall at diagnosis.

Breast Cancer in Males

- Predisposing factors: Klinefelter's syndrome, estrogen therapy, elevated endogenous estrogen, previous irradiation, and trauma.
- Infiltrating ductal carcinoma most common histologic type (men lack breast lobules).
- Diagnosis tends to be late, when the patient presents with a mass, nipple retraction, and skin changes.
- Stage by stage, survival is the same as it is in women. However, more men are diagnosed at a later stage.
- Treatment for early-stage cancer involves a modified radical mastectomy and postoperative radiation.
- Sentinel node biopsy and estrogen receptor status may help to stage disease.

Burns

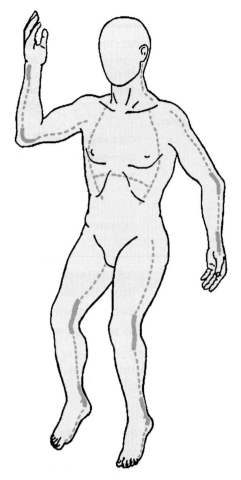

FIGURE 18-2. Locations for escharotomies.

The incisions are placed along the mid-medial lines of the extremities and the thorax (dashed lines). The skin is especially tight along major joints, and decompression at these sites must be complete (solid lines). Neck and digital escharotomies are rarely necessary. (Reproduced, with permission, from Brunicardi FC, Andersen DK, Billiar TR, et al. *Schwartz's Principles of Surgery*, 8th ed. New York: McGraw-Hill, 2004: 194).

> Limit burn excision operations to excision of < 20% BSA at one trip to the OR or to a set time limit of 2 hours.

- Once debridement is complete, the wound is covered with split-thickness skin graft (STSG), full-thickness graft, or biologic dressing.
- Wound closure.
- STSG may be applied when the burn is excised or there is no residual nonviable tissue, no pooled secretions, and surface bacterial count is $< 10^5/cm^2$.
- Autograft should be 0.010–0.015 inches thick:
  - Donor sites may be reharvested (after 2–3 weeks when reepithelialization is complete), but the quality decreases each time as dermis is thinner.
  - Grafts may be meshed at a ratio of 1.5:1 to increase coverage, unless burns are on face or joints.
  - If the risk of mortality is anticipated to be < 50%, first graft hands, feet, face, and joints.
  - If > 50%, graft flat surfaces first to decrease uncovered surface area.

- Biologic dressings: Bilaminate; outer layer with pores to permit water vapor but not liquid or bacterial passage, and inner layer that permits ingrowth of fibrovascular tissue from wound surface.

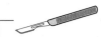

▶ INFECTION

- Infection of a burn wound causes an increase in the depth (thus converts a second-degree burn to a third-degree).
- Biopsy of the wound is the most definitive way to diagnose burn wound infection.
- Burn patients are very prone to pneumonia and catheter-related infections.

TREATMENT

- For invasive infection, use topical antimicrobials (see Table 18-1) and start systemic antibiotics.
- For pseudomonal or pediatric infections, infuse subeschar piperacillin, and plan for emergent operative debridement within 12 hours.
- For candidal infections, start antifungal creams; if that treatment fails, start systemic therapy with amphotericin B.

Burn debridement with the Goulian knife is frequently accompanied by a significant amount of blood loss, which can be minimized by using topical thrombin spray and infiltration with epinephrine or vasopressin.

Infection is more likely in patients with > 30% BSA burn without complete excision or grafting. Apparently infected wounds need to be examined daily and biopsied, including eschar and underlying unburned tissue.

▶ INHALATIONAL INJURY AND CARBON MONOXIDE POISONING

- In closed space burns.
- Carbon monoxide impairs tissue oxygenation by decreasing oxygen-carrying capacity of blood, shifting oxygen-hemoglobin dissociation curve to the left, binding myoglobin and terminal cytochrome oxidase.
- Symptoms do not correlate well with carboxyhemoglobin levels, but levels up to 10% are typically asymptomatic.

SIGNS AND SYMPTOMS

Patients may have hoarse voice, cough, wheeze, bronchorrhea, hypoxemia, carbonaceous sputum, head and neck burns, singed nose hairs.

DIAGNOSIS

- Often delayed but is made with the use of chest x-ray (CXR), bronchoscopy, and ventilation-perfusion (V/Q) scan.
- Measure carboxyhemoglobin with ABG.
- Bronchoscopy reveals edema and ulceration.
- V/Q scanning will demonstrate carbon particle deposition on endobronchial mucosa.

TREATMENT

- Half-life of carbon monoxide decreased from 4 hours on room air to 45–60 minutes with 100% oxygen and 15–20 minutes at 3 atmospheric pressure (hyperbaric oxygen).
- Mild injury: Use warm humidified oxygen and an incentive spirometer.
- Moderate: Repeated bronchoscopy when there is continued mucosal sloughing and the patient is unable to clear it.
- Severe, with progressive hypoxemia: Intubation.

Mortality of burns with inhalational injury is increased compared to burns without inhalational injury.

HIGH-YIELD FACTS

Burns

Carbon monoxide is a colorless, tasteless, odorless gas and has an affinity for hemoglobin 200 times that of oxygen.

Normal carboxyhemoglobin: 3–5% nonsmokers; 7–10% smokers.

Extent of damage from electrical injury depends on both current density and tissue conduction. The surface wound usually underestimates the extent of damage to deeper tissues.

5 Ps of compartment syndrome:
- **Pain**
- **Paresthesia**
- **Pallor**
- **Pulselessness**
- **Poikilothermia**

Strong acid burns may leave a deceptively healthy appearance of tan smooth skin.

COMPLICATIONS

Most commonly, pneumonia.

► ELECTRICAL INJURY

DEFINITION

- Extent of injury depends on voltage of current:
  - Up to 1000 volts—increased resistance limits further passage of current and heating of tissue.
  - More than 1000 volts—passage of current is not limited and tissue injury can continue.
  - Deeper tissue may be more severely injured because it cools more slowly.

MECHANISM

- Tissue damaged via conversion to thermal energy.
- Damage occurs in skin and underlying tissues along the course of current.
- Skin at the point of contact is often severely charred.

SIGNS AND SYMPTOMS

- Charring at point of contact.
- Myoglobinuria (with muscle damage).
- Hyperkalemia (due to tissue necrosis).
- High-voltage or lightning injury may cause cardiac arrest.
- Neuropathy (immediately following injury, likely to resolve over time).
- Compartment syndrome: Swelling of injured extremity with pain, paresthesia, pallor, pulselessness, poikilothermia.

TREATMENT

- Patients with loss of consciousness or abnormal ECG require cardiac monitoring for 48 hours even if there are no further arrhythmias or ECG changes.
- Electrical injury is more likely than other types of burn injury to necessitate fasciotomy because deep tissue edema may be extensive, causing compartment syndrome.

LATE COMPLICATIONS

- Delayed hemorrhage because of inadequate wound exploration, debridement, or exposure of vessel.
- Cataracts.

► CHEMICAL INJURY

MECHANISM

- General: Protein denaturation and precipitation, with release of thermal energy.
- Liquefaction necrosis (alkali).
- Delipidation (petroleum products).
- Vesicle formation (vesicant gas).

SEVERITY

Determined by:

- Concentration
- Amount of agent in contact.
- Duration of contact (tissue injury continues to occur as long as the agent remains in contact with the skin).

PRIORITIES IN TREATMENT

- Remove all clothing to prevent further contact.
- Copious water lavage: Irrigation should continue for at least 30 minutes for acid burns, and longer for alkali burns (because they penetrate deeper into the tissue).
- Check pulmonary status (for edema, mucosal desquamation, bronchospasm).

Chemical wound irrigation should be with water only. Attempts to neutralize the agent may cause further release of heat, thereby causing further damage.

▶ **NUTRITION OF BURN PATIENTS**

- Enteral route preferred (total parenteral nutrition [TPN] only if enteral is not possible).
- Early feeding recommended.
- High calorie (30–35 Kcal/kg/day) and high protein (1.5–2 g/kg/day) requirements.

▶ **BURN SCAR CANCER**

- Rare long-term complication of burn scars (can occur in scars of any origin).
- Called Marjolin's ulcer.
- Usually squamous cell carcinoma, which metastasizes via lymph nodes.
- Diagnosis made by biopsy.
- **Treatment:** Wide excision.

HIGH-YIELD FACTS

Burns

HIGH-YIELD FACTS

Burns

High-Yield Facts for Surgical Electives

SECTION III

High-Yield Facts
for Surgical Electives

Anesthesia

The **8 Ps** of rapid-sequence intubation:

Prepare = equipment
Pretreat = drugs
Position = sniffing position
Preoxygenate = 100% O_2
Pressure = Sellick
Paralyze = drugs
Placement of the tube
Position of the tube =
   confirm by two methods

Actually seeing the tube pass between the vocal cords (direct visualization) is the best method to confirm endotracheal tube (ETT) placement. The next best method is end-tidal CO_2.

Definition

- Drug-induced loss of consciousness during which patients are not arousable, even by painful stimulation.
- Ability to independently maintain ventilatory function is often impaired; therefore, airway assistance by way of intubation, laryngeal mask airway, or other adjunct is usually necessary.

Stages of Anesthesia

Anesthetic drug effects can be divided into four stages of increasing depth of central nervous system depression:

Stage I: Analgesia stage
Stage II: Excitement stage
Stage III: Surgical anesthesia stage
Stage IV: Medullary depression stage

ASA Classification of Surgical Patients

See Table 19-1.

Induction

INTRAVENOUS ANESTHETICS

Intravenous agents are the most common way of inducing patients (see Table 19-2).

INHALED ANESTHETICS

See Table 19-3.

TABLE 19-1. ASA Physical Status Classification System and Expected Mortality

P1	A normal healthy patient (mortality: 0.1%)
P2	A patient with mild systemic disease (mortality: 0.2%)
P3	A patient with severe systemic disease (mortality: 1.8%)
P4	A patient with severe systemic disease that is a constant threat to life (mortality: 7.8%)
P5	A moribund patient who is not expected to survive without the operation (mortality: 9.4%)
P6	A declared brain-dead patient whose organs are being removed for donor purposes

Reproduced, with permission, from Brunicardi FC, Andersen DK, Billiar TR, et al. *Schwartz's Principles of Surgery*, 8th ed. New York: McGraw-Hill, 2004: 1860.

TABLE 19-2. Intravenous Induction Agents

INDUCTION AGENT	ONSET OF ACTION	DURATION OF ACTION	IV PUSH DOSE	CONTRAINDICATIONS/CAVEATS
Thiopental	< 1 min	5–10 min	3.0–5.0 mg/kg	Hypotension, asthma
Methohexital	< 1 min	5–10 min	1.0–2.0 mg/kg	Seizures, hypotension, asthma
Etomidate	< 1 min	5 min	0.3 mg/kg	Age < 10, pregnant/lactating
Fentanyl	2–4 min	45 min	2–5 μg/kg	Hypotension
Midazolam	30 sec	6–15 min	0.05–0.1 mg/kg (6 mos–5 yrs) 0.025–0.05 mg/kg (6–12 yrs) 5–10 mg (adults)	▪ Narrow-angle glaucoma ▪ Decrease dosage in elderly and patients receiving concurrent erythromycin or drugs that inhibit P_{450} system
Ketamine	1 min	10–20 min	1.0–1.5 mg/kg	Head trauma, elevated intracranial pressure
Propofol	40 sec	3–6 min	2–2.5 mg/kg	▪ Propofol comes as a lipid emulsion ▪ Use with caution in patients with disorders of lipid metabolism ▪ Use of aseptic technique especially important to prevent sepsis (emulsion is a great growth medium!)

Neuromuscular Blockade

- It is important to realize that muscle relaxation does not ensure unconsciousness, amnesia, or analgesia.
- Postsynaptic receptors: Located in the neuromuscular junction, they are the site of action of neuromuscular blockers, blocking acetylcholine transmission.
- Depolarizing muscle relaxants (succinylcholine) act as acetylcholine (ACh) receptor agonists, whereas nondepolarizing muscle relaxants (pancuronium, vecuronium, atracurium) function as competitive antagonists.
- Atracurium and cis-atracurium undergo degradation in plasma at physiological pH and temperature by organ-independent Hofmann elimination and so can be used in patients with hepatic and renal dysfunction.
- Anticholinesterases prevent breakdown of ACh, thus allowing ACh to compete more effectively with the paralyzing agents. Can be used to "reverse" neuromuscular blockade of nondepolarizing agents (at end of surgery).

Maintenance

Involves use of inhalational agents (e.g., nitrous oxide, isoflurane, sevoflurane, desflurane) and IV agents (e.g., opiates, ketamine, propofol).

Succinylcholine is contraindicated in the following situations:
- Hyperkalemia
- Burns
- Rhabdomyolysis
- Narrow-angle glaucoma
- Guillain-Barré syndrome
- Malignant hyperthermia
- Other special neuropathies

Nitrous oxide can diffuse into closed spaces/lumens, causing expansion of bowel or worsening of pneumothorax.

HIGH-YIELD FACTS

Anesthesia

TABLE 19-3. Properties of Inhaled Anesthetics

Anesthetic	Blood:Gas Partition Coefficient[a]	Brain:Blood Partition Coefficient[a]	Minimal Alveolar Conc (MAC) (%)[b]	Metabolism	Comments
Nitrous oxide	0.47	1.1	> 100	None	Incomplete anesthetic; rapid onset and recovery
Desflurane	0.42	1.3	6–7	< 0.05%	Low volatility; poor induction agent; rapid recovery
Sevoflurane	0.69	1.7	2.0	2–5% (fluoride)	Rapid onset and recovery; unstable in soda-lime
Isoflurane	1.40	2.6	1.40	< 2%	Medium rate of onset and recovery
Enflurane	1.80	1.4	1.7	8%	Medium rate of onset and recovery
Halothane	2.30	2.9	0.75	> 40%	Medium rate of onset and recovery
Methoxyflurane	12	2.0	0.16	> 70% (fluoride)	Very slow onset and recovery

[a] Partition coefficients (at 37° C) are from multiple literature sources.

[b] MAC is the anesthetic concentration that produces immobility in 50% of patients exposed to a noxious stimulus.

Reproduced, with permission, from Katzung BG. *Basic and Clinical Pharmacology,* 10th ed. New York: McGraw-Hill, 2007: 398.

During emergence, patient is at risk for aspiration and for laryngospasm (involuntary spasm of laryngeal musculature, resulting in the inability to ventilate the patient).

Halothane hepatitis is an immune-mediated hepatotoxicity associated with use of halothane (an inhalational anesthetic). Incidence is 1/22,000 to 1/35,000.

Emergence

- Return of patient to an awake state.
- Patient should have full muscle strength and protective airway reflexes before extubation.

Airway: Due to anatomy of pediatric airway, intubation can be more challenging (see Table 19-4).

TABLE 19-4. Ways Pediatric Airway Differs from Adult

Larger occiput
Large tongue
Larynx is higher up (C3 vs. C4–5) and funnel shaped so narrowest portion of airway is beyond what you see!
Vocal cords are at a slant and more anterior

Anatomy

- Subarachnoid space lies between arachnoid and pia mater, which contains cerebrospinal fluid (CSF).
- Spinal cord ends at L1–L2.
- Iliac crests are at level of L4.

Spinal Anesthesia

- For surgeries of lower extremities, lower abdomen, genitourinary, and anal region.
- Insert needle at L3–L4 or L4–L5 (at this level cauda equina is present and spinal cord has already ended).

Epidural Anesthesia

- Indicated for same surgeries as with spinal anesthesia.
- Differs from spinal anesthesia in that needle is placed in epidural space (outside of CSF); commonly an indwelling catheter is left in place.
- With catheter, can have continuous anesthesia (can periodically bolus the catheter for prolonged surgeries).
- Takes longer to obtain effect and requires higher dosages than spinal anesthesia.
- Technically more difficult and requires more time to place than spinal anesthesia.

COMPLICATIONS

See Table 19-5.

TABLE 19-5. Complications of Spinal and Epidural Anesthesia

COMPLICATION	SPINAL	EPIDURAL
Hypotension (from sympathetic nervous system blockade)	More common	Less common
Nausea (from unopposed parasympathetic activity)	More common	Less common
Postspinal headache (due to CSF leak)	Less common	Occurs only with inadvertent dural puncture during epidural placement
Urinary retention	Common	Common
Backache	Common	Common
Permanent neurologic injury	Very rare	Very rare
Epidural abscess or hematoma	N/A	Rare

Platelet dysfunction is a qualitative defect that affects bleeding time only. Does not affect prothrombin time (PT) or partial thromboplastin time (PTT).

It is important to limit intraoperative fluid replacement in ESRD to prevent risk of pulmonary congestion.

Infants and children are not just small adults; their physiology is dramatically different, affecting their anesthetic management during surgery.

Remember, the narrowest part of a child's airway is at the glottic opening, beyond what is visualized with a laryngoscope.

Obstetric patients are at increased risk for aspiration when general anesthesia is undertaken.

Spinal anesthesia is generally used for surgeries lasting no more than 2–3 hours, since the anesthetic is injected only once.

Think of spinal anesthesia as placing needle closer (deeper) to spinal canal than epidural anesthesia.

Amide anesthetics have "i" before "caine" (e.g., prilocaine, lidocaine, bupivacaine).

Do not use epinephrine in these areas: **SPF-10**
Scrotum
Penis
Fingers
Toes
Ears
Nose

Local Anesthesia

- Used for local infiltration of operative site, during spinal or epidural anesthesia, and peripheral nerve blocks.
- Classification: Ester or amide anesthetic.
- Mechanism of action: Through blockade of sodium channels.
- Myelinated fibers: More susceptible to blockade.
- Sensory fibers: More readily blocked than motor nerves (dose needed for motor blockade is usually double that needed for sensory block).
- Nonionized form: Needed to cross nerve sheath while the ionized form is the active form.
- Acidosis: Local tissue acidosis as from infection increases ionized drug form and limits anesthetic activity of the drug. Therefore, local infiltration into an area of infection may not produce adequate analgesia.
- Epinephrine: Adding this to the local anesthetic prolongs duration of action by vasoconstriction. Avoid epinephrine in areas with lack of collateral blood flow.
- Toxicity: Initially central nervous system (CNS) effects (tinnitus, restlessness, vertigo, seizures), then cardiovascular effects (hypotension, PR prolongation, QRS widening, dysrhythmias).

► MALIGNANT HYPERTHERMIA

DEFINITION

Autosomal dominant inherited hypermetabolic syndrome occurring after exposure to an anesthetic agent (very rare, but life threatening).

ETIOLOGY

Impaired reuptake of calcium by sarcoplasmic reticulum in muscles.

SIGNS AND SYMPTOMS

- Tachycardia, ventricular dysrhythmias
- Hyperthermia
- Hypercarbia, acidosis
- Hypoxemia
- Muscle rigidity

TREATMENT

- Discontinue anesthetics.
- Benzodiazepines (work fastest to control hypermetabolic state).
- Dantrolene sodium (a calcium channel blocker considered more definitive treatment, but onset of action takes about 30 minutes).

Vascular Surgery

Layers of Arterial Wall

- **Intima:** One layer of endothelial cells overlying a matrix of collagen and elastin.
- **Media:** Thick layer of smooth muscle cells, collagen, and elastic fibers.
- **Adventitia:** Collagen and elastin, important component to wall strength.

Types of Arteries

- **Elastic:** Major vessels, including aorta, subclavian, carotid, pulmonary arteries.
- **Muscular:** Branches from elastic arteries: Radial, femoral, coronary, cerebral.
- **Arterioles:** Terminal branches to capillary beds.

Venous Anatomy

- Also three layers, but adventitia is most prominent, and intima and media are generally thin.
- Valves prevent reflux.

► **VASCULAR PHYSICAL EXAM**

Inspection

Signs of vascular insufficiency:

- Hairless, shiny skin.
- Change of skin color—darkening, mottling, reddening, blanching.
- Nail changes.
- Presence of ulcers or gangrene.
- Edema, erythema.

Auscultation

Auscultation for bruits: Carotid, abdomen, common femoral artery (CFA).

Palpation

- Temperature: Cool extremities worrisome for poor circulation.
- Edema.

PULSATILE MASSES

- Pulsations of normal aorta are palpable in thin people.
- Examine abdomen with both hands around epigastrium and periumbilical area for abdominal aortic aneurysm (AAA).
- Easily palpable pulses in either lower quadrant indicate distal aortic or common iliac aneurysm.

If you are not sure whether pulse is palpable, count out pulses with second person palpating an easier artery such as the radial artery. If pulsations are simultaneous, you are likely palpating pulse accurately.

Contrast contains iodine and is renally excreted. Therefore, you should use < 200 cc of dye, and use with caution in patients with renal dysfunction. Ask patients about iodine and shellfish allergies.

EXTREMITY PULSES

- Include brachial, radial, ulnar, femoral, popliteal, dorsalis pedis (DP), posterior tibial.
- Patient should be reclining in supine position, with full exposure of abdomen and legs.
- Legs should be in gentle extension with feet supported.
- To examine pedal pulses, sit at foot of table facing patient.
- Common femoral artery: Found halfway from pubic tubercle to anterior superior iliac spine.
- Popliteal artery: Place both hands in the middle of the fossa, with fingertips parallel longways (fossa: area between pes anserinus tendon laterally, medial head of gastrocnemius and biceps tendon medially, and biceps and lateral head of gastrocnemius laterally).
- Pedal pulses:
  - DP found between proximal first and second metatarsal (slight dorsiflexion may facilitate).
  - Posterior tibial found posterior to medial malleolus.

▶ DIAGNOSTIC TESTS

Doppler

Relates average flow velocity to frequency shift.

Duplex

Combines real-time ultrasound with Doppler analysis.

Plethysmography

Measures volume change in organ or body region:
- Pulse volume recording (PVR): Used with Doppler to assess perfusion of distal extremities, assuming change in volume corresponds to change in arterial pressure; useful to predict healing of ulcers and amputations.
- Other types of plethysmography (seldom used):
  - Ocular plethysmography
  - *Impedance plethysmography*
  - *Photoplethysmography*

Segmental Blood Pressure Measurement

- **Ankle-brachial index (ABI):** Systolic blood pressure (SBP) ankle (via Doppler) / highest SBP in upper extremities.
  - ≥ 1: Normal
  - 0.5–0.7: Claudication
  - ≤ 0.3: Ischemic rest pain, gangrene

- Penile-brachial index (PBI): Used to help determine whether cause of impotence is vascular.
  - PBI < 0.6 indicates likely vascular etiology.
  - Misleading results associated with:
    - Diabetic patients, as calcification of vessels makes them less compressible, thereby elevating results falsely.
    - Collateral flow in long-standing insufficiency may artificially improve results.

Arteriography

- Use of contrast dye with fluoroscopy to delineate arteries.
- Risks: Hemorrhage, allergic reaction to dye, thrombosis of puncture site, embolization of clot, renal dysfunction.
- Dose-independent reactions to dye: Asthma, laryngeal edema, spasm, cardiovascular (CV) collapse.
- **Complications:**
  - Neurologic deficits secondary to emboli.
  - Bleeding: Hematoma, hemorrhage at site.
  - Decreased pulses compared to pre-angio: If resolves within 1 hour, may be due to spasm; otherwise, consider arterial injury, clot.
- Postprocedure:
  - Maintain patient supine for at least 6 hours.
  - Check puncture site for hematoma or false aneurysm.
  - Follow neurologic exam, including mental status.
  - Maintain well-hydrated state.

Digital Subtraction Angiography (DSA)

Dye is injected into vein or artery, and computerized fluoroscopy subtracts bone and soft tissue, so that only arterial system is visible.

Spiral Computed Tomography (CT)

Especially useful for AAA.

Magnetic Resonance Angiography (MRA)

- Allows good visualization of patent distal vessels with minimal flow; also useful for evaluation of carotid bifurcation and abdominal aorta.
- Advantage: No contrast used.
- Gadolinium causes allergic reactions in fewer patients.
- Disadvantage: cost, limited ability to visualize arterial calcification.

▶ ACUTE ARTERIAL OCCLUSION

ETIOLOGY

- Embolization: From heart or any proximal artery.
- Trauma: Posterior knee dislocation, long-bone fracture, penetrating trauma.

A pseudoaneurysm does not contain all three layers of the arterial wall.

Typical scenario: You are asked to see a patient with bleeding from an angiogram puncture site. She has an oozing, pulsatile expanding mass in her groin at the puncture site. *Think:* Expanding hematoma. Maintain direct pressure for 30 minutes. If bleeding continues, wound exploration may be indicated.

Arterial occlusion progresses to irreversible ischemia in 6–8 hours, depending on collateral circulation.

Given Poiseuille's law, in which the formula includes radius to the fourth power, note that radius is the most important determinant of flow.

The 6 P's of acute arterial insufficiency:
Pain
Pulselessness
Pallor
Paresthesia
Paralysis
Poikilothermia

Typical scenario: You are asked to localize a lesion on a patient. You can palpate a femoral pulse but no popliteal or pedal pulses on the right side. Left-sided pulses are present. *Think:* Localize lesion to the vessel above site where pulse is first lost. The lesion is likely to be in the superficial femoral artery (SFA). Tissue ischemia will extend one joint level distal to segment of artery occluded.

Sites commonly affected by embolism:
- Lower extremity: 70% (CFA 34%, popliteal 14%)
- Upper extremity: 13%
- Cerebral circulation: 10%
- Visceral circulation: 5–10%
- Aorta: 9%
- Common iliac artery: 14%

- Iatrogenic (catheter related).
- Thrombosis: Atherosclerosis, aneurysm.

SIGNS AND SYMPTOMS OF ACUTE ARTERIAL INSUFFICIENCY

- Paresthesia and paralysis are most important signs because nerves are most sensitive to ischemia. Secondarily, there will be loss of muscle function.
- Pain may not exist in diabetics with neuropathy or if rapidly progressive ischemia occurs with anesthesia.
- Earliest sign in lower extremity will be along distribution of peroneal nerve, with hypesthesia, no great toe dorsiflexion, foot drop.
- Progression in muscle damage: Muscles soft, then doughy, then stiff/hard.
- Once skin is mottled and no longer blanches, tissue ischemia is irreversible. Color change indicates extravasation of blood from capillaries into dermis.

DIFFERENTIAL DIAGNOSIS

- Nerve root compression
- Deep venous thrombosis (DVT)
- Infection

DIAGNOSIS

- If diagnosis is certain (i.e., cold, newly pulseless, painful extremity), no further workup is required. Patient should be promptly taken to OR.
- Typically, ABI and/or angiography are performed to confirm the site of the lesion. Currently, on-table angiography is an option in some centers.

Embolism

- Must find source of embolism and reason.
- Too large diameter artery: Usually of cardiac origin to CFA.
- Patient may have chronic atrial fibrillation or history of myocardial infarction (MI) or valvular disease (mitral stenosis, with valvular vegetation or mural thrombus).
- Atheroembolism: From aorta, iliac, or femoral vessels to distal vessels.
- "Blue toe" syndrome.
- Likely to have palpable pedal pulses anyway because at least one proximal vessel is likely still patent.
- Suspect atheroembolism in patients with no history of peripheral vascular disease (PVD), with digital ischemia and palpable pulses.

TREATMENT

- See below.
- Address primary problem (i.e., atrial fibrillation).

Thrombosis

- Usually underlying stenosis from atherosclerosis.
- May occur in hypercoagulable states, especially with repeated mild trauma.

- Effects of thrombus vary greatly from no symptoms to severe ischemia depending on extent of collateral circulation.
- All patients should have an angiogram unless ischemia is severe and rapidly progressive.
- Cause suggested by history of PVD, popliteal, or aortic aneurysm.
- On exam, patient may have evidence of PVD such as skin changes or lack of distal pulses on contralateral side.

TREATMENT

- Thrombectomy or grafting (most common).
- Thrombolytic therapy.
- Success rate: 60–80%.
- Mechanism: Activation of plasmin system causes fibrinolysis and clot dissolution.
- Agents:
    - Streptokinase: Bacterial origin (antigenic), binds plasminogen to make plasmin, not often used.
    - Urokinase: From renal parenchyma, directly activates plasminogen, not currently available in the United States.
    - Tissue plasminogen activator (tPA): From vascular endothelium, directly activates plasminogen.
    - Reteplase: Recombinant tPA, catalyzes cleavage of endogenous plasminogen to form plasmin.
- Indications: Acute occlusion of native vessel or graft.
- Contraindications: History of gastrointestinal (GI) or intracerebral lesion, pregnancy, any contraindication to angiography.
- Method: Catheter placed proximally, diagnostic angiogram performed, catheter advanced into clot, thrombolytic agent administered.

COMPLICATIONS

- Intracerebral bleed, catheter site bleed (both infrequent).
- Patient may ultimately require operation to fix underlying problem.

▶ CHRONIC ISCHEMIA

PRESENTATION

- Claudication.
- Rest pain.
- Gangrene.
- Most commonly affects infrarenal aorta, iliac arteries, SFA at adductor canal.

RISK FACTORS

- Systolic hypertension (HTN)
- Cigarette smoking
- Hyperlipidemia
- Diabetes

Any patient with PVD is likely to have cardiac disease as well and will require appropriate preoperative or preprocedure medical stabilization and/or optimization.

Thrombolytic therapy for acute thrombotic occlusion is not done if severe ischemia is present, as it takes time to dissolve clot.

If chronic ischemia occurs at locations other than infrarenal aorta, iliacs, or SFA, the patient is likely to have a comorbid disease, such as diabetes (increased risk at profunda femoris and tibial vessels) or an inflammatory disorder (increased risk at axillary arteries).

Aortoiliac Disease

TYPES

- Localized disease of aorta and common iliac disease (10%).
- Localized disease of external iliac artery (25%).
- Multisegmental disease, including infrainguinal (65%).

DIFFERENTIAL DIAGNOSIS

Nerve root compression (lumbosacral) secondary to disc herniation or spinal stenosis.

DIAGNOSTIC TESTS

- Femoral-brachial pressure ratio.
- Penile-brachial index.
- Angiogram.
- Axillobifemoral has better patency rates and is often used for unilateral disease.
- Indicated when patient is extremely high risk for medical complications following intra-abdominal surgery or if graft from prior operation is infected.

TREATMENT

- Aortofemoral bypass:
  - Five-year patency 90%, 10-year patency 75%.
  - Better patency rates than aortoiliac bypass.
- Aortoiliac endarterectomy: Acceptable for localized atherosclerotic disease when distal vessel is normal.
- Extra-anatomic bypass:
  - Best option: Femoral-femoral bypass (5-year patency 50–75%).
  - Other options: Axillofemoral, axillobifemoral—used in high-risk patients for intra-abdominal surgery (elderly, hostile abdomen, abdominal infection).
- Percutaneous transluminal angioplasty (PTA): Indicated for short, non-occluding lesions with less extensive atherosclerosis.
- Five-year patency rate is 90% with secondary interventions.

COMPLICATIONS

- Hemorrhage.
- Thrombosis of reconstruction.
- Distal embolization.
- Ischemic colitis.
- Paraplegia from lumbar vessel ischemia.
- Sexual dysfunction (if operation involved abdominal aorta).

Infrainguinal Disease

- Most commonly affects SFA at adductor canal.
- Patients have decreased life expectancy regardless of treatment and outcome.
- Ulcers:
  - Arterial insufficiency: Lateral ankle and foot, pale, no granulation tissue.

Leriche syndrome is indicative of aortoiliac disease and presents with claudication, impotence, and decreased (or absent) femoral pulses.

- Venous insufficiency: Medial malleolus, pink, granulation tissue, other stigmata of venous disease.

DIAGNOSTIC TESTS

- Doppler
- ABI
- PVRs
- Angiogram

MANAGEMENT

- Nonoperative:
  - Smoking cessation, increase exercise tolerance, medication.
  - Pentoxifylline: Decreases viscosity, increases flow; unpredictable relief of symptoms but proven to increase microvascular flow.
  - Cilostazol: Type III phosphodiesterase inhibitor, reduces platelet aggregation and increases vasodilation. Can be more effective than pentoxifylline.
- Operative:
  - Revascularization requires adequate inflow, outflow, and conduit.
  - Bypass (femoral-popliteal): Uses polytetrafluoroethylene (PTFE) or saphenous vein, reversed or in situ—reversed saphenous vein graft (RSVG) best patency.
  - Endarterectomy: Limited to short lesions of SFA at adductor canal or origin of profunda.

> Patients presenting with rest pain, ulcers, or gangrene most likely have multisegmental disease.

> ABI is likely to be artificially elevated in a diabetic patient because the vessels are generally less compressible than normal. PVRs are more useful because results are not affected by compressibility of vessels.

Upper Extremity Disease

- Compared to lower extremity, more often due to vasospasm or arteritis.
- Palpate pulses: Axillary, radial, ulnar, brachial.
- Subclavian steal syndrome.
- Nonhemispheric cerebrovascular symptoms with mild arm claudication due to decreased flow to posterior cerebral artery (PCA) when blood flows retrograde through vertebral artery to SCA.
- If patient has neurologic symptoms, then carotid stenosis is present as well.
- Cause is proximal SCA lesion.
- Angiogram shows flow reversal in vertebral artery.
- Operate for:
  - Incapacitating claudication.
  - Emboli to hand or to posterior cerebral circulation.
  - Symptoms of subclavian steal (if also carotid symptoms, fix carotid first).

> In situ bypass requires cutting of the valves so that blood flows from proximal to distal.

Carotid Artery Stenosis

GENERAL

- Differentiate based on asymptomatic or symptomatic.
- Asymptomatic: No history of transient ischemic attack (TIA)-like symptoms.
- Symptomatic history of:
  - Amaurosis fugax—transient blindness due to occlusion of the ophthalmic artery (favorite question of surgeons!).
  - Middle cerebral artery (MCA) syndrome.

Typical scenario: An 83-year-old female with a history of diabetes, HTN, and atherosclerosis presents with painless, monocular vision loss that lasted a few minutes and has now completely resolved. She has no other neurologic deficits. *Think:* Amaurosis fugax.

A carotid bruit detected in isolation is not a reliable indicator of carotid stenosis. In the presence of symptoms suggestive of stroke, a carotid bruit is highly correlated with significant stenosis.

- Anterior cerebral artery (ACA) syndrome.
- Syncope is not considered "symptomatic" because unilateral carotid occlusion rarely results in impairment of consciousness.

EVALUATION

Duplex Doppler Ultrasound
- Detects increased flow in stenotic lesions.
- Not reliable in very high-grade stenoses.
- Near-complete stenosis results in "trickle" flow.
- May be mistaken for complete occlusion.
- Cannot assess carotids above the mandible.

MRA
- Detects functional flow.
- Can estimate plaque thickness.
- Can evaluate intracranial vasculature.
- May not resolve trickle flow.

Carotid Angiogram
- Gold standard.
- Reveals trickle flow.
- Cannot discern thickness of plaque.

TREATMENT

- Medical therapy: Aspirin, aspirin plus dipyridamole, clopidogrel.
- Control of underlying medical conditions (HTN, diabetes mellitus, hyperlipidemia).
- Smoking cessation.
- Surgical therapy—carotid endarterectomy (CEA):
  - Indications: Ipsilateral neurologic symptoms with carotid artery stenosis or asymptomatic with > 70% carotid stenosis.
  - CEA has been shown to be more effective than aspirin alone in preventing subsequent strokes in all symptomatic patients. It is superior to medical management alone in asymptomatic females with > 70% stenosis and in asymptomatic males with > 60% stenosis.
  - Emergency CEA may be indicated in symptomatic cases of recent onset with angiographically proven occlusion or loss of a known previous bruit.
- Procedure:
  - Patient is maintained on aspirin preoperatively.
  - Timing is generally 4–6 weeks after CVA.
  - Intraoperative electroencephalogram (EEG) and sensory evoked potentials routinely monitored in case ischemia develops.
  - The surgeon must ensure complete dissection of the plaque in order to prevent remnant plaque rupture with subsequent embolic stroke.
  - After intraoperative ICA occlusion, measurement of retrograde flow from opposite circulation ("stump pressure") should yield mean arterial pressure (MAP) > 50 mmHg. ICA shunt may be indicated if the stump pressure is < 50 mmHg.

- Risks/complications:
  - Operative mortality: 1–5%.
  - Vagus is the most common nerve injured (during clamping of the common carotid).
  - Hoarseness—recurrent laryngeal nerve injury.
  - Horner syndrome—injury to sympathetic plexus coursing along with carotids.
  - Partial tongue paresis (hypoglossal nerve injury).
  - Hematoma causing airway compromise.
  - Cerebral hyperperfusion syndrome.
  - Unilateral headache due to poor autoregulation.
  - Seizures.
  - Carotid occlusion (100% stenosis) of chronic nature usually has little benefit from surgical intervention. Typically, slowly progressive carotid stenosis affords development of alternative collateralization to the anterior cerebral circulation (e.g., through external carotid artery [ECA] anastomoses).

Only superficial layers should be closed primarily after CEA. Closure of deep fascia creates an enclosed space capable of retaining hematoma under high pressures. Should an arterial leak develop, the airway may be rapidly compromised.

Carotid artery dissection must always be in your differential in a patient presenting with neurological deficits of the head after a traumatic episode.

▶ **AMPUTATIONS**

INDICATIONS

- Nonviable extremity that has become infected.
- Irreparable vascular injury with irreversible ischemia (traumatic or atraumatic).
- Cancer.
- Elderly patient with infection who is not a candidate for surgical revascularization.

TYPES OF AMPUTATIONS

- **Toe:** For gangrene or osteomyelitis distal to proximal interphalangeal joint (PIP) without proximal cellulitis, necrosis, or edema.
- Transmetatarsal: For necrosis between level of transmetatarsal incision and PIP, often interdigital crease necrosis.
- Syme's: Amputation at base of tibia and fibula. For terminal arterial disease of distal foot—not done very often, requires palpable posterior tibialis pulse.
- Below-knee amputation (BKA) (most common level for nonviable foot): For ischemia up to malleoli.
  - Likely to adapt well to prosthesis.
  - Contraindicated if gangrene more proximal than ankle, or if patient has hip or knee contractures.
  - Likely to fail when there is no femoral pulse.
- Above-knee amputation (AKA): For gangrene above below-knee level, for contractures at knee or hip, and for elderly nonambulatory patients.
- Best chance of healing, particularly in PVD patients.
- Hip disarticulation: For extensive lower extremity ischemia, proximal gangrene, tumor, extensive trauma.
- Poor outcome when performed for PVD.
- Upper extremity amputations: More commonly performed for trauma or tumor.
  - Digital, forearm, upper arm.
  - Leave as much as possible, unless for tumor.

If patient has popliteal pulse, BKA has 90–97% success rate. Without palpable popliteal pulse, success rate is about 82%.

Longer stump is more functional.

BASIC PRINCIPLES

1. Patient should be medically stabilized first when possible.
2. Select level of amputation for PVD:
   - Use PVRs and ABI to help predict chance of healing.
   - At proposed level, infection is controlled, skin looks good, without proximal dependent rubor, proximal pain, and with a venous filling time < 20 seconds.
   - If for cancer, wide excision necessary.
   - If status post trauma or for PVD, remaining tissue level must be acceptably healthy.
   - Consider length of stump in regard to ease of fitting/using prosthesis.
   - Consider overall condition of patient.
3. Determination of closure:
   - Standard: Flaps constructed to close over bone.
   - Guillotine (in situation of sepsis): Level is lower than that eventually desired. Stump left open for dressing changes until sepsis is resolved, at which time completion amputation is performed.
4. Postoperative care:
   - Dressing left in place for at least 3 days unless patient becomes febrile or has profuse bleeding through dressing.
   - Rehabilitation.

► CHRONIC VENOUS DISEASE: OBSTRUCTION AND INCOMPETENCE

BASICS

- Postphlebitic syndrome: After DVT, many patients (50%) get chronic venous insufficiency due to valvular incompetence of recanalized veins.
- Up to 50% of patients with signs and symptoms of venous insufficiency have no documented history of DVT.

PRESENTATION

- Pain and swelling in affected leg.
- Findings on exam include induration, swelling, skin darkening, and possibly ulcers.

TREATMENT

- Goals:
  - Alleviate symptoms.
  - Heal any ulcers that exist.
  - Prevent development of new ulcers.
- Nonoperative:
  - Compression stockings.
  - Leg elevation.
  - Ulcer treatment: Bed rest, antibiotics when cellulitis present, thromboembolism deterrents (TEDs), Unna's boots, dressings.
  - Generalized skin care, with antifungal creams when appropriate, moisturizer for eczema.
- Operative:
- Indications: Severe symptoms, failure of conservative measurements, recurrent ulcers.

When the patient is compliant and therapy is properly done, 85% of ulcers heal, but may recur.

HIGH-YIELD FACTS

Vascular Surgery

- Options:
  - **Ligation** of responsible perforators (usually around medial malleolus).
  - Valvuloplasty (leads to symptomatic improvement in 60–80%).
  - Venous reconstruction with grafting (not popular).

▶ ANEURYSM

Definition

- An irreversible dilatation of an artery to at least 1.5 times its normal caliber.
- True aneurysm: Involves all layers of arterial wall.
- False aneurysm: Involves only a portion of wall, or involves surrounding tissue.

Varieties of Aneurysm

- Degenerative—due to atherosclerosis, the most common type of aneurysm:
  - Intima replaced by fibrin.
  - Media fragmented with decreased elasticity.
  - Imbalance in elastin metabolism, between elastase and α_1-antithrombin.
- Traumatic—due to iatrogenic, catheter-related injury, or to penetrating trauma:
  - Results in focal defect in wall; hemorrhage controlled by surrounding tissue.
  - Formation of fibrous capsule.
- Poststenotic—from Bernoulli's principle, occurs distal to cervical rib in thoracic outlet syndrome, distal to coarctation of aorta, or to aortic or pulmonary valvular stenosis.
- Dissecting—blood travels through an intimal defect, creating a false passageway between the intima and the inner two thirds of the media:
  - If ruptures externally, patient exsanguinates.
  - Risk factors: HTN, Marfan's syndrome, Ehlers-Danlos syndrome, cystic medial necrosis, blunt trauma, cannulation during cardiopulmonary bypass.
- Mycotic—infected.
- Anastomotic—separation between graft and native artery, with formation of sac and fibrous capsule, often in CFA status post aortofemoral bypass:
  - Painless, pulsatile, groin mass.
  - Diagnose with duplex for peripheral aneurysms, and CT for abdominal aneurysms, or angiogram.

Abdominal Aortic Aneurysm (AAA)

- Fusiform dilatation of abdominal aorta more than 1.5 times its normal diameter.
- Incidence: 2% of elderly population (9 times more common in males than females).

Unna's boots: Similar to a cast, this is a wrap soaked usually in Calamine lotion and applied to the leg; it lasts until the patient takes a shower.

- Seventy-five percent are asymptomatic at diagnosis.
- Risk factors for rupture: Diastolic HTN, initially large size at diagnosis, chronic obstructive pulmonary disease (COPD).

Size at which AAA is considered for surgical repair: 5 cm.

INDICATIONS FOR REPAIR

- Size at which the risk of rupture exceeds the risk of mortality from the operation (generally about 2–5%).
- Increasing size.
- Consider factors that increase risk of rupture (diastolic HTN, COPD).
- Pain over AAA site.

DIAGNOSIS

- Exam: Periumbilical palpable pulsatile mass.
- CT: Provides information about character, wall thickness, and location with respect to renal arteries, presence of leak or rupture.
- Magnetic resonance imaging (MRI): Provides more details than CT or ultrasound (US) about the lumen, surface anatomy, neck, relationship to renal arteries.
- US: Used more frequently to follow aneurysm size over time than to assess in acute phase (see Figure 20-1).
- Angiogram: Defines vascular anatomy and is especially important in cases of mesenteric ischemia, HTN, renal dysfunction, horseshoe kidney, claudication.

PREOPERATIVE ASSESSMENT

- Includes assessment of carotid disease and cardiac, pulmonary, renal, and hepatic systems.
- Cardiac workup and optimization:
  - No history of coronary artery disease (CAD): 1–3% chance of MI, pulmonary edema, or cardiac death perioperatively.
  - Known CAD, risks increase to 5–10%.
  - Steps to minimize risk:
    - No cardiac history, normal electrocardiogram (ECG): No further workup.

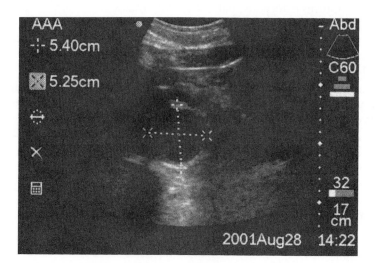

FIGURE 20-1.   AAA on ultrasonography. Aortic diameter is 5.40 cm.

- Known but stable CAD: Echocardiogram/dipyridimole or thallium.
  - If abnormal, consider preoperative revascularization.
- Clinically severe CAD: Definite need for revascularization.
- If percutaneous, may proceed immediately with AAA repair.
- If coronary artery bypass graft (CABG), wait 4–6 weeks.

OPERATIVE PLAN (ELECTIVE)

- Open repair:
  - Approach: Transperitoneal or retroperitoneal.
    - Retroperitoneal approach: Avoids formation of intra-abdominal adhesions, does not interfere with any GI or genitourinary (GU) stoma that may exist, is better tolerated in COPD patients, and provides better suprarenal exposure.
- Endovascular repair (EVAAAR):
  - Endovascular system consists of the graft, stents, and a delivery mechanism.
  - Problems include immediate thrombosis and leakage at anatomic sites.
- Should be considered in patients who are elderly and/or have high operative risk due to a multitude of medical comorbidities.
- Benefits compared to open repair: Shorter procedural time, hospital stay, and recovery time; recent evidence suggests improved mortality.

EMERGENT REPAIR OF RUPTURED AAA

- Higher-risk operation.
- **Signs and symptoms:** Abdominal pain, severe back or flank pain, cardiovascular collapse.
- **Differential diagnosis:** Perforated peptic ulcer, renal or biliary colic, ruptured intervertebral disk.
- **Treatment:**
  - In an unstable patient with known AAA: Proceed to OR immediately—"mobilize the team."
  - In a stable patient, without history of AAA: CT first, then OR as needed.
  - OR:
    1. Team scrubs and preps/drapes.
    2. Only then is anesthesia induced, as surgeon has knife in hand. (Anesthesia causes vasodilatation, which may worsen hypotension.)
    3. Right angle retractor used to compress supraceliac aorta against vertebrae so patient can be resuscitated by anesthesia.
    4. Retractor replaced with supraceliac clamp.
    5. AAA repaired.

COMPLICATIONS OF AAA REPAIR

- Renal failure: 6% elective, 75% ruptured—acute tubular necrosis (ruptured) or atheroemboli (elective).
- Ischemic colitis (5%): Bloody diarrhea, elevated white blood count (WBC), peritonitis.
- Spinal cord ischemia: Disruption of artery of Adamkiewicz.
- EVAAAR: 20–25% will develop endoleak (flow outside graft lumen but inside aneurysm sac).

Graft is placed within the lumen of the aorta, and the vessels walls are closed around it. The aneurysm is not resected.

- Mortality for ruptured AAA is 90%.
- Of those who reach the hospital alive, mortality is still 50%.
- Mortality is further increased in patients with history of CAD, hypotension on arrival, and renal insufficiency, and is also increased by inexperienced surgical team.

Typical scenario: You are called to the emergency department to see a 65-year-old male with a history of AAA, for which he is followed by the vascular service. He now complains of abdominal pain and reports syncope at home. *Think:* Syncope and abdominal pain or hypotension in a patient with known AAA is presumed to be rupture unless proven otherwise. Notify the OR and mobilize your team.

Other Aneurysms

ILIAC ARTERY

- Common iliac artery, 90%; hypogastric artery, 10%.
- Hypogastric artery aneurysms may cause a pulsatile mass palpable on digital rectal examination.
- Resection indicated when > 3 cm, otherwise 6-month follow-up indicated.
- Common iliac artery (CIA) aneurysm is treated with interposition graft.

POPLITEAL ARTERY

- Most common peripheral aneurysm.
- Fifty to seventy-five percent of cases are bilateral aneurysms.
- Untreated, 60% will lead to thrombosis or distal embolization, and 20% to amputation.
- Diagnosis established on exam, and using US and angiography.
- Operation indicated if no serious comorbidity: Excision and interposition graft with RSVG or ligation and bypass.

FEMORAL ARTERY

- Uncommon.
- On exam, mass, local pain, venous obstruction, embolism, thrombosis.
- Whether symptomatic or not, resection and graft indicated once > 2.5 cm.

In pregnant women, iliac artery aneurysms are associated with fibromuscular dysplasia.

External iliac artery is never involved when the cause is atherosclerosis.

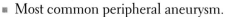

▶ DIABETIC DISEASE

LOCATION

- Usually spares aortoiliac vessels.
- Affects distal profunda femoris, popliteal, tibial, and digital arteries of the foot.
- Small vessels affected: Microangiopathy occurs with intimal and basement membrane thickening.
- Large vessels affected with atherosclerosis and calcification of media.

PROBLEMS

- Diabetic neuropathy: Causes motor and sensory deficits as well as high arch deformity in the foot that increases pressure on tarsal heads (atrophy of intrinsic muscles).
- Arteriopathy.
- Infection: Likely to be worse—gram negatives, gram positives, and anaerobes all potential culprits, in particular *Peptococcus, Proteus, Bacteroides.*

TREATMENT

Revascularization indicated when ulcers occur if there are significant vessels to use in repair. (See above information for further details that apply to diabetic and nondiabetic patients.)

One third of patients with unilateral popliteal artery aneurysms will have AAAs.

Patients with bilateral popliteal artery aneurysms have a 50% chance of concurrent AAA.

ABI in a diabetic patient may be falsely elevated secondary to vessel calcification.

Anatomy

- Superficial: Greater and lesser saphenous veins.
- Deep: Veins follow arteries and have same names (popliteal, superficial femoral vein [SFV], distal femoral vein [DFV], common femoral vein [CFV], external iliac vein [EIV]).
- Perforators: Connect deep and superficial.

The diabetic patient may be unaware of skin or other minor injuries. Classic site of infection: Over metatarsal heads on plantar aspect of foot.

Physiology

- Systemic veins contain two thirds of circulating volume.
- Further from heart, there are more valves.
- Venous return depends on respiration: Inspiration causes descent of diaphragm, increased intra-abdominal pressure, and decreased venous return.
- Venous return generated by the relationship among contraction of the heart, static filling pressure, and gravity.
- Virchow's triad: Stasis, blood abnormality, vessel endothelium injury (factors allowing thrombosis to occur).

Perforators adjacent to medial malleolus are responsible for stasis ulcers when they become incompetent.

Deep Venous Thrombosis (DVT)

- Stasis leads to thrombin formation, which leads to platelet aggregation.
- Endothelial injury and/or a hypercoagulable state may contribute.
- Screening warranted for younger patients or those with repeated occurrences.
- Check prothrombin time (PT), partial thromboplastin time (PTT), WBC, hematocrit (Hct), erythrocyte sedimentation rate (ESR), platelets.
- For extremely high-risk patients, also check homocysteine level, antiphospholipid (APL) antibodies, proteins C and S, antithrombin III (AT III), activated protein C resistance (APC-r), platelet aggregation, mutant factor V Leiden, prothrombin gene mutation (factor II).
- Also check CT scan of the chest, abdomen, and pelvis to look for malignancy if patient has no other risk factors for DVT.

The superficial femoral vein is actually a deep vein.

About one third of apparently healthy patients with DVTs of unknown cause will be diagnosed with a malignancy within 2 years.

RISK FACTORS

Acquired
- Central venous line placement.
- Congestive heart failure (CHF) and MI (20–40%): Passive congestion and increased blood viscosity.
- Joint replacement operation (15–30%): Femoral vein trauma, long OR, postop immobility.
- Fractures of hip, pelvis, proximal femur (35–60%): Endothelial damage.
- Laparoscopic surgery (7–10%): Intra-abdominal pressure > pressure of venous return from legs.
- Prior DVT (five times): Scarring, valvular damage, decreased muscle pumping, stasis.

HIGH-YIELD FACTS

Vascular Surgery

- Hormone replacement therapy (HRT) (two to six times): Increases coagulation factors, and decreases protein S, antithrombin III (AT III), and fibrinolytic activity.
- Other: Trauma patients, malignancy, obesity, pregnancy, sepsis, prolonged immobility.

Congenital

- Antiphospholipid antibody syndrome (APS): Antibodies change normal endothelial function.
- AT III deficiency.
- Plasminogen deficiency: Decreased fibrinolysis.
- Dysfibrinogenemia: Fibrin resistance to plasmin proteolysis, abnormal fibrinogen, defective thrombin binding, increased blood viscosity.
- Factor V Leiden/APC-r: Factor Va resistant to degradation by APC; hyperviscosity syndrome.
- Lupus anticoagulant: Exact mechanism unknown.
- Protein C and S deficiency: Factors V and VIII are not appropriately inactivated.
- Prothrombin gene mutation (factor II).

Central line placement is responsible for one third of upper extremity DVTs.

Two thirds of DVTs are asymptomatic.

DIAGNOSIS

- Exam: Calf tenderness, swelling, Homan's sign (not very reliable).
- Duplex: Demonstrates thrombus, assesses compressibility of veins, analyzes venous flow.

PROPHYLAXIS

- TEDs (compression stockings): Increase velocity of venous flow, reduce venous wall distention, and enhance valvular function.
- Sequential compression devices: Reduce incidence of DVT by up to 75% when used properly.
- Pharmacologic: Subcutaneous heparin, low-molecular-weight heparin.

TREATMENT

- Bed rest until pain and swelling subside.
- Lower extremity elevation.
- Anticoagulation (period of 6 months for first DVT).
- Elastic stockings once ambulating.
- Consider fibinolytics for large thrombi.

LONG-TERM OUTCOME

Recurrent DVT: 18% at 2 years, 30% at 8 years.

Postphlebitic Syndrome

- Occurs in 24%.
- Risk of recurrent DVT then increased six times.
- Symptoms: Edema, pain, aches, fatigue, skin discoloration, scarring, ulcers.

Superficial Venous Thrombosis (SVT)

- Usually a noninfected, localized inflammatory reaction.
- **Signs and symptoms:** Swelling, pain, erythema, tenderness.
- **Diagnosis:** Duplex ultrasonography to rule out associated DVT.
- **Treatment:**
  - Nonsteroidal anti-inflammatory drugs (NSAIDs) as needed until symptoms resolve (about 2–3 weeks).
  - Use elastic stockings.
  - Consider anticoagulation for involvement of saphenofemoral junction.

▶ VASCULAR TRAUMA

Clues to Vascular Injury in the Trauma Patient

- Pulsatile or expanding hematoma.
- Pulsatile bleeding.
- Bruit/thrill.
- End-organ ischemia.
- Unexplained shock.
- Likely location.
- Injury to adjacent nerve.
- Extremity fractures with weak or absent pulses.

Use direct pressure to control bleeding. Tourniquets are really only a last resort.

A Few Facts

- Carotid artery injury with hematoma can affect cranial nerves IX, X, XI, and XII.
- All zones in neck injury are likely to have vascular injury.
- Limb loss secondary to arterial injury associated with lower extremity fracture > 40%.
- Twenty percent of patients with penetrating abdominal trauma will have major vascular injury.

HIGH-YIELD FACTS IN

Pediatric Surgery

Inflammatory masses are the most common congenital neck lesions. Common causes:
- Lymphadenopathy
- Cervical adenitis
- Hematoma
- Benign tumors (lipoma)

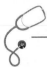

Life-threatening causes of congenital neck lesions:
- Hematoma secondary to trauma.
- Subcutaneous emphysema plus airway injury.
- Non-Hodgkin's lymphoma with mediastinal mass causing airway compromise.

Paragangliomas in the neck (i.e., carotid body tumors) are rare; they originate from neural crest cells. Like all paragangliomas, the Rule of 10 applies: 10% familial, 10% catecholamine-secreting, and 10% malignant.

▶ FLUID MANAGEMENT

Maintenance fluid calculation:
- First 10 kg: 4 cc/kg
- Second 10 kg: 2 cc/kg
- Every additional kilogram past 20 kg: 1 cc/kg
- Minimal urine output: 1–2 mL/kg/hr

▶ NECK MASSES/LESIONS

TYPES

- Congenital
- Inflammatory
- Neoplastic

LOCATION

Location is key in diagnosis.
- **Midline:**
  - Thyroglossal duct remnants
  - Submental lymph node
  - Goiter
- **Lateral:**
  - Branchial cyst
  - Lymphadenitis
  - Lymphoma
  - Carotid body tumor (paraganglioma)
- **Midline or lateral:**
  - Cystic hygroma
  - Dermoid cyst
- **Bilateral:**
  - Cervical lymphadenitis

Thyroglossal Duct Cyst and Sinus

DEFINITION

Midline neck mass that arises from a remnant of the diverticulum that forms when primitive thyroid tissue migrates from the foramen cecum at the base of tongue down toward the hyoid bone.

SIGNS AND SYMPTOMS

- Most commonly present as infection.
- Usually painless, smooth, mobile, and cystic.

DIAGNOSIS

Ultrasound (US).

TREATMENT

- Antibiotics for infection.
- Radionuclide scans prior to surgery to rule out ectopic thyroid gland.

- Sistrunk procedure: Complete excision of cyst and sinus tract with resection of central portion of hyoid bone, necessary to prevent recurrence of cyst formation and infection.
- Follow-up screening for hypothyroidism.

Branchial Cleft Cyst and Sinus

DEFINITION

Remnants of the four branchial clefts in the anterior neck that can form cysts or sinus tracts leading through to the skin.

SIGNS AND SYMPTOMS

- Lateral neck mass that may present with drainage.
- Most common form is second branchial cleft cyst that present at the anterior border of sternocleidomastoid muscle.
- Usually painless.
- Fluctuant, mobile, and nontender.

DIAGNOSIS

US.

TREATMENT

- Complete excision of cyst and entire tract.
- Antibiotics if infected.

Cystic Hygroma

DEFINITION

Congenital lymphangioma.

SIGNS AND SYMPTOMS

- Most are identified at birth.
- May be recognized after injury or upper respiratory infection.
- Painless, soft, and mobile.
- Transilluminate brightly.
- May compress trachea or spread into the floor of mouth, causing upper airway obstruction.
- Do not regress spontaneously.

DIAGNOSIS

Computed tomography (CT) scan (extent and involvement of surrounding structures).

TREATMENT

Surgical excision is necessary to prevent enlargement and possible airway compromise.

Thyroglossal duct cysts elevate with swallowing and tongue protrusion, while branchial cleft cysts and dermoid cysts do not move.

Branchial cleft cysts may not present until adulthood and may become evident only with infection and inflammation.
Probing a branchial cyst can cause infection.

Cystic hygroma is the most common lymphatic malformation in children and is most commonly found at the floor of the oropharynx.

Pectus Excavatum

DEFINITION

Abnormal asymmetric development of costal cartilages causing posterior distortion (caving in) of the sternum and xiphoid.

SIGNS AND SYMPTOMS

- Abnormal "funnel chest" appearance.
- May cause respiratory compromise and exertional dyspnea.
- Occasionally associated with mitral valve prolapse.

TREATMENT

- Surgery at 6 years of age or older.
- Osteotomy to remove abnormal cartilage with a temporary substernal strut to stabilize sternum until new cartilage forms.
- Alternatively: *Nuss procedure*—only strut placement with no osteotomy.

Pectus Carinatum

DEFINITION

Abnormal asymmetric growth of costal cartilages, causing anterior distortion of sternum and xiphoid; less common than pectus excavatum.

SIGNS AND SYMPTOMS

- Abnormal "pigeon chest" appearance.
- Usually asymptomatic.

TREATMENT

- Brace to correct deformity, can be used up to 18 years of age.
- Surgery (osteotomy) after 6 years of age, usually for cosmetic purposes to avoid psychological distress in children not willing to wear braces.

Tracheoesophageal (TE) Malformations

DEFINITION

Failure of complete separation of trachea from esophagus. Can occur with or without esophageal atresia and usually involves a tracheoesophageal fistula.

EMBRYOLOGY

Esophagus and trachea originate from a single diverticulum and divide at fifth week of gestation.

EPIDEMIOLOGY

- One in 3500 births.
- Most commonly "type C" (esophageal atresia with a distal TE fistula).

SIGNS AND SYMPTOMS

- Respiratory distress or choking following first feeding.
- Excess drooling and salivation.

Most common malformation with esophageal atresia is a TE fistula (95%).

AXR: Absence of air in stomach. *Think:* Esophageal atresia without fistula.

TYPES (FIGURE 21-1)

- Pure esophageal atresia.
- Esophageal atresia with proximal TE fistula.
- Esophageal atresia with distal TE fistula.
- Esophageal atresia with proximal and distal fistulas.
- "H-Type"—no esophageal atresia with TE fistula.

DIAGNOSIS

- Esophageal atresia becomes evident within the first few hours of life because of severity of symptoms, inability to pass feeding tube.
- Chest x-ray (CXR): Tube to end or coil in the region of thoracic inlet.
- Abdominal x-ray (AXR).
- Contrast x-ray studies.

TREATMENT

- Decompress blind esophageal pouch and control oral secretions with sump tube on constant suction.
- Parenteral prophylactic antibiotics.
- Evaluate for other anomalies (primarily cardiac and renal)—cardiac echo to define aortic arch.
- If cardiac and respiratory stable, may repair surgically.
- Surgical repair:
  - Ligation of fistula and insertion of gastrostomy tube.
  - Anastomosis of two ends of esophagus.

Congenital Diaphragmatic Hernia

DEFINITION

Patent pleuroperitoneal canal through the diaphragm leading to pulmonary hyperplasia of the restricted ipsilateral lung and respiratory distress. May result in pulmonary hypertension.

Fifty percent of infants with esophageal atresia have associated anomalies. Most commonly part of **VACTERL** constellation of anomalies:

- **Vertebral**
- **Anorectal**
- **Cardiac**
- **TracheoEsophageal fistula**
- **Renal**
- **Limb**

TE malformations also associated with:

- Polyhydramnios
- Preterm birth
- Small for gestational age

H-type fistula most likely to be seen in emergency department in older children who present with recurrent pneumonias (others usually picked up earlier, while infant is still in hospital).

Typical scenario: An infant has excessive oral secretions, choking, and apneic episodes during feedings. *Think:* TE malformation.

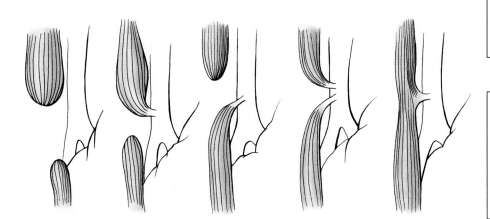

FIGURE 21-1. Five different forms of TE fistula.

(Reproduced, with permission, from Brunicardi FC, Andersen DK, Billiar TR, et al. *Schwartz's Principles of Surgery*, 8th ed. New York: McGraw-Hill, 2004: 1481).

- Total parenteral nutrition (TPN).
- Surgical correction and closure of abdomen.

PROGNOSIS

- Greater than 90% survival rate, postsurgical.
- Twenty percent of cases are complicated by necrotizing enterocolitis (NEC).

Omphalocele

DEFINITION

- Herniation of abdominal contents (often including the liver) into the base of the umbilical cord.
- Protective membrane present.
- Elements of the umbilical cord course individually over the sac and come together at its apex to form a normal-appearing umbilical cord.

EPIDEMIOLOGY

- One in 5000 live births.
- More common in babies born to mothers < 20 years old and > 40 years old.

ASSOCIATED ANOMALIES

- Beckwith-Wiedemann syndrome (gigantism, macroglossia, umbilical defect, hypoglycemia).
- Trisomy 13 and 18.
- Pentalogy of Cantrell (omphalocele, diaphragmatic hernia, cleft sternum, absent pericardium, intracardiac defects).
- Exstrophy of the bladder or cloaca.

TYPES

- Small: Contains only intestine.
- Large: Contains liver, spleen, and gastrointestinal (GI) tract.

TREATMENT

- Ruptured sac:
  - Similar to gastroschisis treatment.
  - Emergent surgical correction.
- Intact sac:
  - Less urgent.
  - Timing of surgery depends on size of defect, size of infant, and presence of other anomalies.

PROGNOSIS

Dependent on presence of other anomalies.

No difference has been shown in outcomes for gastrochisis or omphalocele whether infant is delivered vaginally or via C-section.

Seven percent have coexistent intestinal atresia—important to search for this at surgery.

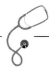

Ruptured omphalocele may be confused with gastroschisis, but the former does not have an intact umbilical cord at the level of abdominal wall.

Inguinal Hernia

DEFINITION

Protrusion of a viscus or part of a viscus through an abnormal weakening in the abdominal wall and through the inguinal canal. In children, most commonly an indirect inguinal hernia from a processus vaginalis that has remained patent.

EPIDEMIOLOGY

- One to five percent of newborns.
- Male-to-female ratio: 4:1.
- Higher incidence in premature infants (30%).
- Indirect hernias are more common on the right side because of the right testicle descends later.

SIGNS AND SYMPTOMS

Bulge in the groin, scrotum, or labia, especially with increased intra-abdominal pressure (coughing, crying, straining, and blowing up a balloon).

DIAGNOSIS

- Physical exam shows firm mass that can slip through the internal inguinal ring.
- Important to differentiate from a hydrocele, which does not extend to the internal ring.
- "Silk glove sign": After hernia is reduced, sac and thickened spermatic cord can be palpated and rolled underneath the examiner's finger.

TREATMENT

- Operative repair:
    - Should be repaired shortly after diagnosis except in premature infants.
    - Unlike adults, pediatric cases are usually not repaired with a mesh. In pediatrics, high ligation of the hernial sac (herniotomy) is performed without repair of the abdominal wall.
- Reasons to operate:
    - Major risks include incarceration of a loop of bowel, an ovary, or a fallopian tube.
    - Fifteen to thirty percent of hernias are incarcerated.
    - Increased risk of incarceration in first few months of life.

If a Meckel's diverticulum is found within a hernia sac, it is called a Littre's hernia.

Correction of inguinal hernia is the most frequent surgical intervention in children.

In females and males < 1 year old, the risk of bilateral hernias is greater and the contralateral side should be explored. The other side can be visualized by a laparoscope placed through the hernia sac (transinguinally).

Indirect inguinal hernias are located lateral to the inferior epigastric vessels (and direct are medial).

▶ **GASTROINTESTINAL DEFECTS**

Pyloric Stenosis

DEFINITION

Narrowing of the pyloric canal due to hypertrophy of the musculature.

EPIDEMIOLOGY

- One in 250 births.
- Male-to-female ratio: 4:1.

Hypokalemic, hypochloremic metabolic alkalosis with paradoxical aciduria is seen in pyloric stenosis.

Pyloric stenosis:
- **Children of affected parents have a 7% chance of disease.**
- **Most common in firstborn male.**

Optimal time of surgery for biliary atresia is < 8 weeks of age.

Biliary atresia accounts for 90% of extrahepatic obstruction in neonates. Of all causes of neonatal jaundice, biliary atresia is the most common indication for surgery.

CAUSES

Unknown.

SIGNS AND SYMPTOMS

- Usually evident between 2 weeks and 2 months old.
- Nonbilious vomiting, progressing from increasingly frequent regurgitation to projectile.
- Hungry after vomiting.
- Dehydration.
- Midepigastric mass ("olive").
- Visible peristaltic wave (left to right).
- Hypochloremic metabolic alkalosis with paradoxic aciduria.

DIAGNOSIS

- Ultrasound (90% sensitivity):
  - Elongated pyloric channel (> 14 mm)
  - Thickened pyloric wall (> 4 mm)
- Radiographic contrast series:
  - **String sign**—from elongated pyloric channel.
  - Shoulder sign—bulge of pyloric muscle into the antrum.
  - Double track sign—parallel streaks of barium in the narrow channel.

TREATMENT

- Correction of fluid and electrolyte and acid-base balance.
- IV fluid 5% dextrose in normal saline plus potassium chloride 3–5 mEq/kg.
- Surgical correction: *Ramstedt pyloromyotomy*—dividing the circular fibers of the pylorus without entering the gastic lumen.

Biliary Atresia

DEFINITION

Obliteration of the entire extrahepatic biliary tree at or above the porta hepatis.

SIGNS AND SYMPTOMS

- Neonatal jaundice (beyond first week).
- Hyperbilirubinemia.
- High γ-glutamyl transpeptidase (GGT) level.
- Signs of portal hypertension (hepatosplenomegaly, ascites).

DIAGNOSIS

- Radioisotope scanning
- Ultrasound
- Direct bilirubin:
  - Greater than 2 mg/dL
  - Greater than 10% of total bilirubin

TREATMENT

- Laparotomy, liver biopsy, and operative cholangiography should be done in any suspicious case.

- Correctable type:
  - Blind-ending cystic dilation of the common hepatic duct.
  - Repaired by direct anastomosis with Roux-en-Y loop of jejunum.
- Noncorrectable type: Kasai procedure—hepatoportoenterostomy (anastomosis between the porta hepatis and the small intestines to drain bile from liver).
- Postoperative treatment:
  - Prophylactic antibiotics
  - Phenobarbital
  - Liver transplantation

Malrotation and Midgut Volvulus

DEFINITION

- Incomplete rotation of the intestine during fetal development.
- May cause complete or partial duodenal obstruction.

EMBRYOLOGY

- Midgut = duodenum to mid-transverse colon.
- Develops extraperitoneally and migrates intraperitoneally at 12 weeks.
- During this migration, the midgut rotates 270° counterclockwise around the superior mesenteric artery (SMA).
- Problem results from abnormal fixation of the mesentery of the bowel.

SIGNS AND SYMPTOMS

- Acute onset of bilious vomiting
- Abdominal distention
- Lethargy
- Skin mottling
- Hypovolemia
- Bloody stool (late sign)

Acute onset of bilious vomiting in an infant is malrotation and volvulus until proven otherwise!

DIAGNOSIS

- AXR:
  - Presence of bowel loops overriding liver.
  - Air in stomach and in duodenum (double bubble sign).
  - No gas in GI tract distal to volvulus.
- Upper GI series: Duodenal C-loop does not extend to the left (stops at level of duodenum).
- Barium enema: Cecum located in right upper quadrant (RUQ).

TREATMENT

- Surgical emergency (can lead to intestinal infarction and death if surgery is delayed).
- *Ladd procedure:*
  - Reduced with counterclockwise rotation.
  - Ligation of Ladd's bands (abnormal fibrous bands attached to cecum and causing obstruction).
  - Appendectomy—because cecum remains in RUQ, changing position of appendix and making appendicitis harder to diagnose.

Malrotation without volvulus may present with intermittent vomiting and abdominal distention.

Duodenal atresia is the most common type of intestinal atresia. Most common site of atresia is at the ampulla of Vater.

Passage of meconium does not rule out intestinal atresia.

Differential diagnosis includes volvulus and annular pancreas.

Since malrotation/volvulus has the same radiographic double bubble sign, get upper GI for confirmation.

Most common cause of acute intestinal obstruction under 2 years of age. Most common site is ileocolic (90%).

Intussusception and link with rotavirus vaccine led to withdrawal of vaccine from the market.

PROGNOSIS

Ten percent chance of recurrent volvulus.

Intestinal Atresia

DEFINITION

Failure of the duodenum to recanalize during early fetal life.

ASSOCIATED CONDITIONS

- Down syndrome
- Esophageal atresia
- Imperforate anus
- Small for gestational age
- Polyhydramnios

SIGNS AND SYMPTOMS

- Bilious vomiting
- Abdominal distention

DIAGNOSIS

Plain abdominal film:

- Dilated bowel proximal to obstruction.
- "Double bubble" sign (air in stomach and duodenum).

TREATMENT

- Fluid resuscitation.
- Gastric decompression.
- Broad-spectrum antibiotics.
- Duodenal atresia: Side-to-side anastomosis (avoids injury to bile and pancreatic duct).
- Jejunoileal atresia: End-to-end anastomosis.

Intussusception

DEFINITION

Invagination of one portion of the bowel into itself—proximal portion usually drawn into distal portion by peristalsis.

EPIDEMIOLOGY

- Incidence 1–4 in 1000 live births.
- Male-to-female ratio: 2:1–4:1.
- Peak incidence 5–12 months.
- Age range: 2 months to 5 years

CAUSES

- Idiopathic.
- "Lead point" (or focus) caused by:
  - Hypertrophied Peyer's patches from viral infection (enterovirus in summer, rotavirus in winter).

- In older children:
  - Meckel's diverticulum
  - Polyp
  - Lymphoma
  - Henoch-Schönlein purpura
  - Cystic fibrosis

SIGNS AND SYMPTOMS

- Classic triad:
  - Intermittent colicky abdominal pain
  - Bilious vomiting
  - Currant jelly stool
- Neurologic signs:
  - Lethargy
  - Shock-like state
  - Seizure-like activity
  - Apnea
- RUQ mass:
  - Sausage shaped
  - Ill defined
  - Dance's sign—absence of bowel in right lower quadrant (RLQ)

DIAGNOSIS

- AXR:
  - Paucity of bowel gas.
  - Loss of visualization of the tip of liver.
  - "Target sign"—two concentric circles of fat density.
- US:
  - "Target" or "donut" sign—single hypoechoic ring with hyperechoic center.
  - "Pseudo-kidney" sign—superimposed hypoechoic (edematous walls of bowel) and hyperechoic (areas of compressed mucosa) layers.
  - Barium enema.

TREATMENT

- Correct dehydration.
- NG tube for decompression.
- Hydrostatic reduction.
- Barium enema:
  - Cervix-like mass.
  - Coiled spring appearance on the evacuation film.
- Contraindications:
  - Peritonitis
  - Perforation
  - Profound shock
- Air enema:
  - Decreased radiation
  - Fewer complications

RECURRENCE

- With radiologic reduction: 7–10%.
- With surgical reduction: 2–5%.

Intussusception
- Classic triad is present in only 20% of cases.
- Absence of currant jelly stool does not exclude the diagnosis.
- Neurologic signs may delay the diagnosis.

Barium enema for intussusception is both diagnostic and therapeutic. Rule of **3s:**
- Barium column should not exceed a height of **3** feet.
- No more than **3** attempts.
- Only **3** minutes/ attempt.

Meckel's Diverticulum

DEFINITION

Persistence of the omphalomesenteric (vitelline) duct (should disappear by seventh week of gestation):

- Arises from the antimesenteric border of ileum.
- Contains heterotopic epithelium (gastric, colonic, or pancreatic).
- A true diverticulum in that it contains all layers of bowel wall.

EPIDEMIOLOGY

- Two percent incidence.
- More common in males.
- Usually presents in children < 2 years old.

SIGNS AND SYMPTOMS

- Intermittent painless rectal bleeding.
- Intestinal obstruction.
- Diverticulitis.

DIAGNOSIS

Meckel's scan (scintigraphy) has 85% sensitivity and 95% specificity. Uptake can be enhanced with cimetidine, glucagon, or gastrin.

TREATMENT

Surgical: Diverticular resection with transverse closure of the enterotomy. If base is thickened then segmental resection of small bowel adjacent to the diverticulum.

Imperforate Anus

DEFINITION

Lack of an anal opening of proper location or size.

CAUSES

Results from a failure of the urinary and hindgut systems to separate.

ASSOCIATED ANOMALIES

VACTERL anomalies (**V**ertebral, **A**norectal, **C**ardiac, **T**racheo**E**sophageal malformations, **R**enal, **L**imb).

TYPES

High and low: Classification depends on whether the rectum ends above (high) or below (low) the puborectalis sling.

TREATMENT

- Colostomy for high lesions.
- Perineal anoplasty or dilatation of fistula for low lesions.

PROGNOSIS

The higher the lesion, the poorer the prognosis.

Hirschsprung's Disease (Congenital Aganglionosis Coli)

DEFINITION

Congenital absence of ganglion cells in the Auerbach (myenteric) and Meissner (submucosal) plexi that results in intestinal obstruction.

Hirschsprung's disease is the most common cause of lower intestinal obstruction in the neonate.

EPIDEMIOLOGY

- Occurs in 1 in 5000–8000 live births.
- Male-to-female ratio: 4:1.
- Family history.

TYPES

- Rectosigmoid (75%)
- Entire colon (10%)

SIGNS AND SYMPTOMS

In neonatal period:

- Ninety-five percent present as delayed passage of meconium (> 24 hours).
- Rectal examination.
- An empty vault that is not dilated.
- Explosive release of feces.
- Most ominous presentation is enterocolitis.
- Presentation later in childhood:
- Bilous vomiting.
- Chronic constipation.
- Abdominal distention.
- Failure to thrive.

DIAGNOSIS

- AXR to look for evidence of obstruction.
- Barium enema to look for transition zone (may not be present until 1–2 weeks of age).
- Rectal biopsy for definitive diagnosis (confirm absence of ganglion cells).

TREATMENT

Surgical repair:

- Temporary colostomy proximal to transition zone at diagnosis.
- Definitive repair when the infant is 6–12 months old.
- Closure of colostomy 1–3 months postoperatively.

Necrotizing Enterocolitis (NEC)

DEFINITION

Serious intestinal injury and necrosis following a combination of vascular, mucosal, and toxic insults to a relatively immature gut.

Typical scenario: A premature infant born at 33 weeks' gestation now at 1 week of age has developed feeding intolerance, is febrile, and has hematochezia and a distended belly. *Think:* Necrotizing enterocolitis.

NEC is the most common GI emergency for infants.

Pneumoperitoneum (free air) on an AXR of an infant with suspected NEC is an indication for immediate surgery!

EPIDEMIOLOGY

- Occurs in 1–3 in 1000 live births.
- Predominantly a disorder of preterm infants; incidence increases with decreasing gestational age.
- Increased incidence with congenital heart disease, severe intrauterine growth retardation (IUGR), sepsis, gastroschisis, and other neonatal disorders.

SIGNS AND SYMPTOMS

Presentation is similar to sepsis.

- Systemic:
  - Lethargy
  - Feeding intolerance
  - Fever
  - Hypothermia
  - Hypotension
  - Apneic spells
- GI:
- Abdominal distention, tenderness
- Vomiting
- Bloody diarrhea
- Hematochezia

DIAGNOSIS

- AXR: Pneumatosis intestinalis (gas within the bowel wall).
- Lateral decubitus or cross-table lateral:
  - Probable NEC:
    - Thickened bowel loop
    - Fixed position loops on serial films
    - Ascites
  - Definite NEC:
    - Intramural gas
    - Portal gas
    - Pneumoperitoneum/free air (denotes perforation)

TREATMENT

- Nothing by mouth.
- Bowel decompression.
- Antibiotics/sepsis evaluation.
- TPN.
- Monitor vital signs and abdominal girth.
- Monitor fluid intake and output.
- Definite indication for surgical resection:
  - Perforation.
  - Full-thickness necrosis of bowel.
- Possible indications:
  - Ascites.
  - Deterioration with medical management.
  - Intestinal obstruction.

PROGNOSIS

Variable (depends on extent of injury). Overall > 95% survival rate.

Wilms' Tumor

DEFINITION

Nephroblastoma—originates intrarenally.

EPIDEMIOLOGY

- Most common intra-abdominal malignancy in childhood.
- Usual presentation between 2 and 4 years; very rapidly growing.

ASSOCIATED CONDITIONS

- WAGR syndrome (**W**ilms' tumor, **A**niridia, **G**enitourinary anomalies, mental **R**etardation).
- Beckwith-Weidemann syndrome (hemihypertrophy, macroglossia, organomegaly).
- Denys-Drash syndrome (Wilms' tumor, pseudohermaphroditism, and glomerulopathy).

SIGNS AND SYMPTOMS

Triad:

- Flank mass
- Hematuria
- Hypertension

DIAGNOSIS

- CT scan with contrast (metastasis—nodal enlargement and liver nodule).
- CXR or CT scan (lung metastasis).
- Intravenous urography (intrarenal solid mass).
- Ultrasound of abdomen (extension into renal vein and inferior vena cava [IVC]).

STAGES

I: Involves only kidney.
II: Invades capsule and possibly perirenal fat.
III: No hematogenous metastasis, not completely resectable.
IV: Hematogenous metastasis to lung, brain, distal nodes.
V: Involves both kidneys.

TREATMENT

- Surgical resection of tumor, exploration of abdomen, evaluation of contralateral kidney.
- Chemotherapy + radiotherapy (for later stages).
- Ninety percent survival rate.

Neuroblastoma

DEFINITION

- Arises from neural crest cells.
- May arise in adrenal medulla, sympathetic ganglia, and organ of Zuckerman (para-aortic ganglia).

Presence of abdominal mass in infant or child is always abnormal and requires evaluation.

Wilms' tumor is associated with aniridia, Beckwith-Wiedemann syndrome, hemihypertophy, neurofibromatosis, horseshoe kidney.

Beckwith-Wiedemann syndrome consists of omphalocele, macrosomia, organomegaly, macroglossia, Wilms' tumor, and neonatal hypoglycemia.

Lung is the most common site of metastasis.

Most common tumor to metastasize to the orbit, causing proptosis in the affected eye.

More than 50% have metastases when first seen.

Neuroblastoma can cross the midline, while Wilms' tumor does not.

Better prognosis for neuroblastomas with younger age (< 1 year old), fewer N-myc proto-oncogene copies.

EPIDEMIOLOGY

- Most common solid tumor in infants (> 33% < 1 year old, 80% < 5 years old).
- Most common solid tumor of childhood outside of central nervous system.
- Abdominal tumors are most common presentation: 65% in adrenal gland.
- Thoracic tumors are next most common presentation.

SIGNS AND SYMPTOMS

- Abdominal pain and mass.
- Fever, failure to thrive, diarrhea, and lethargy.
- Neurological symptoms (ataxia, opsomyoclonus).
- Hypertension (25%).

DIAGNOSIS

- Urine: Raised catecholamines (vanillylmandelic acid [VMA], homovanillic acid [HVA]).
- Intravenous pyelography (inferior displacement of opacified calyces—"drooping lily sign").
- CT abdomen with contrast.

STAGES

I: Tumor is limited to one organ, completely resectable.
II: Tumor does not cross midline.
III: Crosses midline.
IV: Distant metastases.

TREATMENT

- Stage I: Resection.
- Stages II and III: Resection and chemotherapy.
- Stage IV: Resection and aggressive chemo/radiotherapy.

Ear, Nose, and Throat Surgery

Anatomy

EXTERNAL EAR

See Figure 22-1.

- **Auricle funnels sound waves into external auditory canal (EAC).**
- External auditory canal: The outer one third is cartilaginous; the inner two thirds is osseous.
- Tympanic membrane (TM) is divided into two parts: Pars flacida superiorly and pars tensa inferiorly. Pars tensa composed of three layers—outer epithelial, middle fibrous, and inner mucous membrane. Pars flaccida lacks middle fibrous layer. The surrounding fibrous peripheral support is called the annulus. TM is attached to the malleus medially, and conducts sound waves from external ear to middle ear.

MIDDLE EAR

Contains the eustacian tube orifice, ossicles, and entrance to the mastoid cavity:

- The eustachian tube connects the nasopharynx to the anterior wall of the middle ear cavity. It serves to equalize middle ear pressure to atmospheric pressure. It is opened by contraction of two muscles: The adenoids are in close proximity to nasopharyngeal opening of tube.
- Mastoid air cells communicate with the middle ear cavity via the aditus antrum, which lies on the posterosuperior wall of the cavity.
- Ossicles: Tympanic membrane → malleus → incus → stapes → oval window → perilymph of scala vestibuli of the inner ear. The ossicles serve as a lever arm to amplify sound. The malleus is fused to the tympanic membrane internally, and with the incus medially. Tensor tympani muscle is attached to the manubrium of the malleus. The **incus**

External ear embryologically forms from six hillocks, parts of the first and second branchial arches. Failure of the hillocks to fuse result in auricular pits and sinuses, which are prone to repeated infection that may necessitate their removal.

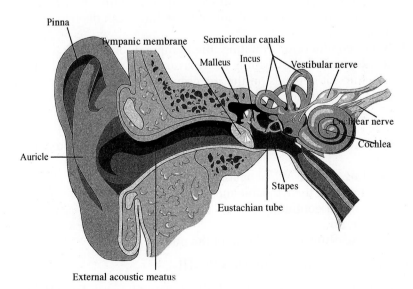

FIGURE 22-1. Anatomy of the ear.

The tensor tympani makes tympanic membrane taut and amplifies sounds; the stapedius pulls the head of the stapes back and decreases sound intensity.

The stimulating electrode in a cochlear implant is placed in the scala tympani.

articulates with the other two ossicles. No muscular attachments. The neck of the **stapes** serves as the attachment for the stapedius muscle, innervated by the stapedial branch of CN VII. The footplate of the stapes is attached to the oval window.

INNER EAR

The inner ear labyrinth consists of a bony labyrinth encompassing the membrous labyrinth and organs of hearing and balance.

- **Acoustic apparatus:** Composed of the cochlea, which consists of the scala vestibuli and scala tympani, both of which are filled with perilymph. The oval window transmits vibrations to the scala vestibuli at the base of the cochlea, which, via the helicotrema at the apex of the cochlea, transmits the pressure waves to the scala tympani. The scala tympani transmits the waves to the round window, where they are dissipated. The scala media, which contains the spiral organ of Corti, is the sensory portion of the inner ear and is filled with endolymph. The inner and outer hair cells in the organ of Corti transmit signals to the cochlear nerve (CN VIII). The neuroepithelium in the cochlea is arranged in a ribbon-like structure along the entire length of the cochlea, with tonotopic organization of sounds—higher frequencies are represented at the base of the cochlea, lower frequencies at the apex.
- **Vestibular apparatus:** Includes the vestibule (utricle and saccule) and semicircular canals, which provide input concerning gravitational pull/linear acceleration and angular acceleration, respectively. Cells in the neuroepithelial regions stimulate the vestibular nerve (cranial nerve [CN] VIII) and provide information about balance. The utricle and saccule as well as the semicircular ducts are filled with endolymph.

Physiology

EVALUATION OF HEARING

Sound waves can reach the cochlea in two ways:

- **Air conduction,** using the ear canal, tympanic membrane, and middle ear structures. Pathology at any of these levels can decrease air conduction.
- **Bone conduction,** vibrating the temporal bone and therefore the cochlea, which lies within it, bypassing the external and middle ear structures; it depends on the integrity of cochlear structures, CN VIII, and central auditory pathways.

Causes of **conductive** hearing loss (CHL):

- Obstruction of external auditory meatus by cerumen, foreign body, or debris.
- Swelling of the EAC, neoplasms, or stenosis of the canal.
- Perforation of the tympanic membrane.
- Ossicular discontinuity.
- Otosclerosis.
- Fluid, scarring, or neoplasms of the middle ear.

Causes of **sensorineural** hearing loss (SNHL):

- Damage to the hair cells of the organ of Corti by intense noise, barotrauma, viral infections (e.g., human herpesvirus), or ototoxic drugs (e.g., aminoglycosides).

- Presbyacusis (normal hearing deterioration with aging).
- Iatrogenic.
- Temporal bone fractures.
- Meningitis.
- Cochlear otosclerosis.
- Ménière's disease (see later discussion).
- Acoustic neuromas (schwannomas).

FUNCTIONAL TESTING

- **Weber test:** A 512-Hz fork is placed on the skull vertex; the patient is asked to which side the tone lateralizes. In conductive hearing loss, the sound lateralizes to the affected ear. In sensorineural hearing loss, the sound lateralizes to the unaffected ear.
- **Rinne test:** Compares the ability to hear by air conduction to that of bone conduction. A vibrating tuning fork is placed on the patient's mastoid process, and the patient is asked to indicate if they hear the sound and when it stops. The tuning fork is then placed at the EAC. Normally, sound is heard louder by air conduction than by bone, called a *positive* Rinne test, but with conductive hearing loss, bone conduction is louder, and thus the Rinne test is *negative*. With sensorineural hearing loss, this test is normal, although technically both bone and air sound perceptions are reduced.

The right ear is referred to as AD, the left ear as AS, both as AU.

Pathology

OTITIS MEDIA

Acute otitis media (AOM), recurrent AOM, chronic otitis media.

DEFINITION

- Inflammation of the lining of the middle ear cleft along with a bacterial infection.
- More common in children.
- Eustachian tube dysfunction and a preceding upper respiratory infection are the most documented etiologic factors precipitating AOM.
- Common bacterial pathogens include *Streptococcus pneumoniae*, *Haemophilus influenzae*, and *Moraxella catarrhalis*.

SIGNS AND SYMPTOMS

Otalgia, ear pulling, and systemic symptoms including fever, anorexia, vomiting, and diarrhea.

DIAGNOSIS

On otoscopic exam, the TM appears to be bulging, red, and immobile on pneumatic otoscopy.

TREATMENT

- Symptom control and analgesia, antibiotic therapy, and prevention of complications.
- For cases of recurrent AOM (more than three episodes of AOM in a 6- to 12-month period) antibiotic prophylaxis is recommended.
- A myringotomy with or without tympanostomy tubes may be recommended if the AOM is not responsive to antibiotics.

COMPLICATIONS

Complications of otitis media include TM perforation, hearing loss, and infection or inflammation of the temporal bone or intracranial cavity.

OTITIS MEDIA WITH EFFUSION (OME)

DEFINITION

Fluid collection in the middle ear cleft without the pain and fever associated with AOM.

SIGNS AND SYMPTOMS

Children usually present with hearing loss and speech delay.

DIAGNOSIS

Otoscopic examination reveals decreased TM mobility, opacity, and, occasionally, evidence of an air-liquid interface behind the TM (air bubbles).

TREATMENT

- There is a clear indication for treatment of children with chronic OME with **myringotomy and tympanostomy tubes** if:
    - There is evidence of change significantly decreased hearing to "conductive hearing loss."
    - The child is at high risk for speech and language delay (craniofacial disorders, cleft palate).
    - The child has a current delay.
    - There are recurrent bouts of AOM superimposed on OME.
    - There is evidence of structural changes to the TM.
- An adeniodectomy may be performed simultaneously in select patients to improve eustachian tube function.

OTITIS EXTERNA

DEFINITION

- Generalized inflammation involving the EAC skin.
- Can be infectious or eczematous.
- Organisms include hemolytic *Streptococcus*, *Candida*, *Staphylococcus*, and *Pseudomonas*.
- **Malignant otitis externa** in immunocompromised patients (e.g., elderly diabetics) is usually caused by *Pseudomonas* spp. and can have more extensive complications (e.g. osteomyelitis).

SIGNS AND SYMPTOMS

- Ear pain, redness, tenderness, weeping, and otorrhea.
- It is often difficult to examine the ear due to pain.

TREATMENT

- Analgesia to control the pain.
- Topical antibiotics +/– topical steroid cream.
- Systemic antibiotics for severe cases only.

CHOLESTEATOMA

DEFINITION

- Benign but invasive tumor of the middle ear/mastoid caused by overgrowth of displaced keratinizing epithelium.
- Can be **acquired** or **congenital**.

SIGNS AND SYMPTOMS

- Foul otorrhea, aural fullness or pressure, hearing loss.
- May cause CHL, SNHL, or CN VII injury or have intracranial extension.

DIAGNOSIS

- Diagnosis is made by noting an area of retraction filled with debris on otoscopic examination.
- Evaluation with computed tomographic (CT) scan and audiologic testing.

TREATMENT

Surgery is the definitive treatment, necessary to eradicate disease and prevent recurrence. It is sometimes performed in two stages to allow assessment for residual disease in the mastoid and middle ear (i.e., second-look procedure).

ACOUSTIC NEUROMA (VESTIBULAR SCHWANNOMA)

DEFINITION

- Benign tumor that arise in the cerebellopontine angle of the internal auditory canal.
- Associated with neurofibromatosis types I and II.

SIGNS AND SYMPTOMS

- The most common clinical singular is progressive asymmetric SNHL, followed by tinnitus and balance disturbance.
- Slow growing and nonmetastatic. They do, however, compress adjacent tissue as they grow, usually the vestibular and cochlear nerve within the internal auditory canal (IAC), but can compress the brain stem and facial nerve once they outgrow that space.

DIAGNOSIS

Audiogram shows unilateral SNHL.

TREATMENT

- Surgery or radiation therapy: Surgical approaches include translabyrinthine, middle cranial fossa and retrosigmoid/suboccipital.
- Watchful waiting is appropriate for patients who are not good surgical candidates.

TINNITUS

DEFINITION

The sensation of sounds originating inside the ear, "ringing in the ears."

SIGNS AND SYMPTOMS

- Usually described as a buzzing, hissing, or ringing sound; can be continuous or intermittent, unilateral or bilateral, and may be more noticeable when there is little background noise.
- Pulsatile tinnitus may be associated with a vascular tumor of the inner ear or an aneurysm.

DIAGNOSIS

- An audiogram is neccessary.
- Adjunctive to that are radiologic imaging and serologic studies.

TREATMENT

- Management of tinnitus can be difficult.
- Counseling the patient about the benign nature of the disease if there is no identified pathological cause.
- Tinnitus retraining therapy includes white noise generators, masking, and techniques for reduction in tinnitus intrusiveness.
- Some patients respond to a short course of antidepressants or anxiolytics for the associated anxiety.

VERTIGO

DEFINITION

- Illusory sensation of rotation or of rotation of objects around oneself, usually described as spinning.
- Can be central or peripheral in nature.
- When of otologic origin, the vertigo may be accompanied by other signs of otologic disease, including tinnitus and hearing loss.

DIAGNOSIS

- A full otologic examination and cranial nerve exam needs to be done, including examination for nystagmus, cerebellar screening tests, and examination of gait and balance. Positional testing for onset of vertigo sensation may be warranted.
- Other special investigations include audiometry, electronystagmography (for evaluation of nystagmus), and cold and warm caloric testing to test the input and symmetry of the vestibular system.

PERIPHERAL CAUSES

- Acute unilateral vestibular failure: Vertigo is of sudden onset. Vestibular therapy is available, and education about what precipitates the attacks (rapid head turning) and how to avoid them.
- Ménière's disease: Characterized by recurrent vertigo, tinnitus, aural fullness, and fluctuating SNHL. Caused by endolymphatic hydrops. Treatment includes diuretics and surgical placement of an endolymphatic shunt for severe cases.
- Benign paroxysmal positional vertigo (BPPV): Vertigo that occurs when the head is in a specific position; due to the displacement of otolith crystals from the crista of the posterior semicircular canal. Vertigo classically lasts < 2 minutes.
- Labyrinthitis: An infection in the labyrinth; can be a complication of middle ear disease.

Classic time frames for vertigo episodes:
Minutes: BPPV
Hours: Ménière's disease
Days: Labyrinthitis

The facial nerve innervates the muscles of facial expression; the digastric, sty-lohyoid, and stapedius muscles; as well as sensation to the anterior two thirds of the tongue and autonomic fibers for taste and to the salivary glands.

- **The circuitous path that the nerve takes has six segments:** *intracranial, meatal, labyrinthine, tympanic, mastoid,* and *extratemporal.*
- It courses through the parotid gland on its way, and splits into five portions that innervate the face: *temporal, zygomatic, buccal, marginal mandibular,* and *cervical.*

Extracranial branches of the facial nerve: The **Zebra Bit My Cookie**
Temporal
Zygomatic
Buccal
Marginal mandibular
Cervical
The posterior auricular branch comes off of the facial nerve before it splits into these five branches.

Facial Nerve Paralysis

- Trauma.
- Iatrogenic injury.
- Injury related to temporal bone fractures.
- Viral infection (herpes zoster oticus [Ramsay Hunt syndrome]).
- Lyme disease.
- Bacterial infection (malignant otitis externa).
- Systemic disease (Guillain-Barré syndrome, mononucleosis, sarcoidosis).

IDIOPATHIC FACIAL NERVE PARALYSIS: BELL'S PALSY

DEFINITION

- The most common form of paralysis.
- Ten percent of patients experience recurrent paralysis.
- Although the etiology is idiopathic, some suggest that the paralysis may result from a cycle of ischemic/inflammatory events of the nerve in the bony canal.
- There is no degeneration of the nerve.

Lesions of the upper motor neuron tract of the facial nerve spare the forehead, as the upper motor neurons innervate the face bilaterally. Lesion of the lower motor neuron (past the geniculate ganglion) involve the entire ipsilateral side of the face.

SIGNS AND SYMPTOMS

- Occurs as a unilateral facial weakness of sudden onset that resolves spontaneously.
- There should be no signs of concurrent central nervous system (CNS) or ear disease.
- Sixty percent of patients experience a viral prodrome, and 60% experience facial, neck, or ear numbness or pain prior to the palsy.
- Symptoms usually improve within about 6 months, completely by 12 months.

DIAGNOSIS

Evaluation includes a history and physical, an audiogram, and electrophysiologic testing of the nerve. If thought to be Bell's palsy and not due to some other cause, radiologic imaging is not recommended.

TREATMENT

- A course of steroids early in the disease process help shorten recovery time and serve as an analgesic.
- Surgical intervention with decompression of the nerve remains controversial.

The scale used to measure facial nerve function is called the **House-Brackman scale.** A score of 1 indicates complete function; 6 indicates complete loss of function.

HIGH-YIELD FACTS

Ear, Nose, and Throat

Anatomy

- **External structure:** Paired nasal bones, midline septum, paired upper and lower lateral cartilages, soft tissue.
- **Internal structure:** The nasal cavity opens to the face through the nares (nostrils). Its axis is at a right angle to the face. Posteriorly, the choana communicate with the nasopharynx.
  - The internal nose is divided into two sides, bound medially by the nasal septum, composed of multiple cartilages and bony structures.
    - Anterior: Quadrangular cartilage.
    - Posterior: Perpendicular plate of the ethmoid and vomer.
    - Inferior: Maxillary spine.
    - The septum is covered by perichondrium and periosteum, which is then covered by nasal mucosa (respiratory epithelium).
  - The lateral border of the nasal cavities consists of three bony ridges called *turbinates*, which each cover an area called a *meatus*. Each meatus contains *ostia*, which drain the paranasal sinuses. The superior and middle turbinates are parts of the ethmoid bone; the inferior turbinate is an independent bone.
  - Four paranasal sinuses: Air spaces in the bony structure of the face that communicate with the nasal cavity via various ostia.
    - Paired maxillary sinuses laterally.
    - Ethmoids and sphenoids superoposteriorly.
    - Frontal sinuses superiorly.

Only the maxillary and ethmoid sinuses are present at birth.

Structure	Opening
Sphenoethmoidal recess	Sphenoid sinus
Superior meatus	Posterior ethmoidal air cells
Middle meatus	Frontal sinus, maxillary sinus, middle ethmoidal air cells, anterior ethmoidal air cells—osteomeatal complex
Inferior meatus	Nasolacrimal duct

BLOOD SUPPLY

Both the *internal carotid system*, via the anterior and *posterior ethmoidal arteries*, and the *external carotid system*, via the *internal maxillary/sphenopalatine artery*, supply the nasal cavity and paranasal sinuses. The facial artery also supplies the *anterior* nose.

NERVE SUPPLY

Sympathetic autonomic innervation has a vasoconstrictive effect; **parasympathetic** fibers function in vasomotor stimulation.

Physiology

- **Nasal respiration:** Humidification, warming, and filtration of inhaled air and substances.
- **Olfaction.**
- **Phonation:** Normal voice depends on contribution of nasal resonance; disorders can give rise to hypo- or hypernasal speech.

- **Anterior rhinoscopy:** Using a nasal speculum. Allows visualization of the anterior portion of the nose, septum, and turbinates.
- **Nasal endoscopy:** Using a flexible or rigid scope. Provides diagnostic information, with attention to color, edema, discharge of nasal mucosa; allows for visualization of masses or abnormalities. Also allows for visualization of the nasopharynx, oropharynx, and hypopharynx/larynx.
- **Imaging:** Plain radiographic imaging of sinuses is of limited value. CT imaging has better resolution of structures, can evaluate for mucosal disease, provides a good "road map" for surgery. Can evaluate for septal deviation, polyps, masses, the osteomeatal complex, ethmoid air cells.

The nasal cavity is usually decongested and topically anesthetized prior to endoscopy (Afrin and lidocaine).

Sinus Disease

ACUTE BACTERIAL RHINOSINUSITIS

DEFINITION

- Infection of the paranasal sinuses/nasal mucosa, usually preceded by an upper respiratory infection (URI), allergy, trauma, or dental infection.
- Impaired immune function predisposes to recurrent disease.
- Usually bilateral.
- Causative organisms include *S. pneumoniae*, *H. influenzae*, and *M. catarrhalis*.

Topical decongestants must be used with caution. If used for more than 3 days, rebound congestion, or rhinitis medicamentosa develops, which causes worsening of symptoms.

SIGNS AND SYMPTOMS

Diagnosed after persistence of viral infection beyond 10 days, with severe or worsening symptoms, including maxillofacial pain, fever, dental pain, otalgia, malaise, and increased nasal drainage.

TREATMENT

- Medical management is with antibiotic therapy. Middle meatus culture or maxillary sinus aspiration can guide antibiotic treatment.
- Adjunctively, relief is provided with nasal saline irrigation, systemic decongestants, topical decongestants, and antihistamines if there is an allergic component.
- For treatment failure, a more comprehensive diagnostic workup is warranted, including imaging.

CHRONIC SINUSITIS

DEFINITION

Defined by sinusitis symptoms for > 3 months.

MANAGEMENT

- Patient receives maximal antibiotic therapy for 4–6 weeks prior to imaging studies, which often demonstrates anatomic variants predisposing the patients to osteomeatal compromise. Medical therapy often fails, and surgical therapy is necessary.
- **Functional endoscopic sinus surgery (FESS)** is the procedure of choice to promote natural drainage and aeration of the sinuses by opening up the osteomeatal complex.

ALLERGIC SINUSITIS

DEFINITION

- Includes both year-round (perennial) allergies and seasonal allergies.
- An immunoglobulin E (IgE)-mediated type 1 hypersensitivity reaction to allergens occurs.

SIGNS AND SYMPTOMS

- Symptoms include nasal obstruction, congestion, rhinorrhea and post-nasal drip, nasal/ocular/palatal pruritus, anosmia, sneezing, sinus pain, and headaches.
- On examination, the nasal mucosa often appears bluish in color and edematous, with visible clear, watery rhinorrhea.
- Some patients manifest an "allergic salute," a crease in the nose from upward stroking of the nasal tip, or "allergic shiners" under the eyes from lower eyelid venous stasis due to nasal congestion.

DIAGNOSIS

Diagnosis can be made on history and physical exam, although allergy testing is often performed when medical therapy for sinusitis fails.

TREATMENT

- Environmental control for allergens.
- Antihistamines are often used in combination with decongestants and topical nasal steroid sprays.
- Failure of pharmacologic therapy may necessitate allergy immunotherapy/desensitization to allergens if the disease is very disabling.

ACUTE INVASIVE FUNGAL SINUSITIS

DEFINITION

An invasive fungal sinus infection that usually occurs in an immunocompromised (e.g., HIV/AIDS, diabetic) host. A true surgical emergency.

SIGNS AND SYMPTOMS

- Diagnosis can be suggested by symptoms of sinusitis, often attenuated due to immunocompromise.
- Symptoms include fever, nasal ulceration and necrosis (~80% of patients), periorbital and facial swelling, vision impairment, and ophthalmoplegia.

DIAGNOSIS

Sinus aspiration and tissue biopsy need to be performed immediately to detect the presence of fungi (cultures take weeks to grow).

TREATMENT

Treatment includes radical surgical eradication of the disease with wide debridement, systemic antifungal therapy, and correction of the immunocompromise, if possible.

Systemic Diseases of the Nose

WEGENER'S GRANULOMATOSIS

DEFINITION

- Systemic vasculitis.
- Presents with necrotizing granulomas of the upper and lower respiratory tract (including vasculitis and glomerulonephritis).

SIGNS AND SYMPTOMS

Ninety percent of patients have sinonasal complaints.

DIAGNOSIS

- Biopsy shows necrotizing granulomas and vasculitis.
- Elevated erythrocyte sedimentation rate (ESR).
- Positive stain for cytoplasmic antinuclear antibody (c-ANCA) has over 90% specificity and sensitivity for active generalized disease.

TREATMENT

Corticosteroids and cyclophosphamide (or other antimetabolites).

SARCOIDOSIS

DEFINITION

An idiopathic granulomatous inflammatory condition; often affects African-American females.

SIGNS AND SYMPTOMS

- Manifestations often mimic allergic rhinitis, with subsequent crusting, formation of submucosal granulomas, epistaxis, and pain.
- Later, ulceration and cartilage destruction may occur, along with sinus involvement.

DIAGNOSIS

- Diagnostic findings of the disease include hilar adenopathy on chest x-ray (CXR).
- Elevated angiotensin-converting enzyme (ACE) levels.

TREATMENT

Therapy depends on the severity of the disease, and includes intranasal or systemic steroid preparations.

Epistaxis

ETIOLOGY

Local Causes
- Trauma: Nose picking, external trauma, dry mucosa (common in the winter months).
- Barometric pressure changes.
- Sinusitis, URI, allergy.

Ninety-five percent of bleeding occurs in the anterior nasal cavity, and ~90% of those are from Kiesselbach's plexus, a confluence of vessels at the anterior septum. These vessels are prominent and most subject to drying, mechanical trauma, and exposure to irritants.

- Neoplasia.
- Septal perforations (with cocaine use).

Systemic Causes

- Systemic disease: Hypertension, renal disease, hepatic failure, heavy alcohol use.
- Hematologic disease: Hemophilia, coagulopathy, thrombocytopenia.
- Vascular lesions: Arteriosclerosis, hereditary hemorrhagic telangiectasia (Osler-Weber-Rendu disease).
- Medication related: Anticoagulants, NSAIDs.

ASSESSMENT AND TREATMENT

- Identify anterior vs. posterior and left vs. right bleeds by routine nasal speculum examination. Remember personal universal exposure precautions!
- Manage bleed based on severity and location. Decongestant and topical anesthetics help decrease the bleeding and allow for better visualization.
    - Anterior bleeds can usually be controlled with local pressure, pinching the tip of the nose with or without silver nitrate or electrocautery. An anterior nasal pack can be used as well, absorbable vs. nonabsorbable packing material.
    - A posterior bleed may require more vigorous management—posterior packing. The bleeding source can be more easily identified by nasal endoscopy.
- Determine the etiology of the bleed based on history and physical exam (coagulopathy, trauma, neoplasia) and manage that as necessary.
- Failure of appropriately placed packing with continued bleeding may require surgical therapy or sphenopalatine, anterior ethmoidal, or posterior ethmoidal artery ligation.
- Selective arterial embolization by an interventional radiologist is extremely effective as well, however, does carry a low risk for cerebral emboli.

Nasal Masses

Endoscopic examination, radiologic imaging, and surgical biopsy/removal are the mainstay of diagnosis and treatment.

BENIGN MASSES

- **Inflammatory polyps:**
    - An idiopathic, reactive, inflammatory condition of the nasal mucous membranes and sinuses, which often originates on the lateral aspect of the middle meatus.
    - Usually bilateral.
    - Occurs in one third of aspirin-allergic patients.
    - Symptoms include those of nasal obstruction, nonallergic rhinitis, and hypo/anosmia.
    - Treatment of choice is topical corticosteroids.
    - Systemic steroids for severe cases.
    - Surgical options for disease refractory to medical management include nasal polypectomy and FESS.
    - Recurrence is common.

- **Antrochoanal polyps:**
  - Unilateral polyps that originate in the antrum of the maxillary sinus and frequently extend through the maxillary osteum into the middle meatus.
  - Treatment is surgical removal, although they have a propensity for re currence.
- **Juvenile nasopharyngeal angiofibroma (JNA):**
  - A benign but locally aggressive vascular tumor of the nasal cavity, usually found in adolescent males. The cause is unknown.
  - Usually presents with epistaxis and symptoms of nasal congestion.
  - A smooth, lobulated, red-gray mass can be found in the posterolateral nasal cavity.
  - Diagnosis requires a contrast CT or MRI.
  - Treatment is primarily surgical removal.
  - Preoperative embolization can be performed within 72 hours prior to surgery to reduce blood loss.
- **Inverting papilloma** (~50% of nasal respiratory papillomas):
  - A benign nasal tumor that arises from the respiratory mucosa, associated with human papillomavirus, strains 6 and 11.
  - Presents as a unilateral polyp with nasal obstruction, epistaxis, rhinorrhea, sinusitis, and facial pain.
  - Appears as a gray-red bulky polypoid mass that is usually found on the lateral nasal walls.
  - It is called *inverting* because the epithelium usually invades surrounding stromal tissue.
  - Treatment is with surgical resection, usually endoscopically, although there is a significant recurrence rate.
  - There is a 5–10% chance of malignant transformation to squamous cell carcinoma.

Samter's triad: Nasal polyposis and reactive airway disease in a patient with asprin sensitivity.

MALIGNANCIES

- **Carcinoma:**
  - Nasal carcinoma accounts for between 27–35% of head and neck cancer.
  - Exposure to irritants and chemicals is associated with specific nasal carcinomas (hardwood dust with ethmoid sinus cancer, nickel exposure with squamous cell carcinoma, and working in shoe/leather tanning and chemical industry, anaplastic carcinoma of the nose and sinuses).
  - Treatment by en-bloc resection via a craniofacial approach is choice; however, due to extent and spread of the cancer, it is often limited.
  - Radiation therapy (RT) is often used as an adjuvant, with chemotherapy for palliation.
- **Lymphoma:**
  - The most common nonepithelial malignancy of the nose.
  - Usually associated with Epstein-Barr virus (EBV); more common in Asia.
  - Involvement usually includes the maxillary antrum, nasal cavity, and ethmoid sinuses.
  - Radiologic evaluation demonstrates opacification of the sinuses, bony erosion, and occasionally a mass.
  - Fresh biopsy sections need to be sent during surgical removal in order to identify the cancer.

- Combined RT and chemotherapy is the preferred method of treatment, as there is a risk of distant recurrence with RT alone.
- **Melanoma:**
  - Nasal melanoma accounts for ~1% of all melanomas.
  - Patients are usually over the age of 60.
  - On nasal endoscopy, the lesions may appear as a benign polyp, or a dark, fungating neoplasm.
  - Treatment is by surgical resection, with a 5-year survival of about 30%.
- **Esthesioneuroblastoma:**
  - An unusual neuroectodermal tumor that arises from the olfactory epithelium high in the nasal cavity, usually involves the skull base and spreads intracranially through the skull base.
  - Symptoms include anosmia, along with other symptoms of nasal obstruction.
  - Treatment is surgical, via a craniofacial approach.
  - RT is used when there are close or positive margins, recurrent disease, and high-grade lesions.
  - Survival is 78% at 5 years and about 60–70% at 10 years.
- **Sinonasal undifferentiated carcinoma (SNUC):**
  - A rare malignancy that usually presents with nasal obstruction, proptosis, epistaxis, rhinorrhea, and facial pain, and neurologic symptoms, which include CN palsies, headache, and impaired mentation.
  - Local disease invasion (sinuses, cranial fossa) is common, and onset of symptoms is usually rapid.
  - Treatment is not standardized as this malignancy is rare; however, it is usually multimodal.
  - Poor prognosis.

Anatomy

- The oral cavity begins at the vermillion border of the lips, ends at the junction of the soft and hard palate superiorly and at the circumvallate papillae of the tongue.
- It includes the lips, buccal mucosa, superior and inferior alveolar ridges, part of the tongue, hard palate, and floor of the mouth.
- The salivary ducts terminate into the oral cavity, including the parotid Stensen's ducts lateral to the second maxillary molars, the submandibular Wharton's duct onto the floor of mouth, along with multiple sublingual duct orifices that drain into the floor of mouth as well.
- The tongue is included in the oral cavity; the frenulum is a fold of mucosa that is anteriorly attached to the tongue that attaches it to the floor of mouth mucosa.
- The oropharynx begins at the junction of hard and soft palate superiorly and the circumvallate papillae on the tongue, and extends to the valeculae).
- The oropharynx contains a ring of lymphoid tissue called Waldeyer's ring. It consists of the adenoids superoposteriorly, the palatine tonsils laterally, and the lingual tonsil at the base of the tongue.

BLOOD SUPPLY

- The palate is supplied by small branches of the descending palatine artery, a branch of the maxillary artery.

- Vascular supply to tongue is via the lingual artery (a branch of the external carotid) and respective vein.
- The tonsils are supplied by the tonsilar and ascending palatine branches of the facial artery, by a branch of the lingual artery, by the ascending pharyngeal artery, and the lesser descending palatine branch of the maxillary artery.

NERVE SUPPLY

- The anterior two thirds of the tongue has somatic sensory innervation from CN V_3, and taste is via the chorda tympani (CN VII). The posterior one third of the tongue is innervated by CN IX (gag reflex) for sensory and taste.
- The muscles of the pharynx are innervated by CN X, except for the tensor veli palatini, which is innervated by CN V_3, and the stylopharyngeus, which is innervated by CN IX. Sensory innervation to the pharynx is by CN V_2, IX, and X.
- Sensory innervation to the oral cavity is via V_3.

Physiology

- The primary function of the oral cavity and oropharynx is mastication of food and food delivery to more distal structures.
- Saliva in the mouth lubricates and begins to digest the food.
- The tongue, lips, muscles, and palate move the bolus of food posteriorly into the oropharynx and then down to the esophagus.
- Once the bolus reaches the oropharynx, voluntary control of swallowing is switched to involuntary control to propel the bolus quickly past the closed glottis to the esophagus.
- During this time, the nasopharynx closes with palate elevation, and respiration must cease.

Infections of the Oral Cavity and Oropharynx

PHARYNGITIS

DEFINITION

- Nonspecific pharyngitis is very common.
- *Acute* pharyngitis can be caused by various environmental factors (cold air, irritants, postnasal drip, reflux) or by an infectious agent, usually viral or *Streptococcus*.
- *Chronic* infection is usually a low-grade problem due to recurrent irritation of the mucous membrane (smoking, postnasal drip, reflux).

SIGNS AND SYMPTOMS

- The patient usually complains of an irritated, sore throat, with some pain on swallowing.
- If infectious, there may be lymphadenopathy, and the pharyngeal mucosa can appear red and inflamed with some mucopus.
- Symptoms of *chronic pharyngitis* are similar to that of a sore throat. Treatment involves withdrawing from the atmosphere and eliminating irritants.

TREATMENT

- Treatment is symptomatic if the pharyngitis is mild.
- In more severe cases, antibiotics are prescribed, especially when infected with strep (to prevent the consequences).
- Steam inhalation and topical numbing agents provide some relief for chronic cases.

MONONUCLEOSIS

DEFINITION

- A generalized infection with EBV, of which pharyngotonsillitis is one of the manifestations.
- The virus is spread by droplet transmission.

SIGNS AND SYMPTOMS

- Patients usually complain of a prodromal illness, which is then followed by a severe sore throat, odynophagia, and large bilateral lymphadenopathy.
- The tonsils are often covered by a whitish exudate.
- Other signs of the disease include petechial hemorrhages on the palate, hepatosplenomegaly, and encephalitis.

DIAGNOSIS

Diagnosis is based on the presence of atypical lymphocytes on a peripheral blood smear, and by a positive heterophile antibody test, which is positive in about 90% of patients.

TREATMENT

- Supportive.
- Systemic steroid may be necessary if the patient is having a lot of difficulty breathing.
- Antibiotics should be avoided and a classic diffuse rash occurs when amoxicillin is administered.

PERITONSILLAR ABSCESS

DEFINITION

- Located deep to the tonsillar capsule, usually at the superior pole.
- May be preceded by a pharyngitis.

SIGNS AND SYMPTOMS

Presents with fever, deviation of the tonsil and uvula, pain, soft palate swelling, trismus, and a hot potato voice.

DIAGNOSIS

Clinical examination.

COMPLICATIONS

- Parapharyngeal abscesses if the infection spreads beyond the superior constrictor muscle, bacteremia, endocarditis, mediastinitis, airway obstruction, and aspiration pneumonia.

Indications for tonsillectomy: recurrent tonsillitis (6/yr × 1 year, 5/yr × 2 years, 3/yr × 3 years), upper airway obstruction due to tonsillar hypertrophy (obstructive sleep apnea), recurrent peritonsillar abscess, malignancy.

TREATMENT

Needle drainage, incision and drainage, or tonsillectomy.

Systemic Disease Affecting the Oral Cavity

- **Pernicious anemia:** Vitamin B$_{12}$ deficiency. The tongue may show lobulations or be shiny, smooth, and red.
- **Osler-Weber-Rendu disease (hereditary hemorrhagic telangiectasia):** Angiomatous-appearing lesions on the oral and nasal mucosa and tongue. May be associated with recurrent epistaxis.
- **Nutritional deficiency:** *Pyridoxine* and *nicotinic acid* deficiency present with angular cheilosis; *vitamin C* deficiency with gingivitis and bleeding gums.

Benign Mucosal Lesions

APHTHOUS ULCERATION

DEFINITION

- Ulceration of the oral mucosa.
- They are recurrent, and last between 7 and 10 days.
- The etiology of these ulcers is unknown.

TREATMENT

- Treatment is symptomatic, with use of topical steroid creams or anesthetic agents.
- Any persistent ulcer should be biopsied to rule out a malignant lesion.

LEUKOPLAKIA

DEFINITION

- It is characterized by white patches on the oral mucosa.
- These lesions place the patient at greater risk for developing a carcinoma, as they are often composed of atypical or dysplastic cells.

TREATMENT

Excision.

The HIV/AIDS Patient

Oral mucosal manifestations of the disease include:

- **Oral candida:** Characterized by white patches that can be removed with a gentle scraping and result in punctate bleeding. Topical treatment with Nystatin "swish and swallow."
- **Herpes simplex virus (HSV)** infection.
- **Bacterial** infection/periodontal disease, often with **atypical bacterial strains.**

Ranula

DEFINITION

- A mucocele of the sublingual gland that presents as a cystic mass on the floor of mouth.
- It is called a "plunging ranula" when it penetrates the mylohyoid muscle, and presents as a soft submental neck mass.

TREATMENT

Excision should include the entire sublingual gland to prevent recurrence, with care taken dissecting around the lingual nerve and Wharton's duct.

Obstructive Sleep Apnea (OSA)/Sleep-Disordered Breathing

DEFINITION

- A group of disorders that disrupt sleep.
- Sleep apnea can be central or occur due to obstruction of the airway during sleep, usually a result of adenotonsillar hypertophy, a long uvula, excessive pharyngeal folds, or upper airway collapsibility/resistance.
- When obstructive, there is a normal voluntary effort made to breathe.
- Physiologic hypertrophy is most common in children between the ages of 2 and 5 years; however, congenital syndromes in which the nasopharynx or mandible is small or tongue is large can precipitate this syndrome.
- Obese adults, often with comorbid disease, are usually affected as well.

SIGNS AND SYMPTOMS

- Symptoms include loud snoring and breathing, irregular respirations during sleep, pauses/gasps, arousal, and daytime hypersomnolence.
- Children may have enuresis, behavior disorders, and growth retardation.
- If severe hypoxia or hypercapnia occurs, then pulmonary disease, including pulmonary hypertension, cor pulmonale, dysrhythmias, and sudden death can occur.

DIAGNOSIS

- Physical examination includes upper airway examination for the site of obstruction and signs of obesity.
- Relevant investigations include lateral neck radiography and polysomnography/sleep study (gold standard).

TREATMENT

- Symptoms can sometimes be alleviated with weight loss.
- Continuous positive airway pressure (CPAP) if a useful medical tool and the mainstay of therapy for adults.
- Surgical intervention includes palatopharyngeal surgery of the uvula, tonsils, and soft palate.
- In children, the apnea is usually resolved with an adenotonsillectomy.
- Tracheotomy.

Oral Malignancies

ORAL CAVITY CARCINOMA

DEFINITION

- Carcinoma of the lip, tongue, floor of mouth, gums, palate.
- Risk factors include tobacco smoke, pipes, betel nut chewing, alcohol, and sunlight exposure (cancer of the lip).
- Mostly squamous cell carcinoma (SCC).

SIGNS AND SYMPTOMS

May present with leukoplakia or erythroplakia, mass or ulceration, or as symptoms due to the invasion of other structures (loose teeth, trismus).

DIAGNOSIS

Assessment involves a biopsy, usually in the OR, along with panendoscopy to look for a second primary tumor. Patients also have a CXR and adjunctive imaging to assess the neck and evaluate extent of invasion. Staging with tumor-node-metastases (TNM) system.

TREATMENT

- Early stages are usually treated surgically.
- When advanced, combined modalities are used.
- The oral cavity has a rich lymphatic supply, so elective neck dissection is often recommended.
- As management of regional lymphatic spread is necessary. Therapeutic neck dissection is performed when there is clinically apparent nodal disease.

OROPHARYNGEAL CARCINOMA

DEFINITION

- Ninety percent SCC, keratizing or nonkeratizing (often with submucosal spread).
- Lymphocytic malignancies include lymphoma of the palatine tonsil and base of tongue. May be the first symptom of a systemic lymphoma.

SIGNS AND SYMPTOMS

Jugulodigastric and submental lymph node groups are most commonly affected.

DIAGNOSIS

- Physical examination includes careful assessment of the pharynx and larynx, as second primary tumors are common.
- Use bimanual palpation (especially for base of tongue), nasal endoscopy, and panendoscopy under sedation.

TREATMENT

- Treatment by radiation therapy is preferred, resulting in less morbidity and functional disturbance.
- Combined modalities, including surgery, chemotherapy, and RT are sometimes used as well, depending on where the lesion is (tonsil vs. base of tongue).

- Patients have an increased risk for distant metastasis; large bulky tumors and nodes should be followed closely and carefully for signs of local, regional, and distant recurrence.

Anatomy

- Cartilaginous skeleton includes the cricoid, thyroid, arytenoids, corniculate, and cuneiform cartilages.
- The cricoid cartilage forms a complete ring.
- Superiorly, the hyoid bone forms an important framework for the larynx below it, as it is a major point of attachment for the extrinsic muscles of the larynx (see Figures 22-2 and 22-3).
- The laryngeal cavity is divided by the *true vocal cords* (TVCs):
  - Above them is the **supraglottis,** from the tip of the epiglottis to the apex of the ventricle, halfway between the true and false vocal cords. It includes the epiglottis, arytenoids, aryepiglottic folds, and false vocal cords.
  - The **glottis** is composed of the vocal folds—the middle of the laryngeal ventricle to 1 cm below the vocal folds.
  - The subglottis begins 1 cm below the TVC to the inferior edge of the cricoid cartilage.
- Muscle groups of the larynx are described as either:
  - **Extrinsic:** Depressors and elevators of the larynx, including the stenohyoid, thyrohyoid, omohyoid, geniohyoid, digastric, mylohyoid, and stylohyoid, innervated by cervical nerves, CN V, and CN VII.
  - **Accessory:** Pharyngeal constrictor muscles.

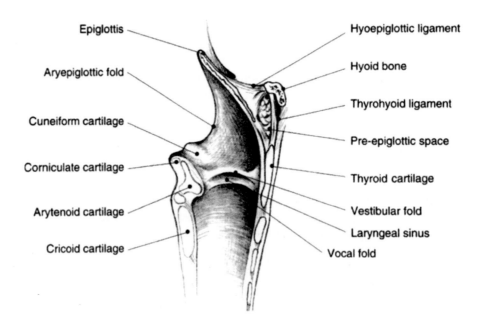

Epiglottis
Aryepiglottic fold
Cuneiform cartilage
Corniculate cartilage
Arytenoid cartilage
Cricoid cartilage

Hyoepiglottic ligament
Hyoid bone
Thyrohyoid ligament
Pre-epiglottic space
Thyroid cartilage
Vestibular fold
Laryngeal sinus
Vocal fold

FIGURE 22-2. **Sagittal section of the larynx demonstrating anatomic divisions of the larynx.**

(Reproduced, with permission, from Lee KJ. *Essential Otolaryngology: Head & Neck Surgery,* 8th ed. New York: McGraw-Hill, 2003: 597.)

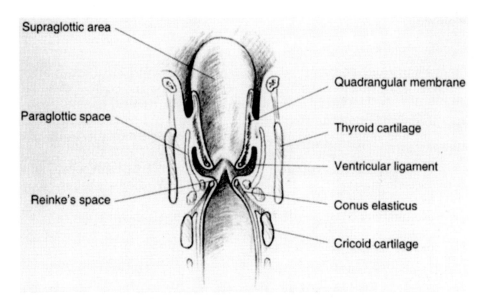

Supraglottic area
Quadrangular membrane
Paraglottic space
Thyroid cartilage
Ventricular ligament
Reinke's space
Conus elasticus
Cricoid cartilage

FIGURE 22-3. **Coronal section of the larynx illustrating barriers to the spread of carcinoma.**

(Reproduced, with permission, from Lee KJ. *Essential Otolaryngology: Head & Neck Surgery*, 8th ed. New York: McGraw-Hill, 2003: 598.)

- **Intrinsic:** Thyroarytenoid, thyroepiglottic, aryepiglottic; muscles of the arytenoids cartilage including the interarytenoid, posterior cricoarytenoid, and lateral cricoarytenoid muscles, which are responsible for abducting and adducting the vocal cords; and the cricothyroid muscle.

LYMPHATIC DRAINAGE

- Drain mainly to the deep cervical group.
- The vocal cords themselves contain very few lymphatic channels, however the supra- and subglottic areas contain extensive lymphatic drainage (important in metastatic tumor spread).

NERVE SUPPLY

Two branches of the vagus nerve (CN X) supply the larynx:

- **Superior laryngeal nerve:** Divides into the external and internal branches.
  - **External:** Supplies motor fibers to the cricothyroid muscle only.
  - **Internal:** Sensory innervation to all areas of the larynx above the glottis.
- **Recurrent laryngeal nerve:** Due to embryonic development, the nerve descends into the thorax on the left side and passes under the aortic arch before it returns to the neck. Provides motor function to all of the intrinsic muscles of the larynx except for the criothyroid muscle; sensory innervation to the laryngeal mucosa below the glottis.

An emergency surgical airway, cricothyroidotomy is created by puncturing through the cricothyroid membrane, situated anteriorly, between the thyroid cartilage and the cricoid cartilage.

Physiology

Functions of the larynx include:

- **Phonation:** The vocal cords act by vibrating. Instrinsic muscles determine the vibratory characteristics such as tension and contour of the vocal cords. The lateral cricoarytenoid and thyroarytenoid muscles adduct the cords, approximating the vocal processes and close the glottis during phonation; the posterior cricoarytenoid muscle primarily abduct the cords, thereby opening the glottis.
- **Protection of the repiratory tract:** The larynx acts as a sphincter—muscles elevate and close the larynx, determine epiglottis position, vocal cord adduction, cough reflex.
- **Respiration:** Muscular dilatation of the laryngeal aperture.

EVALUATION OF THE LARYNX

Indirect laryngoscopy:

- **Mirror examination:** Noninvasive but limited exam of the larynx, headlight illumination of a laryngeal mirror held up against the uvula, reflects an image of the larynx.
- **Flexible fiberoptic examination:** Through the nose.
- **Videostroboscopy:** A large-bore, rigid, 90° fiberoptic endoscope. A camera inside the endoscope continually flashes at a predetermined speed, allowing assessment of vocal fold symmetry, the mucosal wave and subtle lesions.
- **Direct laryngoscopy:** Done in the OR under general anesthesia. A rigid laryngoscope is inserted; one can perform procedures through the scope (biopsy, laser).

Infectious/Inflammatory Lesions of the Larynx

ACUTE LARYNGITIS

DEFINITION

- Infection of the larynx, usually the extension of an upper respiratory infection.
- Most commonly viral (adenovirus, influenza), but superimposed bacterial infection is possible.
- Can occur from smoking, fumes, inhalation, alcohol exposure.
- More problematic in people who use their voice professionally (singers, public speakers, teachers).

SIGNS AND SYMPTOMS

- Symptoms include hoarseness, laryngeal pain and discomfort, irritative cough.
- Examination of the pharynx may reveal pharyngitis, and laryngoscopy may reveal a red, swollen larynx; thickened cords; and an abundance of mucous secretions.

TREATMENT

- Treatment is symptomatic, as laryngitis is usually self-resolving.
- Voice rest, humidification, and increased fluid intake are key.
- Antibiotics may be necessary if there is a superimposed bacterial infection.

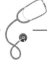

- Stridor: The audible result of turbulent airflow in the larynx/ trachea.
- Inspiratory: Supraglottic pathology
- Expiratory: Tracheal pathology
- Biphasic: Glottic or subglottic pathology

Distinguished from **stertor**, which is generated by pharyngeal obstruction (snoring).

EPIGLOTTITIS

DEFINITION

- A form of acute laryngitis, where the inflammation primarily affects the epiglottis.
- Occurs mainly in children ages 2–7, although with the onset of *H. influenzae* vaccination, cases have virtually disappeared.

SIGNS AND SYMPTOMS

- Rapidly progressing dyspnea, inspiratory stridor—a **medical emergency.**
- Dysphagia, refusal to eat, drooling, dehydration, fever, tachycardia, and restlessness may also be present.
- The voice is described as a "hot potato voice."
- Patients are usually more comfortable sitting up and leaning forward, stenting open the airway.

DIAGNOSIS

- Pediatric patients should be taken to the OR for airway control if there is suspicion of epiglottitis. **Do not** try to visualize the airway, as it can precipitate an episode of extreme respiratory distress.
- Soft tissue radiographs are diagnostic; they show thumbprinting of the epiglottis.

TREATMENT

- Management includes orotracheal intubation or tracheostomy, visualization of the epiglottis under direct laryngoscopy, cultures of the tissue and blood, observation in a monitored care setting, and antibiotic therapy with full coverage for β-lactamase *H. influenzae*.
- Steroids may be used to control the edema and swelling.
- Extubation once the edema and swelling subside (24–48 hours).

SUPRAGLOTTITIS (IN ADULTS)

- Similar to epiglottitis in children, although etiologic agents are more diverse microbiologic organisms, commonly *Streptococcus/Staphylococcus*.
- Potentially fatal as well, as acute swelling of the airway can lead to obstruction.
- Broad-spectrum antibiotic therapy, including coverage for *H. influenzae* as well.

CROUP (ACUTE LARYNGOTRACHEOBRONCHITIS)

DEFINITION

- An acute infection of the lower respiratory tract, extending from the larynx through the bronchial tree.
- More common during the winter season.
- Etiology is usually viral; parainfluenza types are the most common.
- Predominantly affects children ages 1–3.

SIGNS AND SYMPTOMS

- Symptoms begin as those of a common cold, with presence of a cough.
- Hoarseness and stridor follow as swelling increases.
- Retractions and circumoral pallor are indicative of impending airway obstruction.
- Fever, restlessness, dehydration, agitation, tachycardia, and tachypnea may be evident as well.

DIAGNOSIS

An AP film of the neck will reveal subglottic narrowing from the resultant edema—"steeple sign."

TREATMENT

- Hospitalization and antibiotic therapy for β-lactamase-producing organisms.
- Racemic epinephrine via positive pressure.
- Steroids can be helpful, as can airway humifidication and oxygen supplementation.
- Endotracheal intubation is indicated when there are signs of impending airway obstruction.

REINKE'S EDEMA

- Swelling of the vocal cords that results in increased volume of the subepithelial space below the cords.
- Usually occurs in smokers and people who abuse their voice; common in middle-aged women.
- Swelling is bilateral, often has a polypoid appearance.
- In addition to cessation of smoking and voice use, the vocal cords must be stripped in stages for complete resolution.

LARYNGOPHARYNGEAL REFLUX (LPR)

See Esophagus chapter for a more complete discussion of gastrointestinal reflux disease (GERD).

DEFINITION

Acid laryngitis, the most common upper airway manifestation of GERD.

SIGNS AND SYMPTOMS

Patients present with a variety of symptoms, including hoarseness, vocal fatigue, chronic throat clearing, excessive phlegm production, globus sensation, heartburn, and discomfort.

DIAGNOSIS

Complete head and neck exam, fiberoptic laryngoscopy with photographic evidence of erythematous arytenoid mucosa and swelling, ambulatory 24-hour pH probe monitoring, and a barium esophagram.

TREATMENT

- Same as for GERD: Begin with lifestyle and dietary modifications, then advance to antireflux medications.
- Fundoplication surgery if symptoms are severe or persistent.

Benign Lesions of the Vocal Cords

POLYP

DEFINITION

- A pedicled or sessile lesion that occurs on the vocal cords.
- They vary in size and appear as a smooth, glistening body.
- Can overhang the vocal cords, and may be evident on examination only when the patient is asked to cough and the polyp arises from the under-surface of the cords.

SIGNS AND SYMPTOMS

- Presents as long-standing hoarseness.
- Occasionally, they can be large and cause stridor and airway obstruction.

TREATMENT

- Definitive treatment is by lifestyle modifications (smoking, voice abuse), endoscopic removal of the lesion, and stripping of the cords if lesions are bilateral.
- If airway obstruction occurs, tracheotomy or laser debulking of the lesions may be necessary.

CONTACT ULCERS

DEFINITION

- Caused by vocal abuse or laryngeal trauma like coughing or throat clearing, persistent postnasal drip, LPR.
- Most commonly occur on the vocal processes of the arytenoids.

SIGNS AND SYMPTOMS

- Symptoms include hoarseness and pain on phonation.
- Ulceration is noted on examination of the larynx.

TREATMENT

Voice rest, vocal training, eradication of the precipitating factors (antibiotics, decongestion, antireflux medications), and, finally, endoscopic removal.

NODULE ("SINGER'S NODULES")

DEFINITION

- Localized traumatic laryngitis caused by vocal overuse (screaming, harsh talking, faulty singing technique), allergy, URI, sinusitis, smoking, and alcohol.
- Site of injury is usually the epithelium and basement membrane of the vocal cords.

Laryngeal Foreign Bodies
Most commonly food related. Obstruction is usually relieved by the normal reflexes. General anesthesia and rigid bronchoscopy is recommended for removal of the foreign body. If the patient becomes completely obstructed during the removal, the foreign body should be pushed further into the bronchus so that the contralateral lung can be ventilated.

SIGNS AND SYMPTOMS

- Usually presents as hoarseness.
- On exam, nodules are commonly found at the junction of the anterior and middle third of the vocal cords, the area of maximum vibration of the cords.
- Usually bilateral.

TREATMENT

- Behavioral modification, vocal reeducation, voice rest, and therapy.
- Microlaryngoscopic excision if nonresolving.

PAPILLOMA

DEFINITION

- The most common benign tumor of the larynx.
- Bimodal age distribution.
- Causative agent thought to be human papillomavirus (HPV). Certain subtypes of the virus can undergo malignant transformation.
- Can involve any region of the larynx and trachea, as well as the lungs.

SIGNS AND SYMPTOMS

Aphonia or a weak cry in infants, dyspnea and stridor, hoarseness.

TREATMENT

Treatment includes CO_2 laser excision, microdebridement, therapy with interferon, intralesional cidofovir injection, topical application of mitomycin C (an antineoplastic).

VOCAL CORD IMMOBILITY

DEFINITION

- **Congenital:** Cardiovascular lesions that stretch the recurrent laryngeal nerve (RLN).
- **Mechanical fixation:** Laryngeal cancer, rheumatoid arthritis, arytenoid dislocation.
- **Neurological causes:** Stroke, peripheral nerve injury.
- **Iatrogenic:** Birth trauma, thoracic/cardiac or neck surgery (thyroidectomy with injury to the recurrent laryngeal nerve, cervical spine diskectomy/ fusion).
- Paralysis occurs more commonly in adduction.
- Can be unilateral or bilateral.

SIGNS AND SYMPTOMS

- Patients present with a hoarse, breathy voice, usually of rapid onset. May be aspirating or having trouble handling secretions; signs of malignancy if present.
- In a child, unilateral paralysis presents with a weak cry.
- Bilateral paralysis presents with a normal voice or cry, but severe stridor due to airway obstruction and may require emergent airway management.

- Examination involves visualizing the cords during respiration and phonation.
- The postnasal space and chest must be examined for concurrent malignancy causing paralysis, which includes a CXR.
- Panendoscopy; CT to examine the course of the RLN—base of skull to the aortic arch.

TREATMENT

- Treatment is directed at the cause.
- Nonsurgical therapy includes voice therapy.
- Surgical options include vocal fold injection with alloderm, a gel or collagen-based substance (injection thyroplasty), or medialization of the cords by removing a portion of the thyroid cartilage and inserting a shim (Montogomery thyroplasty).
- In cases of severe airway problems, a tracheotomy may be the only way to improve airway function.

SUBGLOTTIC STENOSIS

DEFINITION

- Most commonly a result of prolonged endotracheal intubation.
- Frequently occurs in children (ex-preemies, neonatal intensive care unit [NICU] patients) since the subglottis is the most narrow portion of their airway.
- Can also occur from trauma to the trachea and larynx, neoplastic disease, irradiation, severe infection, or congenital stenosis (hemangioma, subglottic webs and cysts).

SIGNS AND SYMPTOMS

Patients usually present with dyspnea on exertion, wheezing (often misattributed to asthma), nonproductive cough and voice changes, biphasic stridor, and difficulty with extubation; children present with respiratory distress.

DIAGNOSIS

Laryngoscopy, lateral soft tissue films, or CT scan.

TREATMENT

Treatment is either by microlaryngoscopic laser removal, tracheotomy for airway access, or a laryngotracheoplasty.

Laryngeal Cancer

DEFINITION

- Malignant tumors of the larynx and pharynx are usually SCC.
- The most common site for carcinoma in the upper aerodigestive tract.
- As there is an extensive lymphatic supply to the supra- and subglottic regions of the larynx, there is well-defined metastasis to the lymph nodes of the jugular chain or paratracheal regions. The exception to this rule is glottic carcinoma, which presents earlier and has a small likelihood of lymphatic metastasis (owing to the poor lymphatic drainage of the glottis).
- Direct spread and invasion by tumors can occur as well.

- The etiologic factors for most laryngeal SCC are tobacco smoke and alcohol exposure, which act synergistically.

SIGNS AND SYMPTOMS

- The presentation of laryngeal cancer is usually progressive hoarseness due to interference with the vocal cords.
- Other symptoms include dyspnea, dysphagia from pharyngeal involvement, and referred ear pain (an ominous sign).

DIAGNOSIS

- Laryngoscopy must be done on a patient who has a persistent hoarse voice for > 2 weeks if over 40, and after 3–4 weeks if younger, assessing for asymmetry and the extent of any lesions.
- Tumors of the cords appear to be raised and warty in appearance; those of the supraglottis are usually exophytic.
- Vocal cord mobility must be noted.
- The neck is examined for metastatic lymphadenopathy.
- Diagnosis can occur after assessment of the larynx, pharynx, and oral cavity by direct microlaryngoscopy under general anesthesia.
- Depth of invasion and extent of the lesion need to be determined to stage the lesion (TNM classification) and guide treatment.
- Biopsies are taken.

TREATMENT

- Depends on stage and patient characteristics.
- It is either definitive removal or palliative.
- Early tumors are treated by a single modality, usually radiotherapy, and more complicated cases often with a laryngectomy (partial or total depending on the disease state) and postoperative RT.
- Options are available for voice reconstruction (a tracheoesophageal one-way valve) and return of swallowing that allow these patients to have a good quality of life.

▶ SALIVARY GLANDS

Anatomy

PAROTID

- Largest salivary gland; enclosed by deep cervical fascia. Composed of both deep and superficial lobes, separated by a plane of the facial nerve.
- Drains lateral to the second upper molar via Stensen's duct.
- The facial nerve passes through the gland, and divides into its five branches.
- Parasympathetic supply originates in the inferior salivatory nucleus, travels with CN IX to Jacobsen's nerve to the otic ganglion; synapses and fibers are carried on the auriculotemporal nerve of CN V_3.
- Sympathetic fibers come from the superior thoracic nerves and synapse with the superior cervical ganglion. They travel via arterial plexuses and sensory nerves to the gland.

SUBMANDIBULAR

- Drains into the mouth via Wharton's duct, which courses between the sublingual gland and hyoglossus muscle; opens through a small opening lateral to the frenulum on the floor of mouth.
- Parasympathetic supply originates in the superior salivatory nucleus, travels via nervus intermedius of CN VII to the chorda tympani, which then joins the lingual nerve to the submandibular ganglion. Fibers synapse there and travel to the gland.
- Sympathetic supply is the same as for the parotid gland.

SUBLINGUAL

Smallest major salivary gland; lies in a submucosal location on the floor of mouth, and opens there through numerous small ducts called the ducts of Rivinius.

MINOR SALIVARY GLANDS

Between 600 and 1000 distributed all over the oral cavity and oropharynx, mostly on the hard and soft palate.

Physiology

- Parasympathetic stimulation increases saliva secretion; sympathetic slows it down.
- Saliva is high in potassium, low in sodium; it contains substances that begin the breakdown of food, to maintain and protect the oral cavity environment, and immunoglobulin A (IgA).
- Produce between 0.5 and 1.5 L of saliva/day.

RADIOGRAPHIC EVALUATION

- CT/MRI is sometimes performed after injection of contrast medium directly into the ducts.
- Diagnostic ultrasound is also useful but has limitations.
- Fine-needle aspiration (FNA) for diagnosis of tumors vs. inflammatory lesions.

Benign/Systemic Disease

SJÖGREN'S SYNDROME

DEFINITION

- An autoimmune connective tissue disorder that is often associated with rheumatoid arthritis and systemic lupus erythematosus (SLE).
- Patients affected are usually middle-aged, menopausal women.

SIGNS AND SYMPTOMS

Presents with keratoconjunctivitis sicca (dry, itchy eyes), xerostomia, taste changes, enlargement of salivary glands.

DIAGNOSIS

The diagnosis is made clinically: Measurement of salivary flow rates and salivary gland biopsy showing lymphocytic infiltrate and acinar atrophy confirmin suspicions, in addition to relevant rheumatologic tests.

TREATMENT

Treatment for xerostomia and dry eyes is symptomatic: Salivary and lacrimal substitutes.

SIALOLITHIASIS

DEFINITION

- Hydroxyapatite stones in the salivary glands/ducts.
- Most commonly affects the submandibular gland.
- More common in middle-aged men.

SIGNS AND SYMPTOMS

Presents with pain and swelling in the affected area, with symptoms worsening prior to eating.

TREATMENT

- If the stone is in Wharton's duct, it can be surgically removed transorally.
- If it is closer to the hilum of the gland, the gland may need to be removed.

SIALOADENITIS

DEFINITION

- Acute form is due to inflammation of the gland.
- Chronic form is a recurrent, painful enlargement of the gland, caused by salivary stasis.
- Occurs in debilitated and dehydrated patients, after major surgery, trauma, x-ray therapy (XRT).
- Infectious agent is typically *Staphylococcus aureus.*

SIGNS AND SYMPTOMS

Erythema, pain, swelling, and purlent ductal discharge.

TREATMENT

- Acute form: Rehydration, sialogogues, warm compresses, and antibiotics.
- Chronic form: Medication to stimulate secretions, massages of the gland, and hydration.

MUMPS

DEFINITION

Infection with paramyxovirus in children, usually with a history of inadequate immunizations.

SIGNS AND SYMPTOMS

Bilateral painful parotid swelling, trismus, and malaise, along with other systemic manifestations (orchitis, pancreatitis, encephalitis).

DIAGNOSIS

Measurement of antibody titers.

TREATMENT

This condition is usually self-limited, so supportive symptomatic treatment is recommended.

SALIVARY GLAND TUMORS

- FNA may be a useful tool in diagnosis, especially for malignant lesions. CT/MRI imaging in conjunction, especially when planning for surgery.

Benign Tumors

PLEOMORPHIC ADENOMA

- Most common benign tumor; slight predilection for middle-aged women.
- Myoepithelial cells are thought to be the cell of origin.
- There is morphologic diversity: The tumor can be mucoid, chondroid, osseus, or myxoid.
- Slow growing, painless swelling of the gland, usually in the posterior region of the parotid gland.
- Rarely undergoes malignant transformation to carcinoma ex pleomorphic.
- Treatment: Parotidectomy.
- Care must be taken to expose the facial nerve proximal to where it enters the gland, and to follow it forward, dissecting tumor off of the nerve with care to preserve function.

MONOMORPHIC ADENOMA

- A benign tumor with features similar to pleomorphic adenoma, but with only one morphologic cell type present.
- Slow growing and solitary, most often in the parotid gland.

WARTHIN'S TUMOR

- AKA: Papillary cystadenoma lymphomatosum.
- Men > women (5:1); usually in older individuals.
- Often presents as a benign, painless, compressible, slow-growing mass. Can be bilateral in 10%.
- Treatment: Excision of the involved gland.

ONCOCYTOMA

- Benign tumor, mostly in the parotid; accounts for < 1% salivary gland tumors.
- Slow growing and circumscribed, not encapsulated.

Frey's syndrome: Gustatory sweating following parotid surgery, due to cross-reinnervation of the autonomic supply of the parotid gland, now to the overlying skin's sweat glands and blood vessels. Treat with an anticholinergic cream.

Malignant Tumors

MUCOEPIDERMOID CARCINOMA

- Most common malignant tumor of the salivary glands; derived from epithelial cells in the interlobar and intralobar epithelial cells of the gland.
- Can vary from low grade to highly malignant.
- Symptoms: Range from asymptomatic swelling (75%) to pain and facial nerve paralysis.
- Mostly affects the parotid.
- Most commonly induced by prior irradiation.
- Lymph node metastases are common in ~40% of patients.

CARCINOMA EX PLEOMORPHIC

- Usually presents in patients who have undergone resection of a pleomorphic adenoma.
- Pathology shows remnants of benign mixed tumor.

ADENOCARCINOMA

- Twenty percent of salivary tumors and only 4% of parotid tumors are adenocarcinomas.
- Eighty percent of patients are asymptomatic, although 20% have facial nerve paralysis and 15% facial pain due to fixation of the tumor to underlying/overlying structures.
- Arises from the terminal tubules and intercalated or strained duct cells in the gland.
- Many varieties have been described, and are graded as low, intermediate, or high.

ADENOID CYSTIC CARCINOMA

- Origin is the myoepithelial cell.
- Most common malignant tumor of the submandibular and minor salivary glands.
- Malignant but slow growing; most patients are asymptomatic on presentation even though a large percentage of those tumors are fixed to adjacent structures.
- Neurotropic tumor with early distant metastasis.

ACINIC CELL CARCINOMA

- Occurs exclusively in the parotid gland.
- Women > men.
- Pathologically defined by the presence of amyloid.
- Cell of origin in the serous acinar components and the intercalated duct cells.

▶ **NECK**

Anatomy

- The neck is traditionally divided into anterior and posterior triangles (Figure 22-4).

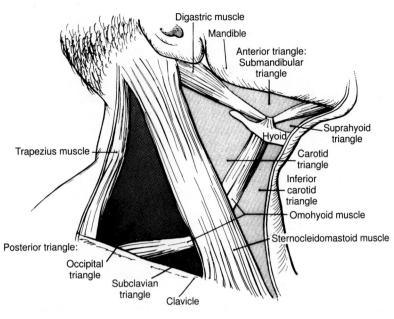

FIGURE 22-4. **Triangles of the neck.**

(Reproduced, with permission, from Lee KJ. *Essential Otolaryngology: Head & Neck Surgery*, 8th ed. New York: McGraw-Hill, 2003: 423.)

- There are two main fascial planes (Figure 22-5):
  - **Superficial cervical fascia:** Encloses the platysma and muscles of facial expression. It begins at the zygoma of the face and extends inferiorly to the clavicle.
  - **Deep cervical fascia:** Composed of four layers:
    1. **Superficial layer/investing fascia:** Encloses the trapezius, sternocleidomastoid (SCM), and strap muscles; submandibular and parotid glands; and the muscles of mastication. Stretches from the mandible to the clavicle.

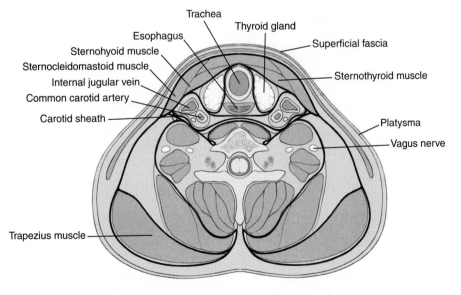

FIGURE 22-5. **Fascial planes of the neck.**

2. **Middle layer/visceral/pretracheal fascia:** Encloses the pharynx, larynx, trachea and esophagus, thyroid/parathyroid glands, buccinator and constrictors, and the strap muscles. It goes from the skull base to the mediastinum. Posteriorly, this fascia forms a midline raphe that connects to the alar layer of the prevertebral fascia.

3. **Deep layer/prevertebral fascia:** Encloses the paraspinous and cervical muscles; goes from skull base to the chest. Anteriorly, there are two layers to this fascia—the prevertebral layer lies anterior to the cervical vertebrae from the skull to the coccyx; anterior to that is the alar layer, which extends from the base of skull to the mediastinum. The danger space lies between the alar and prevertebral layers. Anterior to that is the visceral/buccopharyngeal fascial layer of the middle fascia.

4. **Carotid sheath fascia:** Envelopes the carotid artery, internal jugular vein, CN X. Runs from base of skull to the thorax.

- The spaces formed by the neck fascial layers are potential spaces for an infection to extend to, seed, and spread (Figure 22-6).
- **Above the hyoid bone:**
  - **Parapharyngeal:** Infectious spread from tonsils, pharynx, teeth, parotid gland, and extension from other spaces. Parotid involvement, trismus, fever, and sepsis common with an infection here. Extraoral approach for drainage.
  - **Submandibular.**
  - **Masticator:** Infected when molar teeth infection spreads.
  - **Parotid.**
  - **Peritonsillar:** Loose connective tissue that lies between the tonsillar capsule medially and the superior constrictor laterally. (See section on peritonsillar abscess earlier in this chapter.)
- **Below the hyoid bone:** Visceral space encloses the pharynx, esophagus, larynx, trachea, and thyroid. The prevertebral and retropharyngeal spaces lie posterior to it.

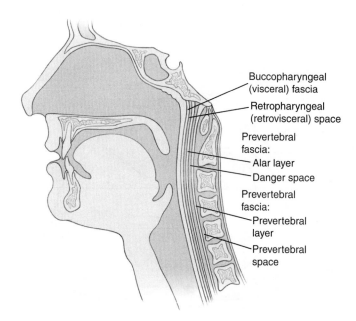

Buccopharyngeal (visceral) fascia

Retropharyngeal (retrovisceral) space

Prevertebral fascia:
Alar layer
Danger space

Prevertebral fascia:
Prevertebral layer
Prevertebral space

FIGURE 22-6. **Fascial layers of the retrovisceral space.**

- **Entire length of the neck:**
    - **Retropharyngeal:** Anterior to the alar layer and posterior to the buccopharyngeal fascia/esophagus and pharynx, an infection from here can spread to the danger space. Contains lymph nodes and connective tissue. The greatest number of LN here are found in children < 4 years old, and accounts for a large number of retropharyngeal abscesses.
    - **Danger/alar space:** Between alar layer and the prevertebral layer of deep cervical fascia. Infection spreads to superior mediastinum.
    - **Prevertebral:** Infection can spread to the coccyx.
    - **Vascular:** Infection of the carotid sheath.

VASCULAR SUPPLY

Carotid and subclavian systems.

NERVE SUPPLY

To the skin: C2–C4.

LYMPHATIC DRAINAGE

- The neck has a rich lymphatic network, and lymphogenous drainage from different sites in the head and neck is highly predictable.
- Lymph node areas are divided into different levels, which become relevant when performing a neck dissection and staging nodal disease.

Congenital Diseases in the Neck

BRANCHIAL APPARATUS ANOMALIES

- The head, neck, and related structures form embryologically from five branchial arches, grooves, and pouches (Table 22-1).
- Anomalies occur when pouches persist as a branchial sinus or a branchial fistula develops between the pouch and groove. A cyst can also develop if part of a groove or pouch becomes separated from the surface and does not resorb and become prone to repeated infections; need to be excised completely.

THYROGLOSSAL DUCT CYST

EMBRYOLOGY/DEFINITION

- The thyroid develops from the foramen cecum at the base of the tongue and migrates down to the root of the neck along the thyroglossal duct.
- A remnant of the embryological migration becomes a thyroglossal duct cyst.

SIGNS AND SYMPTOMS

- Presents as a midline infrahyoid structure.
- The cyst can be at any level along the route of the duct, and usually moves with swallowing and protruding the tongue because of its attachment to the base of tongue.
- These cysts can become infected and drain cutaneously.

TABLE 22-1. The Five Branchial Arches

Arch	Nerve	Bones/Cartilage	Muscles/Vessels	Other
First arch	Mandibular CN V$_3$	Mandible, malleus, incus	Muscles of mastication, tensor tympani, anterior belly of digastric, tensor palatine	The pouch forms the middle ear cavity, and part of the tonsillar fossa and palatine fossa. The groove forms the EAC. A fistula would extend from the skin of the neck to the regions of the eustachian tube.
Second arch	Facial CN VII	Stapes, part of hyoid	Stapedius muscle, facial muscles, buccinators	The pouch forms the tonsillar fossa, palatine tonsil. A fistula would extend from the skin on the lower one third of the neck, anterior to the SCM, to the supratonsillar fossa. These are the **most common** fistulas.
Third arch	Glossopharyngeal CN IX	Part of hyoid bone	Stylopharyngeus, superior and middle constrictors, common and internal carotid artery	The pouch forms the thymus and inferior parathyroid gland
Fourth arch	Vagus CN X/superior laryngeal nerve	Thyroid and cuneiform cartilage	Inferior pharyngeal constrictor, cricopharyngeus, cricothyroid muscle, L aorta, and proximal R subclavian artery	The pouch forms the superior parathyroid glands, ultimobranchial body
Sixth arch	Vagus/CN X—recurrent laryngeal branch	Cricoid, arytenoids, corniculate, and tracheal cartilage	Intrinsic laryngeal muscles, inferior constrictor muscle, and ductus arteriosus	There is no associated pouch

TREATMENT

- Surgical excision of the gland remnant (Sistrunk procedure), provided that ultrasound investigation reveals normal thyroid gland.
- The procedure involves removing the ectopic gland, duct, and central portion of the hyoid bone to minimize the chances of recurrence.

Lymphatic Malformation

Embryology/Definition

A malformation of the lymphatic system results in a multilocular neck mass filled with straw-colored fluid (formerly known as a cystic hygroma).

Signs and Symptoms

Usually presents at birth with extensive neck and facial swelling; may complicate the airway.

Treatment

- Resection is indicated, both functionally and cosmetically.
- Instillation of a sclerosing agent has shown some promise as well.

Infectious/Inflammatory Lesions of the Neck

Deep Neck Infection/Abscess

- Knowledge of facial planes and neck space relationships is key to managing neck infections and preventing morbidity and mortality.
- Common microorganisms are S. *aureus*, *Streptococcus pyogenes*, and anaerobic oral flora.

Lymphadenitis

Definition

- Most frequent cause of neck swelling.
- Usually reactive to an infection in tonsils, teeth, oropharynx, skin, or scalp.

Signs and Symptoms

The involved nodes are usually tender.

Treatment

- Resolves following resolution of the instigating illness, so treatment is directed at the underlying cause of infection.
- Incision and drainage (I&D) for abscess.

Ludwig's Angina

Definition

- Acute cellulitis of the submandibular triangle deep to the mylohyoid muscle.
- Usually arises from an oral cavity infection.

Signs and Symptoms

- Triangle is bound by attachment of the deep cervical fascia to the mandible and hyoid; suppuration that builds up creates a lot of pressure and pain.
- Infection can track posteriorly and potentially cause laryngeal edema.

Treatment

- Aggressive treatment with IV antibiotics is necessary.
- Intubation or tracheostomy may be needed to protect the airway.
- If nonresolving, may need I&D.

Although a neck abscess is usually suppuration of a reactive lymph node, investigation must be taken as to whether the node is infected with mononucleosis, tuberculosis (TB), or lymphoma. FNA of a TB abscess without excision can lead to a persistent draining sinus tract, and a lymphoma must be excised for diagnosis, not just needle biopsied.

RETROPHARYNGEAL ABSCESS

DEFINITION

- Usually results from a suppurating lymph node in the retropharyngeal space.
- Can be secondary to a penetrating pharyngeal injury.
- They can traverse to the danger space and track down to the mediastinum.

SIGNS AND SYMPTOMS

Patients are ill and febrile, dehydrated, complain of dysphagia and pain, and may be stridulous.

DIAGNOSIS

Lateral soft tissue radiography is helpful in diagnosis when there is marked swelling of the prevertebral tissues, and CT can be used to find the exact location of the abscess.

TREATMENT

Drain abscess; maintain airway with an endotracheal tube or a tracheostomy.

TUBERCULOSIS INFECTION

SIGNS AND SYMPTOMS

Can present in the neck as a chronically enlarged lymph node.

DIAGNOSIS

Investigation should include a thorough history, CXR, purified protein derivative (PPD) implantation.

TREATMENT

Definitive treatment is complete excision to prevent the occurrence of a persistent sinus tract.

Malignancy

THYROID/PARATHYROID TUMORS

See Endocrine System chapter.

LYMPHOMA

SIGNS AND SYMPTOMS

- A disease of young and middle-aged adults.
- Usually presents with multiple, slow-growing, rubbery lymph nodes in the neck, which may be the only presenting symptom of the disease.
- Systemic symptoms, including fever and night sweats, imply a worse prognosis.

DIAGNOSIS

Open biopsy of the node. Cellular architecture is important in both diagnosing Hodgkin's vs. non-Hodgkin's lymphoma and determining subtype of each.

TREATMENT

Depends on type and stage, and can include chemotherapy or RT.

METASTATIC LYMPHADENOPATHY

SIGNS AND SYMPTOMS

- Neck mass is the presenting sign of squamous cell carcinoma in the head and neck or other anatomic location.
- Usually presents in older patients with a firm neck mass.

DIAGNOSIS

- FNA, along with panendoscopy of the upper aerodigestive tract is useful for diagnosis.
- Presence of nodal disease significantly affects the stage of disease (TNM staging system).

TREATMENT

Dictated by the location of the primary tumor. A surgical dissection and removal of the neck nodes and associated structures is necessary to pathologically identify and treat the disease.

Neck Dissection
Radical: Removal of all levels of lymph nodes, the SCM, internal jugular vein, and CN XI.
Modified radical: A more selective procedure—removal of all levels of lymph nodes, but preservation of either SCM, internal jugular vein, or CN XI.
Selective: All levels of lymph nodes are not removed.

▶ **REFERENCES**

Lee KJ. *Essential Otolaryngology: Head and Neck Surgery*, 8th ed. New York: McGraw-Hill, 2003.

Burton M. *Hall and Colman's Diseases of the Ear Nose and Throat*, 15th ed. New York: Churchill Livingstone, 2000.

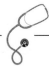

The unknown primary head and neck cancer: Identify based on lymph node presentation pattern and characteristic locations draining to lymphatic groups.

HIGH-YIELD FACTS

Ear, Nose, and Throat

Neurosurgery

Cranial Foramina

- **Optic canal:** Optic nerve and ophthalmic artery.
- **Superior orbital fissure:** Cranial nerves (CN) III, IV, VI, and V_1.
- **Foramen rotundum:** CN V_2.
- **Foramen ovale:** CN V_3.
- **Carotid canal:** Internal carotid artery.
- **Internal acoustic meatus:** CN VII and VIII.
- **Stylomastoid foramen:** CN VII and stylomastoid artery.
- **Jugular foramen:** Internal jugular vein and CN IX–XI.
- **Hypoglossal canal:** CN XII.
- **Foramen spinosum:** Middle meningeal artery and vein.
- **Foramen magnum:** Spinal cord, CN XI (spinal accessory) and vertebral, posterior, and anterior spinal arteries.

▶ CENTRAL NERVOUS SYSTEM (CNS) VASCULATURE

Internal carotid artery (ICA) does not produce branches until it enters the petrous bone, where it gives off geographically occult feeders to the middle and inner ear.

Major ICA Branches Visible with Angiography

Meningohypophyseal, inferolateral trunk, ophthalmic, posterior communicating, anterior choroidal, middle cerebral, anterior cerebral.

Anterior Cerebral Artery (ACA) Branches

Medial lenticulostriates, anterior communication, recurrent artery of Heubner, orbitofrontal, frontopolar, pericallosal, callosomarginal.

Middle Cerebral Artery (MCA) Branches

Lateral lenticulostriates, anterior temporal, posterior cerebral, ascending frontal, lateral orbitofrontal, precentral, central, anterior parietal, posterior parietal, angular.

Vertebral Artery Branches

Posterior meningeal, anterior spinal, posterior inferior cerebellar, vertebrals fuse to form the basilar artery.

Basilar Artery Branches

Anterior inferior cerebellar, pontine perforators, superior cerebellar, posterior cerebral.

Posterior Cerebral Artery Branches

Posterior thalamoperforators, medial posterior choroidal, lateral posterior choroidal, thalamogeniculates, inferior temporals, parieto-occipital, calcarine, posterior pericallosal.

Arterial

Circle of Willis is complete in only approximately one fifth of persons (see Figure 23-1).

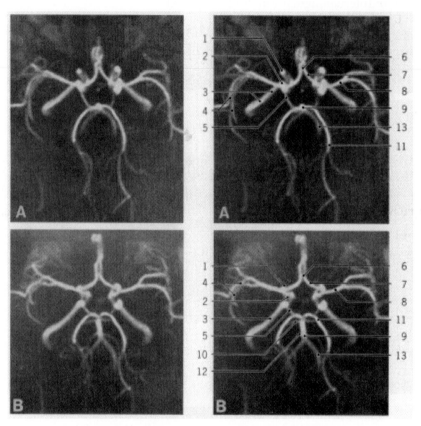

Cerebral arteries, MR angiography, circle of Willis

1: Internal carotid artery, "siphon"
2: Internal carotid artery in cavernous sinus
3: Internal carotid artery in carotid canal
4: Insular branches of middle cerebral artery
5: Posterior communicating artery

6: Anterior communicating artery
7: Anterior cerebral artery
8: Middle cerebral artery
9: Basilar artery
10: Superior cerebellar artery

11: Posterior cerebral artery
12: Anterior inferior cerebral artery (AICA)
13: Vertebral artery

FIGURE 23-1. **MR angiography demonstrating circle of Willis.**

(Reproduced, with permission, from Fleckenstein P, Tranum-Jensen J. *Anatomy and Diagnostic Imaging,* 2nd ed. Philadelphia, PA: WB Saunders, 2001: 244.)

Anatomy and Physiology

SCALP

- The scalp consists of five layers.
- Highly vascular structure, may be the source of major blood loss.

SKULL

- Rigid and inflexible (fixed volume).
- Composed of the cranial vault and base.

BRAIN

- Makes up 80% of intracranial volume.
- Partially compartmentalized by the reflections of dura (falx cerebri and tentorium cerebelli).

CEREBROSPINAL FLUID (CSF)

- Formed primarily by the choroid plexus at a rate of ~500 cc/day with 150 cc of CSF circulating at a given moment.
- Cushions the brain.

CEREBRAL BLOOD FLOW

- Brain receives ~15% of cardiac output.
- Brain responsible for ~20% of total body O_2 consumption.

CEREBRAL PERFUSION PRESSURE (CPP)

- CPP = MAP – ICP.
- MAP = mean arterial blood pressure (avoid systolic blood pressure [SBP] < 90 mmHg).
- ICP = intracranial pressure (ICP > 20 mmHg should be treated).
- Maintaining CPP between 50 and 70 mmHg in nonoperative brain injury is the fundamental treatment.

MONRO-KELLIE HYPOTHESIS

The sum of the volume of the brain, blood, and CSF within the skull must remain constant. Therefore, an increase in one of the above must be offset by decreased volume of the others.

ASSESSMENT

- History.
- Identify mechanism and time of injury, loss of consciousness, concurrent use of drugs or alcohol, medications that may affect pupillary size (e.g., glaucoma medications), past medical history (especially previous head trauma and stroke with their residual effects, and previous eye surgery, which can affect pupillary size and response) and the presence of a "lucid interval."

Layers of the **SCALP**:
Skin
Connective tissue
Aponeurosis (galea)
Loose areolar tissue
Pericranium

CN III runs along the edge of the tentorium cerebelli.

Concept of CPP is important in a hypertensive patient. Lowering the BP too fast will also decrease the CPP, creating a new problem.

Hypotension is usually not caused by isolated head injury. Look for other injuries in this setting.

HIGH-YIELD FACTS

Neurosurgery

Eyes	Open spontaneously	4
	Open to verbal command	3
	Open to pain	2
	No response	1
Best motor response	Obeys verbal command	6
	Localizes pain to painful stimulus	5
	Flexion–withdrawal	4
	Decorticate rigidity	3
	Decerebrate rigidity	2
	No response	1
Best verbal response	Oriented and converses	5
	Disoriented and converses	4
	Inappropriate words	3
	Incomprehensible sounds	2
	No response	1
TOTAL		**15**

FIGURE 23-2. **Glasgow Coma Scale.**

An enlarging pupil with a concurrent decrease in level of consciousness is strongly suggestive of uncal herniation.

VITAL SIGNS

Cushing reflex:

- Brain's attempt to maintain the CPP.
- Hypertension and bradycardia in the setting of increased ICP.

PHYSICAL EXAM

- Search for signs of external trauma such as lacerations, hemotympanum, ecchymoses, and avulsions, as these may be clues to underlying injuries such as depressed or open skull fractures.
- Anisocoria (unequal pupils) is found in a small percentage (10%) of normal people; however, anisocoria in the patient with head trauma is pathologic until proven otherwise.

GLASGOW COMA SCALE (GCS)

The Glasgow Coma Scale may be used as a tool for classifying head injury (see Figure 23-2):

Severe head injury	GCS 8 or less
Moderate head injury	GCS 9–13
Mild head injury	GCS 14 or 15

Skin staples interfere with CT scanning and should therefore not be used until after CT scanning is complete.

DIAGNOSTIC STUDIES

- Assume C-spine injury in head injury patients and immobilize until cleared.
- Skull films have largely been replaced by computed tomographic (CT) scan.
- Indications for head/brain CT:
  1. Neurologic deficit.
  2. Persisting depression or worsening of mental status.
  3. Depressed skull fracture or linear fracture overlying a dural venous sinus or meningeal artery groove (as demonstrated with skull x-rays).

Linear (Nondepressed)

STELLATE

- **Depressed:** Carries a much greater risk of underlying brain injury and complications, such as meningitis and posttraumatic seizures.
- **Basilar:** Signs include periorbital ecchymoses (raccoon's eyes), retroauricular ecchymoses (Battle's sign), otorrhea, rhinorrhea, hemotympanum, and cranial nerve palsies.

Cerebral Concussion

- Transient loss of consciousness that occurs immediately following blunt, nonpenetrating head trauma, caused by impairment of the reticular activating system.
- Recovery is often complete; however, residual effects such as headache may last for some time.

Diffuse Axonal Injury (DAI)

- Caused by microscopic shearing of nerve fibers, scattered microscopic abnormalities.
- Frequently requires intubation, hyperventilation, CPP monitoring, and admission to a neurosurgical intensive care unit (ICU).
- Patients are often comatose for prolonged periods of time.
- Mortality is approximately 33%.

Cerebral Contusion

- Occurs when the brain impacts the skull. May occur directly under the site of impact (coup) or on the contralateral side (contrecoup).
- Patients may have focal deficits; mental status ranges from confusion to coma.

Intracerebral Hemorrhage

Caused by traumatic tearing of intracerebral blood vessels. Difficult to differentiate from a contusion.

Ring test for CSF rhinorrhea (in the presence of epistaxis): Sample of blood from nose placed on filter paper to test for presence of CSF. If present, a large transparent ring will be seen encircling a clot of blood.

Typical scenario: A 20-year-old female has brief loss of consciousness following head injury. She presents to the ED awake but is amnestic for the event and keeps asking the same questions again and again. *Think:* Concussion.

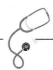

No mass lesion is seen on CT in DAI.

HIGH-YIELD FACTS

Neurosurgery

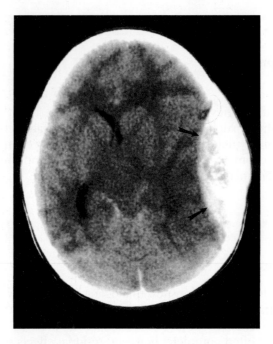

FIGURE 23-3. Epidural hematoma.

Arrows indicate the characteristic lens-shaped lesion. (Reproduced, with permission, from Schwartz SI, Spencer SC, Galloway AC, et al. *Principles of Surgery*, 7th ed. New York: McGraw-Hill, 1999: 1882.)

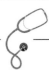

Typical scenario: A 19-year-old male with a head injury has loss of consciousness followed by a brief lucid interval. He presents to the emergency department (ED) in a coma, with an ipsilateral fixed and dilated pupil and contralateral hemiparesis. *Think:* Epidural hematoma.

Acute subdural hematomas have a high mortality — approximately one third to two thirds — mostly due to underlying brain contusion and shear.

Epidural Hematoma

- Collection of blood between the dura and the skull.
- Majority associated with tearing of the middle meningeal artery from an overlying temporal bone fracture.
- Typically biconvex or lenticular in shape (see Figure 23-3).
- Patients may have the classic "lucid interval," where they "talk and die." Requires early neurosurgical involvement and hematoma evacuation.
- Good outcome if promptly treated.

Subdural Hematoma

- Collection of blood below the dura and over the brain (see Figure 23-4). Results from tearing of the bridging veins, usually secondary to an acceleration-deceleration mechanism.
- Classified as acute (< 24 hours), subacute (24 hours–2 weeks), and chronic (> 2 weeks old).
- Acute and subacute subdurals require early neurosurgical involvement.
- Alcoholics and the elderly (patients likely to have brain atrophy), have increased susceptibility.

► MANAGEMENT OF MILD TO MODERATE HEAD TRAUMA

- Safe disposition of the patient depends on multiple factors.
- Any patient with a persisting or worsening decrease in mental status, focal deficits, severe mechanism of injury, penetrating trauma, open or

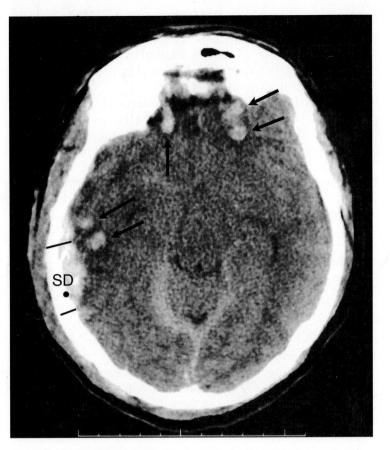

FIGURE 23-4. Subdural hematoma.

depressed skull fracture, or seizures, or who is unreliable or cannot be safely observed at home, should be admitted for observation.

- Patients with mild and sometimes moderate head trauma, brief or no loss of consciousness, no focal deficits, an intact mental status, a normal CT scan, and reliable family members who can adequately observe the patient at home can often be discharged with proper discharge instructions.
- Discharge instructions should include signs and symptoms for family members to watch for, such as persisting or worsening headache, dizziness, vomiting, inequality of pupils, confusion.
- If any of the above signs are found, the patient should be brought to the ED immediately.

When in doubt, admit the patient for observation.

▶ MANAGEMENT OF SEVERE HEAD INJURY (GCS < 9)

- Check airway, breathing, circulation (ABCs).
  - Patient needs intubation by definition.
  - Hyperventilation is not recommended, P_{CO_2} should be maintained at 35 mmHg and $PaO_2 > 60$ mmHg.
- ICP measurement via ventriculostomy should be done in all patients with severe traumatic brain injury and CT scan abnormalities.

Measures to lower ICP:
HIVED
Hyperventilation
Intubation with
  pretreatment and
  sedation
Ventriculostomy (burr
  hole)
Elevate the head of the bed
Diuretics (mannitol)

- Maintain an adequate blood pressure (BP) with isotonic fluids. Avoid systolic blood pressure (SBP) < 90 mmHg.
    - Treatment of increased ICP: > 20 mmHg with mannitol.
    - Maintain CPP between 50 and 70 mmHg (preferably > 60 mmHg).
- Early feeding improves outcome.
- Use sequential compression device for deep venous thrombosis (DVT) prophylaxis.
- Corticosteroids are contraindicated in these patients.
- Consider prophylactic anticonvulsant therapy with phenytoin for 7 days.
- Hypothermia may be beneficial for neurological recovery.
- Treat the pathology whenever possible (e.g., surgical drainage of a hematoma).

Hydrocephalus

Enlargement of the ventricles with excess CSF.

GENERAL

- Prevalence, –1%; congenital incidence, 1 in 1000.
- Three general categories:
    - **Communicating:** Also known as normal-pressure hydrocephalus since flow remains between all the ventricles. Defective absorption by arachnoid granulations in the subarachnoid space.
    - **Noncommunicating (obstructive):** Increased pressure within the ventricular system due to disruption of CSF flow between the ventricles (e.g., aqueductal stenosis, tumor, cyst). May not affect all ventricles depending on the location of the block (e.g., aqueductal stenosis spares the fourth ventricle).
    - **Ex vacuo:** Atrophic parenchymal tissue loss resulting in dilated ventricles. Not pathologic hydrocephalus. (*Example:* Atrophy of caudate nuclei in Huntington's disease causes expansion of the lateral ventricles.)

IMAGING

See Figure 23-5.

ETIOLOGIES

- **Congenital:** Aqueduct stenosis, Dandy-Walker syndrome, Chiari malformation.
- **Acquired:**
    - Hemorrhage: Subarachnoid hemorrhages cause meningeal adhesions.
    - Infectious/inflammatory: Meningitis will cause meningeal adhesions.
    - Obstructing masses.
    - Postoperative (particularly in pediatric posterior fossa procedures).

CLINICAL PRESENTATION

- **Communicating:** Classic triad of gait apraxia, dementia, and incontinence. Gait apraxia is usually first and can have a slow onset.
- **Noncommunicating:** Headache, nausea/vomiting, ataxia, abducens palsy, Parinaud's syndrome.

MacEwen's sign: Tapping on the head of a hydrocephalic infant produces a cracked pot sound.

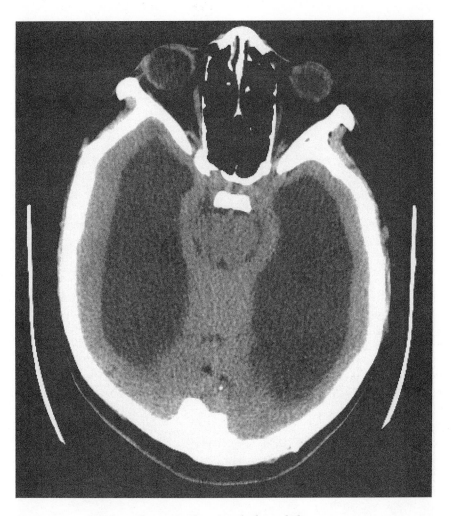

FIGURE 23-5. **Brain CT demonstrating gross hydrocephalus.**

Note massive dilatation of lateral and third ventricles. The fourth ventricle is decompressed. There is a VP shunt tip in the body of the right lateral ventricle. Note deformity of calvarium, which is consistent with long-standing hydrocephalus.

- In children, check for bulging anterior fontanelle, increase in head circumference, irritability, poor feeding, and engorged scalp veins.

TREATMENT

- Acetazolamide to reduce CSF production and furosemide to promote diuresis (both only temporizing).
- Lumbar puncture: Used to quickly relieve CSF pressure. Considerable clinical improvement has high predictive value for success of shunt placement.
- Shunt placement:
    - Most commonly, a ventriculoperitoneal (VP) shunt is placed (see Figure 23-6). Alternatives include ventriculoatrial and ventriculopleural shunts.

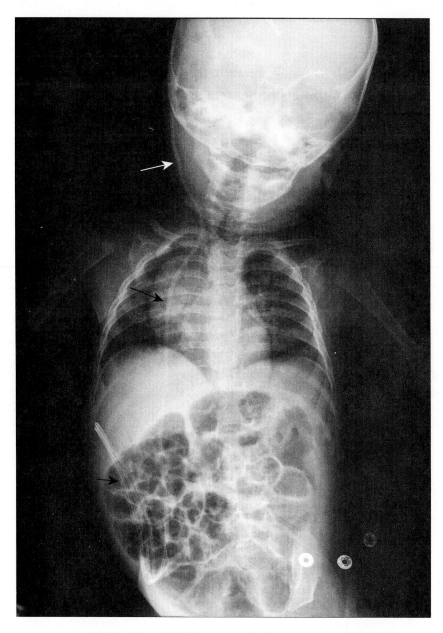

FIGURE 23-6. Plain radiograph ("shunt-o-gram") demonstrating VP shunt catheter coiled in the upper abdomen without evidence of kinks in this 8-month-old girl.

- Shunts are placed similar to an extraventricular drain except that the catheter is subcutaneously tunneled behind the ear, where a valve is attached and placed in the subgaleal space. The catheter is then tunneled over the clavicle and to the destination outsource; peritoneum (VP, most common), atrium (ventriculoatrial), or pleura (ventriculopleural). Ventriculoatrial shunts occasionally cause pulmonary hypertension as a complication.

COMPLICATIONS

- Obstruction (usually proximal).
- Infection: *Staphylococcus.*

- Subdural hematoma.
- Patient growth—possible need for replacement of the distal catheter as the infant/child grows (shunt tip will pull out of peritoneal cavity).

GENERAL

- Most brain tumors present with progressive neurologic deficit, motor weakness, headache, or seizure.
- Tumor headache is usually due to elevated ICP.
- Any new-onset seizure in adulthood should prompt an aggressive search for a brain tumor.

PRESENTATION

- **Posterior fossa mass:** Headache, nausea/vomiting, ataxia, diplopia, Parinaud's syndrome, cranial nerve paresis, rotatory/vertical nystagmus.
- **Supratentorial mass:** Headache, nausea/vomiting, diplopia, Parinaud's syndrome, motor weakness, aphasia, tumor transient ischemic attack (TIA—hemorrhage/vascular compression).
- Dexamethasone may halt/reverse neurologic deterioration caused by vasogenic edema.

Glial Tumor

CNS tumor arising from glial cells (astrocytes or oligodendrocytes).

Astrocytoma

World Health Organization (WHO) grading system for astrocytomas most commonly used:

- Grade 1—pilocytic astrocytoma: In children, consisting of cystic lesions, most often in the cerebellum, brain stem, or hypothalamus. Has good prognosis.
- Grade 2—low-grade astrocytoma: Present at 20–40 years; median survival 5–10 years.
- Grade 3—anaplastic astrocytoma.
- Grade 4—glioblastoma multiforme: Present at 50–70 years; median survival 1–2 years; highly malignant with poor prognosis.

Oligodendroglioma

- Four percent of primary brain tumors.
- Male > female (3:2).
- Mostly occur in middle-aged adults, slow growing.
- Predilection for frontal and temporal lobes (40–70%).
- Uniform cells with round nuclei ("fried egg" appearance).
- May have mixed astrocyte component, here called oligoastrocytomas.

- Most frequently presents with a seizure.
- Surgery for symptomatic lesions, lesions > 5 cm.
- Responds well to chemo.

Ependymoma

- Derived from cells lining the ventricles.
- Six percent of primary brain tumors.
- Most occur in children.
- Fourth ventricle (most common).
- Spinal cord.
- Lateral ventricles.
- Most often there is hydrocephalus.
- Tends to disseminate through CSF ("seeding").
- Surgical resection.
- Radiation if in fourth ventricle or spinal cord.
- Chemotherapy is of little benefit.

Meningioma

- Originates from arachnoid granulations.
- Most common benign brain tumor.
- Fifteen percent of all primary brain tumors.
- Highest incidence in sixth to seventh decades.
- Seen at superior convexities, sphenoid wing, orbital rim, cerebellar tentorium, ventricles.
- Rarely invasive or metastatic; many discovered incidentally.
- Observe with annual CT scans if asymptomatic and < 2 cm.
- Surgical excision if symptomatic.
- External beam radiotherapy/gamma knife if subtotal resection or unresectable.

Pituitary Adenoma

- Ten percent of primary brain tumors.
- Associated with multiple endocrine neoplasia (MEN) syndrome.
- Seen at the sella turcica with parasellar extension.
- May envelop carotid arteries.
- Cell of origin may be chromophobe (null cell or prolactinoma), acidophil (growth hormone [GH], causing acromegaly) or basophil (adrenocorticotropic hormone [ACTH]—Cushing's syndrome).
- Generally slow, progressive enlargement.
- Headache, bitemporal hemianopsia (superior to inferior loss).
- **Prolactinomas (prolactin secreting):**
  - Medical treatment (dopamine agonists).
  - Surgical excision if no response to therapy, through transsphenoidal approach.
- **Acromegaly (growth hormone secreting):**
  - Surgical resection—50% cure.
  - Avoid surgery in asymptomatic eldery patients as there is no survival benefit.
  - Medical therapy with octreotide (somatostatin analogue).

Preop imaging of the spinal neuraxis should be performed to detect CSF seeding.

- **Cushing's disease (cortisol secreting):**
  - Surgery is the treatment of choice—85% cure.
  - Nonfunctional adenomas.
  - Observe if asymptomatic; otherwise, surgical resection.

Neuroma

- Eight to ten percent of primary brain tumors.
- CN VIII affected most frequently (acoustic neuroma).
- Typical extension of acoustic neuroma into cerebellopontine angle with possible compression of CN V, VII, IX, or X.
- Usually unilateral.
- Bilateral CN VIII neuromas pathognomonic for neurofibromatosis type 2 (NF2).
- Unilateral progressive hearing loss (sensorineural), tinnitus, dysequilibrium, possible vertigo.
- Perform pretreatment audiometric and vestibular testing.
- Surgical excision or stereotactic radiosurgery.
- Conventional radiotherapy (RT).

- Unilateral acoustic neuromas are common.
- Symptoms of hearing loss, vertigo, tinnitus.
- Bilateral indicative of NF2.

Craniopharyngioma

- Three percent of primary brain tumors.
- Most occur in childhood.
- Anterior superior pituitary margin, may extend upwards toward third ventricle; may compress optic chiasm or pituitary gland.
- Benign but difficult to cure.
- Arises from remnants of the craniopharyngeal duct or Rathke's pouch.
- Headache and visual disturbance.
- Preop endocrinological evaluation.
- **Treatment:** May be observed; surgical resection if symptomatic.

Hemangioblastoma

- Two percent of primary brain tumors.
- Tend to appear clinically in middle adulthood.
- Associated with Von Hippel–Lindau disease (dominant inheritance).
- Most common adult posterior fossa tumor.
- Spinal cord (70% have associated syringomyelia).
- Benign.
- Ataxia, dizziness, concurrent hepatic, renal, or pancreatic cysts.
- Surgery curative in sporadic cases.
- RT to slow growth if surgically unresectable.

Von Hippel–Lindau Disease
- Autosomal dominant (chromosome 3).
- Multiorgan angiomatosis.
- CNS tumors are benign hemangioblastomas.
- Other organs: Spinal cord, eye, adrenal glands, kidneys, pancreas.
- Tendency for renal cell carcinoma and pheochromocytoma.

Glomus Tumors

Tumors arising from paraganglion cells:

- **Glomus jugulare tumor:** Since located underneath floor of middle ear, typical presentation involves deafness, facial palsy, and possibly a palpable mass anterior to the mastoid eminence.
  - **Treatment:** Surgery with possible radical mastoidectomy followed with RT.

- **Carotid body tumor:** Painless mass below angle of jaw. May affect other cranial nerves in area. Small percentage of patients have experienced TIAs.
  - **Treatment:** Surgery; **no RT.** Possible embolization prior to surgery.

- More than 50% of brain tumors are metastatic in origin.
- Most disseminate hematogenously.
- Incidence of cerebral metastases is increasing.
- Common sources: Bronchogenic lung cancer (40%), breast cancer (19%), melanoma (10%), colon adenocarcinoma (7%).
- Most present with progressive focal neurologic deficit or signs/symptoms of increased ICP.
- Certain metastases are more likely to hemorrhage: Melanoma, renal cell carcinoma, choriocarcinoma.
- Most metastases occur in the cerebral hemispheres at the **gray-white junction** or in the cerebellum.

IMAGING

- CT or magnetic resonance imaging (MRI—preferred).
- Typically, metastases are well circumscribed.
- Usually, significant surrounding edema greater than that seen with primary brain tumors.
- Metastases usually enhance (completely or ring enhancement).

EVALUATION

Search for a primary source:

- Chest x-ray (CXR).
- CT chest/abdomen/pelvis.
- Bone scan, mammogram in women, guaiac for occult blood.

MANAGEMENT

- Biopsy for diagnosis if no other source identified.
- Resect most solitary symptomatic lesions and treat with RT postoperatively.
- If multiple metastases, proceed directly to RT.

A solitary cerebellar mass in an adult is presumed a metastasis until proven otherwise.

Tuberous sclerosis clinical triad:
- Mental retardation
- Adenoma sebaceum (actually perivascular fibromata)
- Seizures

DEFINITIONS

- **Spondylosis:** Degenerative changes in spine; arthritis.
- **Spondylolisthesis:** Subluxation of one vertebral body on another.
- **Spondylolysis:**
  - Fracture or defect in pars interarticularis.
  - Mostly congenital at L5 level (spina bifida occulta).
  - If due to congenital/degenerative etiology generally does not require surgical intervention.
  - Traumatic spondylolysis requires spinal fusion.

HIGH-YIELD FACTS

Neurosurgery

Low Back Pain

See Orthopedics chapter.

GENERAL

- Spinal trauma may involve injury to the spinal column, spinal cord, or both.
- Over 50% of spinal injuries occur in the cervical spine (see Figure 23-7), with the remainder being divided between the thoracic spine, the thoracolumbar junction, and the lumbosacral region.
- As long as the spine is appropriately immobilized, evaluation for spinal injury may be deferred until the patient is stabilized.

ANATOMY

- There are 7 cervical, 12 thoracic, 5 lumbar, 5 sacral, and 4 coccygeal vertebrae.

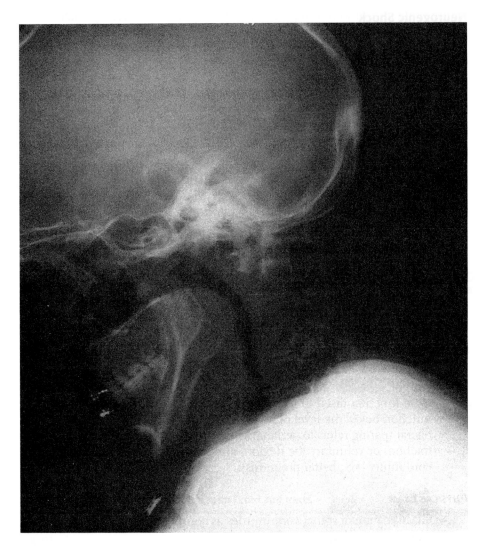

FIGURE 23-7. Atlantoaxial subluxation in a patient with rheumatoid arthritis.

Abdominal injuries frequently coexist with fracture-dislocations.

Median neuropathy due to carpal tunnel syndrome often involves the fingers but spares the palm, unlike compression at the pronator teres (palmar cutaneous branch of median nerve is outside the carpal tunnel).

Rotating head away from affected side with elevation of arm producing paresthesia/pain is suggestive of neurologic TOS. Concomitant reduction of radial pulse suggests vascular TOS.

DISTRACTION OR SEAT-BELT INJURY

- Frequently referred to as a **Chance fracture.**
- Horizontal fracture through the vertebral body, spinous processes, laminae, pedicles, and tearing of the posterior spinous ligament.
- Caused by an acceleration-deceleration injury of a mobile person moving forward into a fixed seat belt.

THORACIC OUTLET SYNDROME (TOS)

- Subclavian artery/vein and brachial plexus pass through a space defined by the clavicle and first rib (thoracic outlet).
- Vascular compromise is more common than neurologic: Unilateral Raynaud's phenomenon, Adson's sign—loss of radial pulse on abduction and external rotation of the arm.
- Can present with T1 sensory loss, wasting of thenar muscles.

ETIOLOGIES

- Fibrous band compressing C8/T1 roots (inferior trunk).
- Elongated C7 transverse process—"cervical rib."

TREATMENT

Surgical lysis of fibrous band or removal of C7 transverse process by either transaxillary or supraclavicular approach to thoracic outlet.

Cardiothoracic Surgery

DEFINITION

Myocardial injury caused by chronic or acute episodes of ischemia.

CAUSES

Disorders that affect coronary blood flow:

- Atherosclerotic coronary artery disease (most common).
- Valvular heart disease.
- Vasculitis.
- Congenital coronary anomalies.
- Aortic dissection with involvement of ostia.

ANATOMY

- **Right coronary dominance** (90% of patients): Right coronary artery (RCA) gives rise to posterior descending artery (PDA).
- **Left coronary dominance** (10%): Left circumflex artery gives rise to posterior descending artery.
- **Codominance:** Occasionally, PDA arises from both the RCA and left coronary artery (LCA).
- Consider how a lesion from either side will affect the posterior and inferior walls.

PATHOPHYSIOLOGY

- Ischemic areas arise from lack of blood flow relative to the metabolic demands of the myocardium.
- The oxygen extraction already being high under normal metabolic conditions (75%), the heart must rely on increased blood flow to meet heightened demand.
- Determinants of demand: Wall tension (vis à vis preload, afterload, wall thickness), heart rate, level of contractility.
- An atherosclerotic plaque impedes flow significantly when coronary cross-sectional area is reduced by 75% (a 50% reduction in diameter).
- Coronary atherosclerotic lesions are usually multifocal, multivessel.
- Plaque rupture is the main cause of escalation of symptoms. Intermittent closure of dynamic plaques underlies symptoms of unstable angina.

Coronary atherosclerosis most common cause of cardiovascular morbidity and mortality in the Western world. Before age 70, men are more commonly affected than women by a ratio of 4:1. After age 70, it is 1:1.

RISK FACTORS

- Hypertension (HTN)
- Smoking
- Hypercholesterolemia
- Obesity
- Diabetes
- Family history

SIGNS AND SYMPTOMS

- Fatigue
- Angina pectoris
- Dyspnea
- Edema
- Palpitations

- Syncope
- Abnormal heart sounds
- Seventy-five percent present with classic angina, 25% present atypically, many have "silent" myocardial infarctions (MIs) (particularly diabetics and elderly).

DIAGNOSIS

- Electrocardiogram (ECG) may reveal ST segment elevations or depressions, inverted T waves, or Q waves.
- Stress test (to look at myocardial response when myocardial demand is increased).
- Echocardiography (localize dyskinetic wall segments, valvular dysfunction, estimate ejection fraction [EF]).
- Cardiac catheterization with angiography and left ventriculography (specifies coronary anatomy and sites of lesions to qualify the severity of the disease and vulnerable areas of myocardium, as well as to provide a road map for surgical or percutaneous intervention).

Severity of heart failure graded by **NYHA Classification**:
Class I—no symptoms (fatigue, dyspnea, palpitations, anginal pain)
Class II—symptoms with severe exertion
Class III—symptoms with mild exertion
Class IV—symptoms at rest

TREATMENT

- Medical—aspirin, β-blockers, calcium channel blockers, angiotensin-converting enzyme (ACE) inhibitors, diuretics, nitrates.
- Percutaneous transluminal coronary angioplasty (PTCA).
- Surgical—coronary artery bypass grafting.

▶ CORONARY ARTERY BYPASS GRAFTING (CABG)

DESCRIPTION

- Bypass of discrete areas of obstruction in coronary vessels using the internal mammary artery (IMA), radial artery, a reversed segment of saphenous vein, inferior epigastric artery, or gastroepiploic artery.
- IMA used in 95% of CABGs, usually to left anterior descending (LAD).
- Three or four grafts are used on average.
- Minimally invasive direct CABG (MIDCAB): Fewer incisions, no cardiopulmonary bypass or cardioplegia is used (performed on a beating heart, limited to single-vessel disease). Minimizes pain, recovery time, and chances of wound infection.
- Port access technique: Endovascular aortic occlusion and cardiopulmonary bypass with cardioplegia allows for broader use of MIDCAB (multivessel disease, combined valve-coronary artery surgery).
- Vessel acronyms:
  - LAD—left anterior descending
  - RCA—right coronary artery
  - LMCA—left main coronary artery
  - LCX—left circumflex artery
  - PDA—posterior descending artery
  - OMn—oblique marginal artery number 1, 2, 3, etc.
  - (L)(R)IMA—(left)(right) internal mammary artery

Diffuse patterns of coronary vessel obstruction, as can occur in diabetes, may not be amenable to CABG.

INDICATIONS

- Mild angina or asymptomatic:
  - LMCA stenosis > 60%.
  - LMCA equivalent: Proximal LAD and LCX stenoses > 70%.

- Leads to pulmonary congestion and pulmonary hypertension, left atrial dilation, atrial fibrillation, reduced cardiac output.

SIGNS AND SYMPTOMS

- Dyspnea, DOE (dyspnea on exertion).
- Rales.
- Cough.
- Hemoptysis.
- Systemic embolism (secondary to stagnation of blood in enlarged left atrium).
- Loud S1, opening snap.
- Accentuated right ventricle precordial thrust.
- Signs of right ventricular (RV) failure.
- Hoarse voice (secondary to enlarged left atrium impinging on recurrent laryngeal nerve).

DIAGNOSIS

- Murmur is mid-diastolic with opening snap, low-pitched rumble.
- Best heard over left sternal border between second and fourth interspace.
- Chest x-ray (CXR) may show straight left heart border secondary to enlarged left atrium and Kerley B lines from pulmonary effusion.
- ECG may show left atrial enlargement, RV hypertrophy, atrial fibrillation.
- Echocardiography demonstrates diseased valve, fish-mouth opening, and decreased cross-sectional area; 2.0 cm^2, moderate stenosis, 1.0 cm^2, severe stenosis (normal mitral valve cross-sectional area 4–6 cm^2).
- Elevated transmitral pressure gradient > 10 mmHg (under normal conditions there is no transvalvular gradient).

TREATMENT

- **Medical:**
  - Asymptomatic patients need only endocarditis prophylaxis.
  - Symptomatic patients are treated with diuretics (to lower left atrial pressure), β-blocking agents, and/or calcium channel blocking agents (to maintain sinus rhythm).
  - Digoxin is helpful in controlling ventricular rate in patients who do go into atrial fibrillation.
  - Anticoagulation for atrial thrombus/fibrillation if present.
  - Percutaneous mitral valve balloon valvuloplasty.
- **Surgical:**
  - Indications for surgery:
    - NYHA Class III or IV symptoms.
    - Atrial fibrillation.
    - Worsening pulmonary hypertension.
    - Systemic embolization.
    - Infective endocarditis.
    - Class II patients > 40 of age.
  - Open commissurotomy:
    - Will suffice in 30–50% of cases.
    - Fused leaflets are incised, calcifications are debrided, problematic chordae are resected, papillary muscle heads may be split, and mitral ring added to prevent regurgitation (annuloplasty).

Remember: Dilation of the left atrium is a major cause of atrial fibrillation.

Auscultatory triad of mitral stenosis:
- Increased first heart sound
- Opening snap
- Apical diastolic rumble

- Valve replacement employed when excessive debridement would be required.
- Percutaneous balloon valvuloplasty not as effective in the long term, possibly because fused chordae cannot be corrected.
- Minimally invasive mitral valve surgery (port access technique) has recently been introduced.

PROGNOSIS

- Ten years after commissurotomy, 7% require valve replacement.
- Yearly reoperation rates are 12% (balloon), 4% (commissurotomy), and 1.2% (valve replacement).
- Five-year survival after mitral valve replacement (MVR) 60–90%, 40–75% after 10 years (varies widely due to effect of risk factors, such as age, NYHA functional status, associated mitral insufficiency, additional need for CABG).

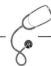

Balloon valvuloplasty in mitral stenosis is an effective intervention, as it has a low incidence of restenosis, in contrast to aortic stenosis, and increases the mitral valve area to 2.0 cm².

Mitral Insufficiency

ETIOLOGY

- Papillary muscle dysfunction from either ischemia or infarction (post-MI papillary muscle rupture causes massive regurgitation).
- Rupture of chordae tendineae (can happen spontaneously in otherwise healthy individuals).
- Valve destruction—scarring from rheumatic heart disease or destruction from endocarditis.
- Prolapse frequently progresses to valvular incompetence.

SIGNS AND SYMPTOMS

- Dyspnea.
- Fatigue.
- Weakness.
- Cough.
- Atrial fibrillation.
- Systemic emboli.
- Leads to pulmonary congestion, right-sided failure, left atrial dilation, atrial fibrillation, and volume overload of left ventricle. Cardiac output increases, then decreases.

DIAGNOSIS

- Murmur is loud, holosystolic, high-pitched, apical radiating to the axilla.
- Wide splitting of S2 with inspiration (widening occurs in severe cases due to premature emptying of LV).
- S3 due to rapid filling of LV by blood regurgitated during systole.
- ECG shows enlarged left atrium.
- Echocardiography demonstrates diseased/prolapsed valve and can be used to quantify mitral regurgitation (MR). The severity of the regurgitation is gauged as a function of the distance from the mitral annulus that the regurgitant jet can be visualized (e.g., into the pulmonary veins) and by the width of the regurgitant jet. The regurgitation is scored on a scale from 1 (mild) to 4 (severe).

Carpentier's functional classification of mitral insufficiency:
Type I—annular dilation or leaflet perforation with normal leaflet motion.
Type II—increased leaflet motion and prolapse.
Type III—restricted leaflet motion.

Two parameters of LV function useful in decision making are EF and end-systolic diameter (ESD). Patients are referred for surgery when the left ventricular EF is < 60% or when the left ventricular ESD is > 45 mm.

TREATMENT

- **Medical:**
  - Not definitive but used until surgery or in poor surgical candidates.
  - Diuretics to reduce volume load, reduce LV diameter (and mitral annulus), and thus reduce regurgitant fraction.
  - Cornerstone of medical management is afterload reduction by vasodilators (mainly ACE inhibitors), thus favoring aortic forward flow.
  - Anticoagulation for atrial fibrillation.
  - Mitral insufficiency has a good prognosis if LV function is preserved, and patient needs closed follow up with serial echocardiograms.
- **Surgical:**
  - Valve replacement or repair.
  - Indications for surgery: Symptoms despite medical management; severe mitral regurgitation with an identified structural abnormality, such as a ruptured chorda tendinea; development of pulmonary hypertension; or evidence of decline in left ventricular contractile function; atrial fibrillation; left atrium > 4.5–5 cm.
- **Mitral valve reconstruction:**
  - Involves resection of redundant areas of leaflets, chordal shortening, and ring annuloplasty (this corrects annular dilatation and stabilizes the repair).
  - Preferable to MVR in degenerative disease; MVR better in advanced deformity not amenable to reconstruction (e.g., due to rheumatic disease).

PROGNOSIS

- Better late survival in nonrheumatic patients undergoing reconstruction vs. replacement.
- Opposite in rheumatic patients.

Aortic Stenosis

ETIOLOGY

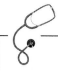

Congenital malformations account for about 50% of aortic valve operations.

- Degenerative calcific disease (idiopathic, older population).
- Congenital stenosis.
- Bicuspid aortic valve.
- Rheumatic heart disease.

PATHOPHYSIOLOGY

Obstruction of flow leads to left ventricular hypertrophy (LVH) (concentric type) and decreased LV compliance, then to LV dilation and congestion.

SIGNS AND SYMPTOMS

Usually asymptomatic early in course. Then:

- Dyspnea
- Angina and syncope—particularly during exercise. Peripheral resistance falls; LV pressure remains the same due to stenotic valve; cardiac output (CO) cannot maintain BP, causing syncope; low blood pressure (BP) to coronary arteries causes angina.
- Heart failure.
- HTN (consider associated aortic coarctation).

- Symptoms are associated with reduction in the aortic valve area from the normal 3–4 cm² to < 1 cm².

DIAGNOSIS

- Forceful apex beat with normally located point of maximal impulse (PMI).
- Loud systolic ejection murmur, crescendo-decrescendo, medium pitched, loudest at second right interspace, radiates to carotids.
- S4 (presystolic gallop) frequently present secondary to reduced LV compliance.
- Paradoxical splitting of S2.
- Narrow pulse pressure.
- ECG may show LV strain pattern.
- Echocardiography demonstrates diseased valve and quantifies severity.
- Calcification of aortic valve may be seen on chest x-ray (CXR).

Mean survival for patients with aortic stenosis and:
Angina: 5 years
Syncope: 2–3 years
Heart failure: 1–2 years

LV strain pattern is ST segment depression and T wave inversion in I, AVL, and left precordial leads.

TREATMENT

- **Medical:**
  - Avoid strenuous activity.
  - Avoid afterload reduction.
- **Surgical:**
  - Indications for surgery:
    - Asymptomatic with high transvalvular gradient (> 50 mmHg) and LVH or declining EF.
    - Presence of symptoms: CHF is an indication of urgent intervention, while angina and syncope warrant elective surgical treatment.
    - Aortic valve area < 0.8 cm².
  - Aortic balloon valvuloplasty produces only temporary improvement as rate of restenosis is very high. Only potential role of valvuloplasty is in aged, frail, and possibly senile patients whose long-term survival is poor.
  - Valve replacement is definitive therapy. Nearly all patients attain symptomatic relief and improvement in EF while resolution of ventricular hypertrophy may require months.
  - Surgical mortality increases exponentially with decreasing LV function. Aortic valve replacement (AVR) in patients with CHF carries a mortality rate of up to 24%.
  - Intra-annular and supra-annular placement of prosthesis (latter for small annulus).
  - Ross procedure for aortic valve replacement: Patient's own pulmonary valve is substituted (autograft), while a cryopreserved homograft (cadaveric) is used to replace the pulmonary valve. No need for anticoagulation, plus good durability (20-year failure rate of 15%).

PROGNOSIS

Ten-year survival after aortic valve replacement > 80% except in high-risk patients (e.g., severely impaired LV function, NYHA Class IV, pulmonary hypertension).

Aortic Regurgitation

ETIOLOGY

- Aortic root dilatation: Idiopathic (correlates with hypertension [HTN] and age), collagen vascular disease, Marfan's syndrome.
- Valvular disease: Rheumatic heart disease, endocarditis.
- Proximal aortic root dissection: Cystic medial necrosis (Marfan's syndrome again), syphilis, HTN, Ehlers-Danlos, Turner syndrome, third trimester.

PATHOPHYSIOLOGY

Leads to LV dilation, eccentric hypertrophy, mitral insufficiency, cardiomegaly, CHF.

SIGNS AND SYMPTOMS

Other conditions with wide pulse pressure:
- **Hyperthyroidism**
- **Anemia**
- **Wet beriberi**
- **Hypertrophic subaortic stenosis**
- **HTN**

- Dyspnea, orthopnea, paroxysmal nocturnal dyspnea.
- Angina (secondary to reduced diastolic coronary blood flow due to elevated LV end-diastolic pressure).
- Left ventricular failure (LVF).
- Wide pulse pressure.
- Bounding "Corrigan" pulse, "pistol shot" femorals, pulsus bisferiens (dicrotic pulse with two palpable waves in systole).
- **Duroziez's sign:** Presence of diastolic femoral bruit when femoral artery is compressed enough to hear a systolic bruit.
- **Hill's sign:** Systolic pressure in the legs > 20 mmHg higher than in the arms.
- **Quincke's sign:** Alternating blushing and blanching of the fingernails when gentle pressure is applied.
- **De Musset's sign:** Bobbing of head with heartbeat.

DIAGNOSIS

- High-pitched, blowing, decrescendo diastolic murmur best heard over second right interspace or third left interspace, accentuated by leaning forward.
- Austin Flint murmur: Observed in severe regurgitation, low-pitched diastolic rumble secondary to regurgitated blood striking the anterior mitral leaflet (similar sound to mitral regurgitation).
- A2 accentuated (due to high pulse pressure in the aorta at the beginning of ventricular diastole).
- Hyperdynamic down and laterally displaced PMI secondary to LV enlargement.
- ECG shows LV hypertrophy.
- Echocardiography demonstrates regurgitant valve.

TREATMENT

- **Medical:**
  - Diuretics and afterload reduction: Afterload reduction achieved by ACE inhibitors. Nifedipine has been shown to delay the need for AVR.
  - Asymptomatic patients should have serial echocardiography to monitor for any systolic dysfunction or decreasing EF.
  - Endocarditis prophylaxis.

- Surgical:
  - Indications for surgery:
    - Asymptomatic with first sign of declining LV function or rapid increase in cardiac size. AVR to be performed before end-systolic dimension exceeds 55 mm.
    - Presence of symptoms.
  - Valve *repair* may be suitable for pure aortic insufficiency (no stenosis and no other valves involved) and in cases of aortic root aneurysm.
  - Valve *replacement* is necessary for severe cases and is the only definitive treatment.

PROGNOSIS

- See Aortic Stenosis section.
- Valvular resection with annuloplasty: 10% reoperation rate at 2 years.

Tricuspid Stenosis

ETIOLOGY

Rheumatic heart disease, congenital, carcinoid.

SIGNS AND SYMPTOMS

- Peripheral edema
- Jugular venous distention (JVD)
- Hepatomegaly, ascites, jaundice

DIAGNOSIS

- Murmur is diastolic, rumbling, low pitched.
- Murmur accentuated with inspiration.
- Accentuated precordial thrust of right ventricle.
- Diastolic thrill at lower left sternal border.
- Best heard over left sternal border between fourth and fifth interspace.
- Echocardiography demonstrates diseased valve and quantifies transvalvular gradient.

A rumbling diastolic murmur can be due to mitral stenosis or tricuspid stenosis. Tricuspid stenosis will increase with inspiration.

TREATMENT

- Valve replacement for most cases.
- Commissurotomy with annuloplasty used for commissural fusion.

Types of Valve Prostheses

MECHANICAL PROSTHESES

- St. Jude.
- Offer greater durability (15-year failure rate 5%), but need for lifelong anticoagulation (with associated risk of hemorrhagic complications).
- A better choice for the young.

BIOPROSTHESES

- Porcine or bovine xenografts.
- Fewer thromboembolic concerns (usually no need for anticoagulation) but less durable (15-year failure rate 50%).

Heart block is a common complication in tricuspid valve replacement due to the close proximity of the conduction bundle to the tricuspid annulus.

- Better choice for the elderly.
- Calcification can complicate use in the young.

TYPES

- **Small cell lung cancer:**
  - Represents 20% of all lung cancers and 80% of centrally located.
  - Neuroendocrine in origin.
  - Sensitive to chemotherapy (cisplatin and etoposide) and x-ray therapy (XRT).
  - Usually nonresectable at time of diagnosis (< 5% candidates for surgery).
  - Five-year survival: Very poor prognosis (2–4 months from diagnosis to death).
  - Only T1, N0, M0 stage has 50% 5-year survival.
- **Non–small cell lung cancer:**
  - Includes squamous cell (SCCA), large cell, and adenocarcinoma (ACA).
  - ACA most common lung cancer (45% of all lung cancers), and 75% are peripherally located.
  - ACA metastasizes earlier than SCCA and more frequently to the central nervous system.
  - SCCA represents 30% of all lung cancers and two thirds are centrally located.
  - Large cell carcinoma accounts for 10% of all lung cancer, tend to occurs peripherally and metastasize relatively early.
  - Chemotherapy for non–small cell cancer (stage II or higher)—carboplatin, paclitaxel.
  - Treated with surgery (debulking).
  - Prognosis varies with stage.

EPIDEMIOLOGY

- Leading cause of cancer death in both men and women in the United States.
- Cases have been decreasing in men but increasing in women.
- Smoking is by far the most important causative factor in the development of lung cancer.

ETIOLOGY

- Smoking
- Passive smoke exposure
- Radon gas exposure
- Asbestos
- Arsenic
- Nickel

SIGNS AND SYMPTOMS

- Cough.
- Hemoptysis.
- Stridor.
- Dyspnea.

SCCA has a rapid mitotic rate, and therefore is sensitive to chemotherapy. Surgery is not indicated.

Two types of cancer share a "s"entral location:
- Small cell
- Squamous cell

Bronchoalveolar cancer, a type of adenocarcinoma, is not linked to smoking, and is more common in women.

- Hoarseness (recurrent laryngeal nerve paralysis).
- Postobstructive pneumonia.
- Dysphagia.
- Associated (paraneoplastic) syndromes (see Table 24-1).

DIAGNOSIS

See section on diagnostic evaluation of a lung mass below.

TREATMENT

The two main types of lung cancer, small cell and non–small cell cancer, have different responses to radiotherapy, chemotherapy, and surgery (see Table 24-2).

Diagnostic Evaluation of a Lung Mass

PLAIN FILM

- Most malignant nodules seen by 0.8–1 cm in diameter (may be seen smaller) (see Figure 24-1).
- Comparison with previous films whenever possible.
- Those nodules stable for 2 years need no further evaluation.
- Those that are new in the last 2 months are unlikely to be malignant.
- Plain film may be the only imaging modality necessary if there is obvious bony metastasis or bulky, contralateral mediastinal adenopathy.
- Will more than likely need computed tomography (CT).

Chronic cough is the most common symptom of lung cancer.

Paraneoplastic Syndromes
Small cell carcinoma: ACTH, ADH.
Squamous cell carcinoma: PTH-related peptide.
ACTH secretion of small cell carcinoma is the most common paraneoplastic syndrome.

HIGH-YIELD FACTS

Cardiothoracic Surgery

TABLE 24-1. Syndromes Associated with Lung Cancer

Horner syndrome	Sympathetic nerve paralysis produces enophthalmos, ptosis, miosis, ipsilateral anhidrosis
Pancoast's syndrome	Superior sulcus tumor injuring the eighth cervical nerve and the first and second thoracic nerves and ribs, causing shoulder pain radiating to arm
Superior vena cava syndrome	Tumor causing obstruction of the superior vena cava and subsequent venous return, producing facial swelling, dyspnea, cough, headaches, epistaxis, syncope. Symptoms worsened with bending forward, and on awakening in the morning
Syndrome of inappropriate antidiuretic hormone (SIADH)	Ectopic arginine vasopressin (AVP) release in the setting of plasma hyposmolality, producing hyponatremia without edema. Also caused by other lung diseases, CNS trauma or infection, and certain medications
Eaton-Lambert syndrome	Presynaptic nerve terminals attacked by antibodies, decreasing acetylcholine release, treated by plasmapheresis and immunosuppression; 40% associated with small cell lung cancer, 20% have other cancer, 40% have no cancer
Trousseau's syndrome	Venous thrombosis associated with metastatic cancer

TABLE 24-2. Distinction between Small and Non–Small Cell Lung Cancer

CHARACTERISTIC	SMALL CELL LUNG CANCER	NON–SMALL CELL LUNG CANCER
Histology	Small dark nuclei, scant cytoplasm	Copious cytoplasm, pleomorphic nuclei
Ectopic peptide production	Gastrin, ACTH, AVP, calcitonin, ANF	PTH
Response to radiotherapy	80–90% will shrink	30–50% will shrink
Response to chemotherapy	Complete regression in 50%	Complete regression in 5%
Surgical resection	Not indicated	Stage I, II, IIIA
Included subtypes	Small cell only	Adenocarcinoma, squamous cell, large cell, bronchoalveolar
5-year survival rate—all stages	5%	11–83%

ACTH, adrenocorticotropic hormone; AVP, arginine vasopressin; ANF, atrial natriuretic factor; PTH, parathyroid hormone.

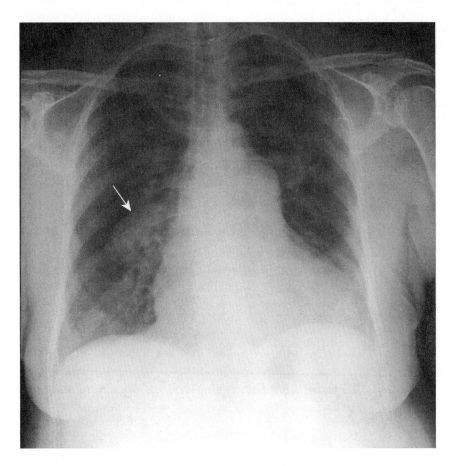

FIGURE 24-1. CXR demonstrating right middle lobe mass suspicious for malignancy.

CT

- Provides better characterization and location of mass as well as detecting mediastinal invasion.
- Should be extended to include liver and adrenal glands as these are frequent sites of metastasis.

BRONCHOSCOPY

- Method of choice of centrally located masses (squamous cell and small cell).
- Specimens can be obtained via direct biopsy of visualized lesions, brushings, washings, or transbronchial needle aspiration (TBNA).
- The most important application of TBNA is staging of mediastinal lymph nodes.
- Risks of this procedure are respiratory arrest, pneumothorax, and bleeding.
- Although this method works well for centrally located lesions, it is poor when it comes to peripheral lung nodules.

TRANSTHORACIC NEEDLE BIOPSY (TNB)

- Method of choice for peripherally located nodules. Most are CT guided.
- Sensitivity: 70–100%.

THORACENTESIS

Test of choice for patients with pleural effusion and suspected malignancy.

Solitary Pulmonary Nodule

- A single small (< 3 cm) intraparenchymal opacity that is reasonably well marginated.
- Most will be benign.
- Benign: Granulomas, hamartomas, or intrapulmonary lymph nodes.
- Malignant: Bronchogenic carcinoma.

Small Cell Lung Cancer

- Seventy percent metastatic at the time of diagnosis.
- Generally considered inoperable for cure.
- Two stages: Limited and extensive.
    - Limited: Confined to a single radiation portal.
    - Extensive: All others.

Non–Small Cell Lung Cancer

- Need to determine resectability: Chest CT and search for distant metastases.
- Malignant pleural effusion precludes curative resection.
- Tumor-node-metastasis (TNM) staging system.

DEFINITION

- **Aneurysm:** Ballooning defect in the vessel wall.
- **Dissection:** Tear of the arterial intima.

TYPES

- **Degenerative:**
  - Due to abnormal collagen metabolism.
  - Seen with Marfan's and Ehlers-Danlos syndromes (usually ascending aortic aneurysms).
- **Atherosclerotic** (usually descending aortic aneurysms): Due to remodeling and dilatation of the aortic wall.

ANATOMIC CLASSIFICATION

- DeBakey type I: Ascending and descending aorta.
- DeBakey type II: Ascending aorta only.
- DeBakey type III: Descending aorta only.
- Stanford A: Ascending aorta (same as DeBakey I/II).
- Stanford B: Descending aorta (same as DeBakey III).
- Ascending aorta and aortic arch aneurysms are worse than descending aortic aneurysms.
- Expansion rate is –0.56 cm/year for arch aneurysms and –0.42 cm/year for descending aorta.

EPIDEMIOLOGY

- Six per 100,000 a year.
- Male-to-female ratio is 2:1.
- Familial clustering.
- Patients tend to be younger than those with abdominal aortic aneurysm (AAA).

SIGNS AND SYMPTOMS OF EXPANSION OR RUPTURE

- "Tearing" or "ripping" chest pain radiating to the back.
- Acute neurologic symptoms (syncope, coma, convulsions, hemiplegia).
- Palpable thrust may be seen in right second or third intercostal space.
- Pulsating sternoclavicular joint may be seen (secondary to swelling at the base of the aorta).
- Hoarseness.
- Stridor.
- Dysphagia.
- New aortic regurgitation murmur.
- Hemoptysis or hematemesis.
- Absent or diminished pulses.

DIAGNOSIS

- **CXR** (Figure 24-2):
  - Widened mediastinum.
  - Abnormal aortic contour.
  - "Calcium sign": Reflects separation of intimal calcification from the adventitial surface.

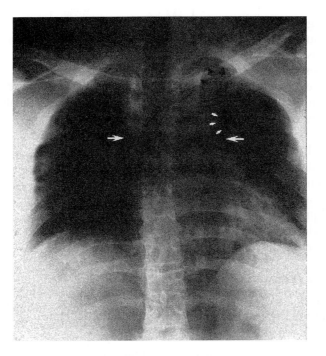

FIGURE 24-2. Thoracic aneurysm diagnosed on CXR.

- **Contrast CT** (Figure 24-3):
  - Sensitivity 85–100%.
  - Specificity 100%.
- **Magnetic resonance imaging (MRI):**
  - Excellent sensitivity and specificity.
  - Gives info about branch vessels that CT does not.
  - No need for contrast.
  - Limited to stable patients.

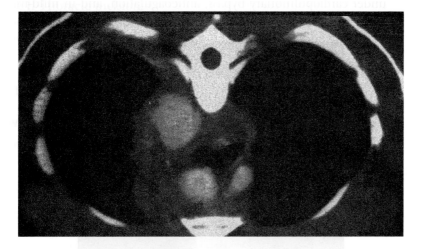

FIGURE 24-3. Thoracic aneurysm on CT.

Transplant

▶ **DEFINITIONS**

Autograft: Donor and recipient are same individual.
Allograft: Donor and recipient belong to same species but have different genetic makeup.
Xenograft: Donor and recipient are of different species.
Orthotopic: Transplant graft placed into its anatomic position.
Heterotopic: Transplant graft placed at different site.

▶ **BRAIN DEATH**

Adult Criteria

1. No cerebral function: Patient is in a deep coma, unresponsive to stimuli.
2. No brain stem function: No evidence on exam of cranial nerve function; lack of reflexes (papillary, corneal, cold water calorics, doll's eyes, gag).
3. No spontaneous breathing: Apnea test.

- **Requirements:** Normothermia, no central nervous system (CNS) depressants or neuromuscular blockers in effect.
- **Suggestions:** Electroencephalogram (EEG), though not legally required; 6-hour observation period prior to performing brain death examination.

Non-Heart-Beating Donors

Applies to patients with cardiac arrest near hospital, and to patients requesting removal of life support or in whom death is expected.

Donor Management

Goal: To optimize organ function avoid hypoxia, hypotension, and fever.

If the patient does not qualify for organ donation, cornea and heart valves may still be used.

▶ **TRANSPLANT IMMUNOLOGY**

Basics

Major histocompatibility complexes (MHCs) present antigens to T cells and are the major target of activated lymphocytes.

MHC I

- Found on all nucleated cells.
- Consists of heavy and light chains, and β_2 microglobulin.
- Encodes cell surface transplant antigens.
- Primary target for CD8 T cells in graft rejection.
- Gene loci: A, B, C.

MHC II

- Found on hematopoietic cells.
- Composed of alpha and beta chains.
- Primary target for T-helper cells.
- Gene loci: DR, DQ, DP.

MHC III

- Encodes complement proteins.
- Not addressed here.
- **B cells** are responsible for antibody-mediated hyperacute rejection when the transplant contains an antigen that the recipient B cells have seen before.

Graft survival is improved with matching for kidney, pancreas, and heart transplants, but is not improved and, in fact, may be worsened for liver transplants. (Human leukocyte antigen [HLA] presents viral peptides to T cells and compatibility may potentiate the inflammatory phase of viral reinfection after transplant, thereby increasing chance of recurrence of original disease.)

Tissue Typing

- Determination of MHC alleles in an individual to minimize differences in histocompatibility.
- Of above alleles, only A, B, and DR are used in tissue typing.
- Of these three genes, DR is most important to match, followed by B and then A, as evidenced by United Network for Organ Sharing (UNOS) data regarding graft survival.

Crossmatch

- Test for preformed cytotoxic antibody in serum of potential recipient.
- Donor lymphocytes are cultured with recipient serum in the presence of complement and dye.
- Lymphocyte destruction is evidenced by uptake of dye, indicating a positive crossmatch.
- A positive crossmatch is generally a contraindication to transplant as hyperacute rejection is likely.

> ► **IMMUNOSUPPRESSION**

Steroids

- Most commonly, prednisone (PO) or methylprednisolone (IV).
- Binds to intracellular receptor, is transported into nucleus—DNA-binding protein that works to limit, ultimately, the inflammatory response by blocking nuclear factor-κB (NF-κB), interleukin-1 (IL-1), tumor necrosis factor-α (TNF-α), interferon, and phospholipase A_2, as well as histamine and prostacyclin.
- Side effects: Impaired glucose tolerance, impaired wound healing, fluid retention, insomnia, depression, nervousness, psychosis.
- Chronic effects: Cushing's syndrome, increased risk for peptic ulcer disease, osteoporosis.

Cyclosporine (CsA)

- Calcineurin inhibitor: CsA binds to cyclophilin and, together, they bind to calcineurin-calmodulin complex, blocking calcium-dependent phosphorylation and activation of NF-AT, thereby preventing transcription of several genes needed for T-cell activation, including IL-2. Put simply, it inhibits T-cell activity.
- P_{450} metabolism: Levels are increased by P_{450} inhibitors such as ketoconazole, erythromycin, calcium channel blockers, and decreased by P_{450} inducers like rifampin, phenobarbital, and phenytoin.
- Side effects: Nephrotoxicity (dose related, based on vasoconstriction of proximal renal arterioles), hemolytic-uremic syndrome (uncommon), hypertension, tremors, headache, paresthesia, depression, confusion, seizures (rare), hypertrichosis, gingival hyperplasia, hepatotoxicity.

Mycophenolate Mofetil (MMF)

- Noncompetitive reversible inhibitor of inosine monophosphate dehydrogenase: Thereby halts purine metabolism, blocks proliferation of T and B cells, suppresses B-cell memory, and inhibits antibody formation.
- Side effects: Mild diarrhea or nausea.

Azathioprine

- Inhibits DNA synthesis by alkylating DNA precursors and depleting cell of adenosine.
- Side effects: Leukopenia, hepatotoxicity.

Tacrolimus (FK-506)

- Drug of choice for liver transplant.
- Calcineurin inhibitor: Works in similar fashion to CsA, but binds initially to FK-binding protein.
- A hundred times more potent than CsA.
- Side effects as for CsA, though more neurotoxic and diabetogenic, and fewer cosmetic effects.

Antithymocyte Globulin (ATG)

- Usually used for treatment of steroid-resistant rejection, but may also be used for induction therapy.
- Polyclonal antihuman γ-globulin extracted from horse sera of horses immunized with thymus lymphocytes.
- Side effects include fever and chills (20%), thrombocytopenia, leukocytopenia, rash (15%).

OKT3

- Monoclonal antibody to CD3, a signal transducer on human T cells, thereby prevents transduction of antigen binding; also downregulates T-cell receptor.
- Used as rescue agent for steroid-resistant rejection and also for induction.
- Side effects: Hypotension, pulmonary edema, cardiac depression.

Azathioprine is not generally used in liver transplant because it is likely to cause hepatotoxicity.

FK-506 and CsA have an additive immunosuppressive effect, but the toxicity may be too much.

Some studies have found up to 40% incidence of posttransplant lymphoproliferative disorder with tacrolimus, and therefore, this drug is used with extreme caution in children.

HIGH-YIELD FACTS

Transplant

Presensitization of the recipient to a donor antigen can result from prior pregnancy, transfusion, or transplant.

Forty to fifty percent of kidney transplant recipients and 70–80% of pancreas transplant recipients will have at least one episode of acute rejection.

Typical scenario: A kidney transplant recipient is seen in the emergency department (ED) for nausea and abdominal pain, fever, and elevated creatinine. *Think:* Acute rejection. Diagnosis may be confirmed by ultrasound-guided biopsy. Pulse steroid treatment is indicated.

Treatment of acute rejection of a kidney transplant (with pulse steroids or OKT3 for SRR) is effective in 90% of cases.

▶ REJECTION

Hyperacute

- **Cause:** Presensitization of recipient to donor antigen.
- **Timing:** *Immediately* following graft reperfusion.
- **Mechanism:** Antibody binds to donor tissue, initiating complement-mediated lysis, which has a procoagulant effect. End result is thrombosis of graft.
- **Prevention:** ABO typing and negative crossmatch prevent hyperacute rejection in > 99% of patients.
- **Treatment:** None (graft removal).
- **Outcome:** Graft failure/loss.

Acute

- **Cause:** Normal T-cell activity (would ultimately affect every allograft were it not for immunosuppression).
- **Timing:** Between postoperative day 5 and postoperative month 6.
- **Mechanism:** T cells bind antigens in one of two ways—directly through T-cell receptor (TCR) or after phagocytosis and presentation of donor tissue, resulting in T-cell infiltration of graft with organ destruction.
- **Diagnosis:** Generally by decreased graft function and by biopsy.
- **Histology:** Lymphocytic infiltrate and/or graft necrosis. Liver rejection also characterized by eosinophilic infiltrate.
- **Prevention:** Minimize mismatch of MHC; usual immunosuppression; monitor for organ dysfunction as signs of rejection that may otherwise be asymptomatic.
- **Treatment:** High-dose steroids; OKT3 or ATG when steroid-resistant rejection (SRR) after 2 days.
- **Outcome:** Ninety to ninety-five percent of transplants are salvaged with treatment.

Chronic

- **Cause:** Cumulative effect of recognition of MHC by recipient immune system.
- **Timing:** Insidious onset over months and years.
- **Mechanism:** Recipient's immune system recognizes donor MHC; other factors not yet understood.
- **Diagnosis:** Biopsy.
- **Histology:** Parenchymal replacement with fibrous tissue, some lymphocytic infiltrate, endothelial destruction.
- **Prevention:** None known.
- **Treatment:** None.
- **Outcome:** Graft failure/loss.

Risk of Malignancy

- Overall incidence in kidney transplant recipients: 6%—lymphoma, skin cancer, genital neoplasms.
- Posttransplant lymphoproliferative disease (PTLD): Caused by Epstein-Barr virus (EBV), leads ultimately to monoclonal B-cell lymphoma/ treatment to lower or stop immunosuppression and restore immunity.

▶ ORGAN PRESERVATION

Maximum Times for Each Organ

- Heart and lungs: Up to 6 hours.
- Small bowel: Up to 12 hours.
- Liver: Up to 24 hours.
- Pancreas: Up to 24 hours.
- Kidney: Up to 48 hours.

▶ KIDNEY TRANSPLANTATION

Background

Most common solid organ to be transplanted.

Causes of End-Stage Renal Disease (ESRD)

- Diabetes
- Hypertension
- Glomerular nephritis
- Congenital anomalies
- Urologic abnormalities
- Dysplasia
- Focal segmental glomerular sclerosis

Types of Donors

- Cadaveric.
- Living:
  - May be related or unrelated.
  - Decreased warm ischemia time.
  - Associated with less delayed graft function and better outcome.
  - Donor mortality: 1/10,000.
  - Living donor evaluation: Rule out potential donors with:
    - Diabetes, hypertension, malignancy, chronic obstructive pulmonary disease (COPD), renal disease.
    - Genitourinary (GU) anomalies assessed by proteinuria > 250 mg/24 hr or creatinine clearance rate (CCr) < 80 mL/min, computed tomography (CT) of urinary tract.

Warm ischemia time should be minimized because it leads to rapid decline in adenosine triphosphate (ATP) and therefore decrease in biosynthetic reactions, a redistribution of electrolytes across cell membranes, and continuation of biodegradation reactions leading to acidosis and ultimately loss of organ viability.

Morbidity and mortality associated with dialysis: A 49-year-old with end-stage renal disease (ESRD) on dialysis has an expected duration of life of 7 years, compared to 30 years for a healthy 49-year-old.

Decreased quality of life in ESRD is associated with time commitment for dialysis and increased number of hospital days.

Cardiovascular disease is responsible for 50% of dialysis patients' deaths, and infection accounts for 15–30%.

Appropriate Recipient

- General health assessment:
  - Identify comorbidities such as heart disease, COPD, and diabetes.
  - Assess ability to handle immunosuppression and compliance.
- Laboratory evaluation consisting of chemistries, complete blood count (CBC), urinalysis, serologies for hepatitis B and C, cytomegalovirus (CMV), and human immunodeficiency virus (HIV).
- Conduct ECG and chest x-ray (CXR).
- Further cardiac workup based on need.
- Psychosocial evaluation regarding compliance.
- May need bilateral nephrectomy for recurrent urinary tract infections (UTIs) or polycystic kidney disease (PCKD).
- See Table 25-1 for contraindications to kidney transplantation.
- The donor kidney is usually placed in the iliac fossa with vascular anastomosis to the iliacs and the native kidney of the recipient need not be removed excepting for PCKD and recurrent UTIs.

Complications Specific to Kidney Transplantation

EARLY COMPLICATIONS

- Delayed graft function.
- Evidenced by oliguria or anuria (assess volume status, ensure that Foley is working; once checked, but still anuric/oliguric, Doppler ultrasound [US] indicated to assess blood flow). If blood flow is adequate, look for urine leak or obstruction at ureterovesicular junction (UVJ) with US or renal scan. Once all workup negative, diagnosis is delayed graft function.
- Management may include dialysis in postoperative period.
- **Graft thrombosis:**
  - Requires immediate reoperation to save transplant.
  - Diagnosis indicated by abrupt cessation of urine output.
  - May assess with Doppler US.
- **Urine leak:**
  - Usually at UVJ.
  - **Diagnosis:** Decreased urine output, lower abdominal pain, scrotal or labial edema, rising creatinine.

> The left kidney is preferred by surgeons because of its longer renal vein, but preoperative imaging studies in the potential donor can identify variants of normal anatomy (like multiple arteries) that may make the right kidney a better choice.

TABLE 25-1. Contraindications to Kidney Transplantation

ABSOLUTE CONTRAINDICATIONS	RELATIVE CONTRAINDICATIONS
Cancer (other than squamous cell or basal cell carcinoma of skin)	Sickle cell disease
Infection (HIV, tuberculosis)	Likely to be noncompliant
Cirrhosis (chronic active)	Ischemic heart disease severe, without possibility of coronary artery bypass graft or angioplasty
Ongoing drug use	

- **Tests:** US with fluid aspiration and analysis, renal scan with extravasation of radioisotope.
- **Treatment:** Reexploration and repair.

LATE COMPLICATIONS

- **Ureteral stricture:**
    - Rising creatinine and hydronephrosis on ultrasound.
    - Distal stricture result of rejection or ischemia; antegrade pyelogram best diagnostic tool.
    - **Treatment:** Balloon dilatation; longer ones require surgical repair.
- Renal artery stenosis:
    - Ten percent of renal transplants within first 6 months.
    - **Presentation:** Hypertension, fluid retention.
    - **Diagnosis:** Angiogram, US, magnetic resonance angiography (MRA).
    - If distal to anastomosis, may be secondary to rejection, atherosclerosis, clamp or other iatrogenic injury. Occurs more frequently with end-to-end anastomoses.
    - **Treatment:** > 80% correctible with angioplasty; others require surgical repair.
    - **Donor complications:** UTI, wound infection, pneumothorax.

▶ PANCREAS TRANSPLANTATION

Indications

Type 1 (insulin-dependent) diabetes mellitus.

Exclusions

- Significant coronary artery disease (CAD).
- Severe peripheral vascular disease (PVD) resulting in amputations.
- Severe visual impairment.
- Untreated malignancy.
- Active infection.
- HIV.

Timing of Operation

- **Pancreas transplant (5%):** For the nonuremic diabetic patient with minimal or no evident nephropathy.
- **Pancreas transplant after kidney transplant (PAK) (7%):** For the uremic diabetic patient with potentially reversible secondary effects, with suitable living related kidney donor available.
- **Simultaneous pancreas and kidney transplants (SPK) (87%):** For the diabetic uremic patient with potentially reversible secondary effects, lacking a suitable living related kidney donor.

Alternatives to whole-organ pancreas transplant is use of insulin pump and islet of Langerhans transplant.

The pancreas transplant is placed in the abdominal cavity rather than in the retroperitoneal space because of a lower incidence of peripancreatic fluid collections and lymphocele.

Pancreas transplant: Expect euglycemia within 12 hours of operation; no postop insulin should be required.

HIGH-YIELD FACTS

Transplant

Consider acute rejection of a pancreas transplant when urinary amylase is consistently decreased by 25%.

Bladder irrigation may help clear up hematuria and prevent clot retention.

UTI is the most common infectious complication after pancreas transplants, especially following bladder-drained SPK transplants.

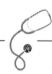

Human leukocyte antigen (HLA) mismatch and preservation time do not have a significant impact on graft survival for pancreas transplants.

Liver transplant outcome is generally better for chronic liver failure patients.

▶ DRAINAGE OPTIONS

- **Bladder drainage:**
    - Advantage: Urinary amylase may be used as a sign of rejection.
    - Up to 25% may require conversion to enteric drainage.
- **Enteric drainage:**
    - Avoidance of postop GU complications that affect 30% of bladder drained patients.
    - Avoidance of chronic dehydration.
    - No need for bicarbonate replacement.
    - Equal efficacy, graft survival, morbidity.
    - In SPK, rejection usually involves pancreas and kidney. May diagnose by creatinine and renal biopsy.

COMPLICATIONS

- Gross hematuria.
- Urinary leak.
- UTI.
- Urethritis.
- Hyperamylasemia.
- Peripancreatic fluid collections on CT and US. Drain if infection is suspected.

▶ LIVER TRANSPLANTATION

INDICATIONS

- Irreversible liver failure.
- **Chronic (more common):**
    - Cirrhosis (posthepatic, alcoholic).
    - Primary and secondary biliary cirrhosis.
    - Primary sclerosing cholangitis.
    - Metabolic defects (α_1-antitrypsin deficiency, amyloidosis, hemochromatosis, sarcoidosis, tyrosinemia, ornithine transcarbinase deficiency, Crigler-Najjar).
    - Malignancy (hepatocellular carcinoma [HCC] or cholangiocarcinoma).
    - Others: Biliary atresia, cystic fibrosis.
- **Acute or fulminant:**
    - Viral or alcoholic hepatitis.
    - Wilson's disease.
    - Hepatotoxic drugs (e.g., acetaminophen overdose).
    - Contraindications.
    - Multisystem organ failure.
    - Severe cardiopulmonary disease.
    - Sepsis secondary to nonhepatic source.
    - Widespread cancer.
    - Noncompliance with medical therapy.
    - Severely impaired neurologic status.

EVALUATION

- The Model for End-Stage Liver Disease (MELD) score is used for adult liver transplant assessment (uses patient's values for bilirubin, international normalized ratio for prothrombin time [INR], and creatinine).
- Preoperative control of:
    - Variceal bleeding: Transjugular intrahepatic portosystemic shunt (TIPS) when needed.
    - Ascites: Diuretics and/or paracentesis.

COMPLICATIONS

- Graft failure: Usually secondary to primary nonfunction, recurrence of disease, biliary or vascular complications (not generally due to rejection).
- Rejection occurs in first 3 months posttransplant with 50% incidence, but is well treated with steroids or antilymphocyte therapy (indicated by elevated liver function tests [LFTs], particularly γ-glutamyl transpeptidase [GGTP]).

> Cancer and alcohol abuse remain controversial indications for liver transplant:
> - Alcoholic liver disease accounts for 75% of liver failure in the United States. Patients have excellent outcome, with low rate of recidivism. Pretransplant abstinence, evidence of support system, and lack of other alcohol-related comorbidities are required.
> - Patients transplanted for liver cancer have worse outcome than patients transplanted for other reasons, but survival is improved compared to cancer patients who are not transplanted (40% 5-year survival).

► SMALL BOWEL TRANSPLANTATION

INDICATIONS

- Adults: Short bowel syndrome, due to Crohn's disease, mesenteric thrombosis, trauma.
- Children: Short bowel syndrome, due to necrotizing enterocolitis, intestinal pseudo-obstruction, gastroschisis, volvulus, intestinal atresia.

OPERATION

- Isolated intestinal failure: Isolated intestinal transplant.
- With liver failure: Liver-intestine combined transplant.
- Sometimes, multivisceral transplant: Liver, stomach, pancreas, duodenum, small intestine, possibly large bowel.
- Stoma usually placed for monitoring and biopsies.

COMPLICATIONS

- Graft-versus-host disease (GVHD): Prevent with immunosuppression, and/or pretreatment of donor.
- Rejection: More difficult to treat than in other organs; newer agents may prove to be more useful than older ones (tacrolimus based).
- Diagnosed by fever, abdominal pain, elevated white count, ileus, gastrointestinal (GI) bleed, positive blood cultures; also by biopsy showing cryptitis, villi shortening, mononuclear infiltrate.

► CARDIAC TRANSPLANTATION

INDICATIONS

- Severe cardiac disability on maximal medical therapy (multiple hospitalizations for congestive heart failure [CHF], New York Hospital Association class III [NYHA III] or IV, or peak oxygen consumption < 15 mL/kg/min).

Typical scenario: A 53-year-old woman who is status post liver transplant calls your office asking what she can take for some musculoskeletal pain. *Think:* Patient is on tacrolimus, which ultimately causes renal insufficiency in most patients. Do not give anything that could potentiate its nephrotoxicity. First-line drug for pain would be acetaminophen, standard doses of which a transplanted liver should be able to tolerate.

Cardiac transplant: Cold ischemic time up to 6 hours may be tolerated, though 3–4 is ideal (2 hours maximum for patients with pulmonary hypertension).

Transplanted heart has increased sensitivity to catecholamines, with increased density of adrenergic receptors with loss of norepinephrine uptake; cardiac output and index remain at low normal, with adequate but abnormal exercise response (increase in heart rate is usually delayed).

- Symptomatic ischemia or recurrent ventricular arrhythmias refractory to usual therapy, with left ventricular ejection fraction (LVEF) < 30%, or with unstable angina and not a candidate for CABG or percutaneous transluminal coronary angioplasty (PTCA).
- All surgical alternatives already excluded.

CONTRAINDICATIONS

- Irreversible, severe, pulmonary, renal, or hepatic dysfunction.
- Unstaged or incompletely staged cancer.
- Psychiatric illness.
- Severe systemic disease.

EVALUATION

Matching/compatibility based on:

1. ABO compatibility.
2. Body size.
3. Donor weight/recipient weight.
4. Phosphoribosylamine (PRA) (if PRA > 5%, crossmatch is done).

COMPLICATIONS

- The most common cause of perioperative death is infection (50%). Other common causes are pulmonary hypertension and nonspecific graft failure.
- **Infection:**
  - Peak incidence: Early postoperative period.
  - Most patients will have an infection at some point in the first 5 postoperative years.
- **Rejection:**
  - At least 75% incidence in first 3 posttransplant months.
  - Diagnosis confirmed by endomyocardial biopsy (via right internal jugular).
- **Histology:** Lymphocyte infiltration and/or myocytic necrosis.
- **Treatment:** Pulse steroids if early on (later in course, mild rejection treated by 3-day increased dose of oral prednisone); refractory rejection treated with ATG or OKT3.
- **Chronic rejection:** Concentric intimal proliferation with smooth muscle hyperplasia yielding atherosclerosis more diffuse than in nontransplanted hearts.
- Prevalence of CAD: 25% at 1 year and 80% at 5 years.
- Yearly angiogram recommended.
- **Cancer:** Increased risk, with immunosuppression, of skin, vulvar, or anal cancer; B-cell lymphoproliferative disorder (BLPD), and cervical intraepithelial neoplasia (CIN).

▶ LUNG TRANSPLANTATION

TYPES OF OPERATIONS AND INDICATIONS

- Single lung for fibrotic lung disease: Pulmonary fibrosis, emphysema, bronchopulmonary dysplasia, primary pulmonary hypertension (without cardiac dysfunction), posttransplant obliterative bronchiolitis.
- Bilateral single lung for cystic fibrosis, bronchiectasis, COPD.

- Heart-lung for pulmonary vascular disease, end-stage lung disease with cardiac dysfunction.
- Lobar lung, to increase donor pool from living related and cadaveric donors.

CONTRAINDICATIONS

- Significant systemic disease, including hepatic or renal disease.
- Active infection.
- Malignancy.
- Noncompliance.
- Current smoking.

EVALUATION

- ABO compatible.
- Infection-free donor and recipient.
- Donor: Good pulmonary gas exchange, no smoking history, similar lung volume, where possible.

COMPLICATIONS

- **Acute rejection:**
  - Sixty to seventy percent incidence in first postoperative month.
  - Diagnosed by clinical parameters: Fever, dyspnea, decreased PaO_2, decreased forced expiratory volume in 1 second (FEV_1), CXR with interstitial infiltrate.
  - Confirm with biopsy via bronchoscopy: Lymphocytic infiltrate to varying degrees.
- **Chronic rejection:**
  - Presents as obliterative bronchiolitis.
  - Twenty to fifty percent of long-term survivors.
  - No treatment.
- **Infection:** Early, predominance of gram-negative bacillus (GNB) infection.
  - **Viral:** CMV, treated with ganciclovir, also EBV.
  - **Fungal:** *Candida, Aspergillus.*
  - **Protozoan:** *Pneumocystis jiroveci* pneumonia.
- **Outcomes:**
  - Kidney transplants have best outcomes, 5-year graft survival for living donor is 81% (90% patient survival) in the United States.
  - Small bowel and lung have the lowest rate of organ survival.

CMV occurs at 75–100% incidence in cardiac transplant patients and has been identified as trigger for graft-related atherosclerosis (treated with ganciclovir and hyperimmune globulin).

HIGH-YIELD FACTS

Transplant

The Genitourinary System

Cryptorchidism increases the risk for cancer. Approximately 10% of testicular tumors (usually seminoma) arise from undescended testes.

Bell-clapper deformity: Insufficient attachment of the testicles to the tunica vaginalis, allowing for a pathologically large degree of rotational freedom. This increases risk of torsion.

Penis

- Made up of three cylindrical bodies (see Figure 26-1):
  - Two corpora cavernosa covered by tunica albuginea, comprising the erectile tissue of the penile shaft.
  - One corpus spongiosum, which surrounds the urethra and expands to form the glans.
  - Buck's fascia surrounds the corpora cavernosa and corpus spongiosum structures.
- Blood supply: Internal pudendal artery. Dorsal veins drain into the pudendal plexus, which in turn drains into pudendal vein.
- Lymphatic drainage: Deep and superficial inguinal nodes.

Scrotum

- Made up of smooth muscle, elastic tissue layers of Darto's fascia, which is a continuation of Scarpa's fascia from the abdominal wall.
- Blood supply: Femoral and internal pudendal artery.
- Lymphatic drainage: Inguinal and femoral nodes.

Testes

- Lie in the scrotum, usually vertically.
- Encased in tunica albigunea except posteriolaterally, where it is attached to the epididymis. This entire unit is then wrapped in the tunica vaginalis, which attaches to the scrotum posterior-inferiorly via the gubernaculum.

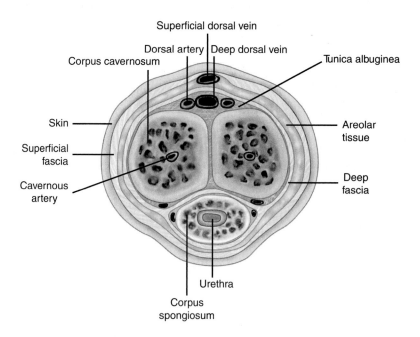

FIGURE 26-1. **Cross-section of the penis.**

(Reproduced, with permission, from Le T, Krause K. *First Aid for the Basic Sciences: Organ Systems.* New York: McGraw-Hill, 2009: 753.)

HIGH-YIELD FACTS

The Genitourinary System

- Vestigial structures: The appendix testis is located in the superior aspect of the testicle, and is of müllerian duct origin. The appendix epididymis is located on the epididymis, and is of wolffian duct origin.
- Blood supply to testis: Gonadal artery, deferential artery and cremasteric vessels. All three travel in the spermatic cord!
- Venous return: Pampiniform plexus, which in turn drains into the gonadal vein.
- Lymphatic drainage: External, common iliac, and periaortic nodes.

Epididymis

- Tubular structure, originating from the wolffian duct.
- Four to five meters in length compressed to an area of about 5 cm.
- Site of sperm maturation and motility.

Vas Deferens

- Originates from the wolffian duct.
- A muscular tube that originates at the epididymis, exiting the scrotum laterally. It then courses into the inguinal canal via the external ring and exits the canal at the internal ring. Here, the vas deferens diverges from the spermatic cord, crossing medially behind the bladder and over the ureters to form the ampulla of vas deferens. It then joins the seminal vesicles to form the paired ejaculatory ducts in the prostatic urethra.
- Spermatic cord contains vas deferens, testicular vessels, cremasteric muscle fibers, and spermatic fasciae.

Prostate

- Originates from the urogenital sinus and matures via dihydrotestosterone stimulation.
- Secretory gland that contributes to seminal fluid, along with seminal vesicles, Cowper's glands, and epididymis.
- Posterior surface easily palpable on digital rectal exam.

Kidneys

- Kidneys, like all urologic organs, are retroperitoneal structures.
- Lie obliquely on psoas muscle and quadratus lumborus.
- Renal hilum consists of (from medial to lateral) vein, artery, and ureter/renal pelvis. Occasionally, there is an accessory artery elsewhere. On the left side, the gonadal vein inserts into the renal vein. However, on the right side, the gonadal vein inserts directly into the inferior vena cava (IVC) (Figure 26-2).
- Surrounded by perirenal fat, both the kidneys and adrenal glands lie within Gerota's fascia.
- The adrenal gland is located superior-medially to the kidney. However, in cases of renal ectopia and agenesis, the adrenal gland remains orthotopic.

Clinical Pearl: Varicoceles are far more common on the left, due to the difference in drainage pattern of each side's gonadal vein (see Kidney section below).

Torsion of the testicular or epididymal appendix can cause extreme pain mimicking torsion of the testes. However, this is a benign entity and is treated with NSAIDs.

Obstruction at the renal pelvis is a common cause of hydronephrosis. This may be caused by a crossing blood vessel to the kidney or a non-gravity-dependent ureteral insertion into the renal pelvis.

A pathologically short intramural ureter predisposes a patient to vesicoureteral reflux.

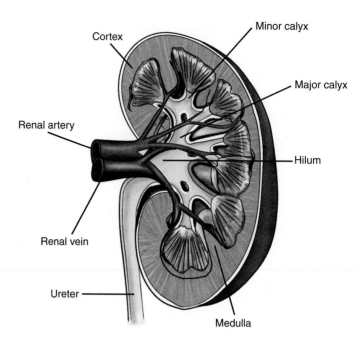

FIGURE 26-2. Gross anatomy of the kidney.

(Reproduced, with permission, from Le T, Krause K. *First Aid for the Basic Sciences: Organ Systems.* New York: McGraw-Hill, 2009: 656.)

Ureters

Ureters course along psoas muscle, cross the iliacs anteriorly at the bifurcation of the external/interal iliac arteries. The ureters then course medially toward the bladder, inserting posteriorly.

Bladder/Urethra

- Bladder consists of detrusor muscle, covered by a urothelial layer. Histologically, this is transitional epithelium.
- Both the detrusor and the bladder neck (internal sphincter) have autonomic innervation. The external (striated) urinary sphincter is under voluntary control.
- In males, the prostatic urethra is located between the internal and external sphincters (this is a common site of adenomatous growth and urinary obstruction).

▶ HEMATURIA

DEFINITION

- Presence of blood in the urine.
- Can be gross or microscopic.
- Normal urine should contain < 3 red blood cells per high power field of spun urine.

- **Pediatric:** Acute urinary tract infection (UTI), glomerular origin, congenital urinary tract abnormality, stones, trauma.
- **Adult/elderly:** Acute UTI, bladder cancer, urolithiasis, benign prostatic hyperplasia.

OTHER CAUSES

- **Upper tract:** Sickle cell disease, collagen vascular disease, renal disease (glomerulonephritis, vascular abnormalities, pyelonephritis, polycystic kidney, granulomatous disease, interstitial nephritis, neoplasm/renal cell carcinoma [RCC]).
- **Lower tract:** Urethritis, stones, cystitis, prostatitis, epididymitis. Mild hematuria is a normal finding in a patient with recent urologic instrumentation (including catheterization).
- Coagulopathy and anticoagulation may unmask (but not cause) hematuria.

In working up microhematuria, assess for the presence of red cell casts, which are present in glomerular bleeding.

False positive on dipstick occurs when myoglobin is present.

What can cause gross hematuria with a dipstick negative for blood? *Think:* Anthocyanin dye in beets and berries, pyridium, rifampin, porphyria, some food colorings.

▶ PRIAPISM

- **Definition:** An erection lasting more than 4 hours, generally not maintained by sexual stimulation.
- Two types: Diagnosed by history and physical and intracorporeal arterial blood gas (ABG)—see below).
    - **High flow:** Not ischemic (pH ~7.4), not painful. May result from arteriovenous (AV) fistula secondary to trauma (usually prior injection/irrigation as treatment for low flow).
- May be erect for days to weeks. Erection not fully turgid and glans generally not engorged. Treated with angioembolization of AV fistula site. Less common than low flow.
- **Low flow:** More common. Painful and entirely erect. Ischemic (pH < ~7.2), so risk of long-term erectile dysfunction, corporal fibrosis, or organ loss in severe cases. Common causes: Intracoporal Caverject (alprostadil) injections, cocaine, trazadone, PDE5 inhibitors (Viagra), sickle cell.
- Initial treatment involves local ice application, IM verapamil and Sudafed. If these fail (and they will!), patients require intracorporeal phenylephrine injections with or without saline irrigation of the corporal. (Remember to monitor hemodynamics closely when giving intracorporeal phenylephrine injections!) All of the above can be used when treating sickle cell priapism, but systemic treatments should be first attempted (i.e., exchange blood transfuse, oxygen administration, aggressive hydration hydroxyurea).

Whereas adult hydroceles gradually enlarge, pediatric hydroceles grow throughout the day and typically disappear overnight as the fluid flows back through the processus vaginalis into the peritoneal cavity.

▶ ACUTE SCROTUM

- **Differential diagnosis:** Testicular torsion, epididymo-orchitis, testicular tumor, peritesticular tumor (rhabdomyosarcoma, leiomyosarcoma, liposarcoma), torsion of testicular appendage, orchitis, trauma to scrotum, hernia, hydrocele, varicocele.
- Testicular torsion is a surgical emergency and must always be considered in the case of acute scrotal mass.

- Roughly 10% of seminomas secrete hCG; 90% of seminomas do not have elevated tumor markers.

CLASSIFICATION AND PATHOLOGY

- Classification is based on the cell type from which the tumor is derived—germinal or stromal.
- Germinal cell tumors comprise 95% of all testicular tumors:
  - Seminomas (pure single-cell tumors) 35% of testicular tumors.
  - Nonseminomas (embryonal cell carcinoma 20%, teratoma 5%, choriocarcinoma < 1%).
  - Combination tumors 40%.
- Tumors of gonadal stroma (1–2%):
  - Leydig cell.
  - Sertoli cell.
  - Primitive gonadal structures.
  - Gonadoblastomas (germinal cell + stromal cell).

STAGING EVALUATION

- To determine whether the cancer is localized to the testis, regional lymphatics or widely metastasized.
- Abdominal and pelvic CT scan to determine the presence of adenopathy or visceral involvement, chest x-ray (CXR) ± chest CT.
- There are many staging systems; however, most include three stages:
  - **Stage I:** No clinical or radiographic evidence of tumor presence beyond the confines of the testis. Markers normalize after orchiectomy.
  - **Stage II:** Retroperitoneal adenopathy on CT scan, subdiaphragmatic disease, and failure of markers to normalize after orchiectomy.
  - **Stage III:** Distant metastases or visceral involvement.

TREATMENT

- **Surgical approach:** High radical inguinal orchiectomy.
- Trans-scrotal biopsy of the testis or a trans-scrotal orchiectomy should not be performed if the diagnosis of testicular cancer is likely because the lymphatic drainage of the testes is different from that of the scrotum; a scrotal incision in the presence of testicular cancer may cause local recurrence, metastasis, and unpredictably lymphatic spread.
- **Early seminoma:** Orchiectomy + retroperitoneal x-ray therapy (XRT).
- **Advanced seminoma:** Orchiectomy, and combination chemotherapy followed by restaging.
- **Stage I nonseminoma:** Orchiectomy + retroperitoneal lymph node dissection (RPLND) or surveillance.
- **Stage II nonseminoma:** The optimal management of this group of patients is controversial. RPLND can be curative but have a high relapse rate. If relapse occurs, chemotherapy can be given as adjunctive therapy. Alternatively, chemotherapy can be given prior to RPLND.
- Advanced stage nonseminoma: Orchiectomy + chemotherapy ± tumor reductive surgery.
- The most commonly used chemotherapeutic regimen: BEP (etoposide, bleomycin, cisplatin).

DEFINITION AND EPIDEMIOLOGY

- One of the most common diseases of the urinary tract.
- Male-to-female ratio of 3:1.
- Familial tendency in stone formation.
- Average risk is 1%/year.
- Tendency for recurrence: Thirty-six percent of patients with a first stone will have another stone within one year, and 50% will recur within years.

ETIOLOGY

- Most common are calcium oxalate or a mixture of calcium (75%).
- Magnesium-ammonium-phosphate stones (struvite) 15%—seen in UTI with urea-splitting bacteria (*Proteus*). May cause staghorn calculi.
- Uric acid stones (15%), which are radiolucent (will not show up on x-ray, but are visible on noncontrast CT).
- Less than 1% are cystine stones (secondary to an inborn error of metabolism).
- Indinivir stones are not visible on CT scan or plain films.

RISK FACTORS

- Poor fluid intake/residence in a hot climate.
- Disease processes that increase free calcium, including bony destruction, multiple myeloma, hyperparathyroidism, osteolytic lesions, and sarcoidosis.
- Prolonged immobilization.
- History of calculus in the past and in family members.
- Drug ingestion (analgesics, alkalis, uricosuric agents, protease inhibitors).
- Prior history of gout/Lesch-Nyhan.
- Underlying gastrointestinal disease/malabsorption (Crohn's, ulcerative colitis, peptic ulcer disease [PUD], gastric bypass surgery).
- In a normal individual, dietary calcium intake is **not** a risk factor.

SIGNS AND SYMPTOMS

- Severe, abrupt onset of colicky pain, which begins in the flank and may radiate toward the groin. In males, the pain may radiate toward the testicle. In females, it may radiate toward the labium majoris.
- Nausea and vomiting. Gastrointestinal (GI) upset may be the only symptom in patients with chronic stones and infection, as seen in xanthogranulomatous pyelonephritis (XGP).
- Fever.
- Abdominal distention from ileus.
- Gross or microhematuria.

DIAGNOSTIC TESTS

- **Urinalysis and culture:**
  - Some patients will have red blood cells (RBCs) in the urine (absence does not rule out stones).

Typical scenario: A 40-year-old man presents with sudden onset left-sided flank pain that he rates a 10/10. He is writhing, unable to stay still or find a comfortable position. *Think:* Renal colic. Check a urine dip for blood and order a noncontrast CT scan.

- White blood cells (WBCs) or bacteria may suggest underlying UTI and should be aggressively treated.
- **Radiographic studies:**
  - Noncontrast abdominal/pelvic CT (Figure 26-3):
    - Fast, requires no IV contrast.
    - Most useful to diagnose small stones (95% sensitivity), hydronephrosis, hydroureter, and perinephric stranding.
    - Useful for revealing other abdominal/pelvic pathology.
    - Study of choice!
  - Plain abdominal film (KUB): Only radiopaque stones > 3 cm will be seen (60–70% specific in the diagnosis of a calculus). However, it is a cheap and quick test to do and is useful in combination with other studies.
  - Renal US: Fast, easy, and relatively inexpensive. Primarily useful in patients who should avoid radiation, such as pregnant women.

MANAGEMENT

- Analgesia with nonsteroidal anti-inflammatory drugs (parenteral ketorolac) and/or opiates.
- IV or PO hydration.
- During passage of a stone, there are four sites where the passage is likely to become arrested. These are narrowest points of the urinary system:
  - Ureteropelvic junction
  - Pelvic brim
  - Iliac crossing
  - Ureterovesical junction
  - Vesicle orifice
- If stone impaction occurs and hydronephrosis develops, decompression of the affected kidney may be necessary to preserve kidney function.

Most stones < 5 mm will pass spontaneously in adults.

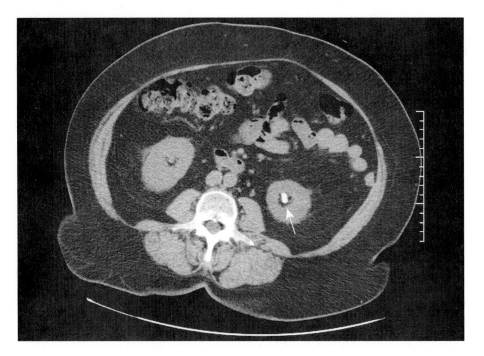

FIGURE 26-3. Noncontrast abdominal CT demonstrating nephrolithiasis (arrow) in the right kidney, which shows up as radiopaque (white).

- For stones unlikely to pass spontaneously:
  - Extracorporeal shockwave lithotripsy (ESWL) is effective for stones (< 1 cm).
  - Ureteroscopy with stone extraction for ureteral calculi and small renal calculi.
  - Percutaneous nephrolithotomy, which establishes a tract from the skin to the collecting system, is used when stones are too large or too hard for lithotripsy.
- Surgical emergency if accompanied by fever and UTI, necessitating stent placement or nephrostomy tube.

▶ BENIGN PROSTATIC HYPERPLASIA

DEFINITION

- Benign prostatic hyperplasia is the most common benign tumor in men.
- Incidence is directly proportional to age, affecting approximately 90% of men > 80.
- The prostate enlarges (within the confines of a tight prostatic capsule) during puberty when it undergoes androgen-mediated growth. It remains stable in size until about the fifth or sixth decade, when its size increases again.

PATHOPHYSIOLOGY

- Hyperplasia begins in the periurethral area, then progresses to the remainder of the gland; hence, the most common initial symptoms are of urinary outflow obstruction.
- Histologically, the hyperplastic tissue is comprised of glandular epithelium, stroma, and smooth muscle.
- As hyperplasia increases with increasing obstruction, frank urinary retention can occur or may be precipitated by extrinsic etiologies, such as infection, anticholinergic drugs, α-agonists, or alcohol.

SIGNS AND SYMPTOMS

- Early symptoms include hesitancy in initiating voiding, weak stream, postvoid dribbling, and the sensation of incomplete emptying.
- As the amount of residual urine increases symptoms may include nocturia, overflow incontinence, and urinary frequency and urgency.

DIAGNOSIS

- Clinical history.
- Digital rectal exam—in hyperplasia, the prostate will be smooth, firm, but enlarged.
- Measurement of postvoid residual urine volume and uroflow.

MANAGEMENT

- **Medical:**
  - 5-α reductase inhibitor (finasteride): Blocks conversion of testosterone to dihydrotestoseterone, may shrink prostatic hyperplasia up to 20%.
  - α-adrenergic antagonists (prazosin, terazosin, tamsulosin) decrease urethral resistance.

Typical scenario: A 65-year-old male who complains of frequent urination at night with difficulty starting the urine stream. Once starting the urine stream, he states he has difficulty stopping the stream. *Think:* Prostatic hyperplasia.

- **Surgical** (it is important to note that these procedures are not cancer surgeries):
  - Transurethral prostatectomy (TURP) for smaller prostates.
  - Open simple prostatectomy for larger prostates.
  - Retrograde ejaculation is a consequence of these surgeries.

▶ PROSTATIC CARCINOMA

DEFINITION

- The most common malignancy in men in the United States.
- Rare before age 50.

RISK FACTORS

- Increasing age
- African-American

Typical scenario: An 87-year-old man presents with a history of prostate cancer presents with low back pain. *Think:* Bony metastases and possibly cord compression.

CLASSIFICATION

- Ninety-five percent are adenocarcinoma. The remaining 5% are squamous, transitional cell, sarcoma, and occasional metastatic tumors.
- Predilection to originate in the peripheral zone and is often multifocal.

SIGNS AND SYMPTOMS

- Most patients are asymptomatic at the time of diagnosis, secondary to widespread use of PSA screening tests. It is important to note, that patients on 5-α reductase inhibitors have artificially reduced PSA levels (up to 50%).
- In symptomatic patients, common symptoms include obstructive or irritative voiding complaints.
- Metastatic disease to the bone may cause bone pain.
- Symptoms in advanced disease may include ureteral obstruction, spinal cord compression, deep venous thrombosis (DVT), and pulmonary emboli.

DIAGNOSIS

- On digital rectal exam (DRE), the prostate is usually hard, nodular, and irregular.
- Prostate-specific antigen (PSA) is the most sensitive test for early detection of prostatic cancer. Following diagnosis, PSA is used to follow progression of disease and response to treatment. However, the PSA is not a specific test. PSA can be elevated in prostatic hyperplasia or prostatitis. Although debate is ongoing, a PSA of 4 in a male over the age of 50 is generally agreed upon as indication for transrectal ultrasonography (TRUS) biopsy.
- **Imaging studies:**
  - TRUS, used for image guided biopsies: Carcinomas appear as hypoechoic densities in the peripheral zone, has very low sensitivity and specificity.
  - MRI or CT may also be helpful in identifying metastasis and lymph node involvement.
- **Biopsy:** Essential in establishing the diagnosis of prostate cancer.

STAGING

- Metastatic spread occurs via:
  - Direct extension (into the seminal vesicles and/or bladder floor).
  - Lymphatic spread to obturator, internal iliac, common iliac, presacral, and periaortic nodes.
  - Hematogenous spread occurs to bone more frequently than viscera.
- Standard staging scheme used is the **tumor-node-metastases (TNM) system.**
- Gleason grading system is based on a histologic evaluation of prostate tissue samples. The Gleason score is the sum of the two most common cell patterns seen in the tissue sample. The patterns can range from 1 (well differentiated) to 5 (poorly differentiated, highly malignant). Overall scores range from 2 to 10. A grade of 2 has the best prognosis, while a grade of 10 represents poorly differentiated tissue and confers the worst prognosis.
- Bony metastasis can contain both osteoblastic components. Axial skeleton is most commonly affected. Skeletal survey has a low sensitivity for detecting bony metastasis. Radionuclide bone scan has a much higher sensitivity and is also useful in monitoring progression and response to therapy.
- CT of abdomen and pelvis is used to assess lymph node involvement.

Ten to fifteen percent of prostate cancer cases may have normal PSA, hence the importance of the DRE.

TREATMENT

- Treatments vary in aggressiveness depending on patient age, health status, and stage/grade of disease. Treatments may include any/all of the following:
  - Watchful waiting/active surveillance.
  - Androgen deprivation therapy: It has been established that prostatic carcinomas are hormonally dependent. Some degree of control can be obtained by hormonal therapy. Androgen deprivation can be achieved via:
    - Surgical castration (bilateral orchiectomy results in 90% reduction in testosterone).
    - Gonadotropin-releasing hormone (GnRH) agonist (leuprolide) therapy.
    - Androgen receptor antagonists (flutamide, bicalutamide).
    - Estrogen administration.
  - Radiation: Can be via XRT or brachytherapy (radioactive seed placement).
  - Radical prostatectomy: May be retropubic (transabdominal), transperineal, laparoscopic, or robotic.
  - Chemotherapy is not very effective, but may be used as a last resort in cases of very advanced, hormone-refractory disease.
  - Combinations of all of the above are commonly used.

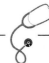

Complications of radiation therapy for prostate cancer:
- Cystitis
- Acute proctitis (diarrhea)
- Urethritis (can lead to strictures)
- Rectal strictures and fistula
- Impotence
- Secondary malignancy

▶ RENAL CELL CARCINOMA (RCC)

ETIOLOGY

- Eighty-five percent of all primary malignant renal neoplasms.
- Peak incidence between 50 and 60 years.
- Male-to-female ratio: 2:1.

- Environmental factors: Cigarette smoking; exposure to cadmium, asbestos, and solvents.
- Hereditary link: Genetic defect linked to translocations between chromosomes 3 and 8.

SIGNS AND SYMPTOMS

- Classic triad of gross hematuria, flank pain, and palpable abdominal mass (seen in 10–15% of cases).
- Most commonly an incidental finding.
- Most often diagnosed via its systemic symptoms: Fatigability, weight loss and cachexia, intermittent fever, and anemia.
- Other symptoms may relate to the production of hormones and hormone-like substances (paraneoplastic syndromes):
  - Hypercalcemia (parathyroid hormone)
  - Galactorrhea (prolactin)
  - Cushing's syndrome (glucocorticoid)

DIAGNOSIS

- It is most important to differentiate cystic from solid lesions.
- Ultrasound has improved the ability to differentiate a solid from a cystic lesion.
- CT is the method of choice for diagnosis and staging of RCC.

STAGING

- **Stage I:** Tumor confined within the kidney parenchyma.
- **Stage II:** Invasion through the kidney capsule, involves perinephric fat but confined within Gerota's fascia.
- **Stage III:** Involvement of regional lymph nodes, ipsilateral renal vein, or vena cava.
- **Stage IV:** Distant metastasis, adjacent organ involvement.

TREATMENT

- Radical nephrectomy is the treatment of choice if there is no evidence of metastasis. Partial nephrectomy (complete resection of mass) is oncologically equal to radical nephrectomy.
- Radiation therapy can be used in the palliation of patients with metastatic RCC.
- There are no standard chemotherapeutic regimens or hormonal therapy for metastatic disease, and these treatments have been employed with limited success.
- Chemotherapeutic agents (sorafenib).

PROGNOSIS

Five-year survival rates:

Stage I: 91–100%
Stage II: 74–96%
Stage III: 59–70%
Stage IV: 16–32%

DEFINITION AND EPIDEMIOLOGY

The lining of the urinary system from the renal pelvis to the urethra is made up of transitional cells. This entire lining is subject to carcinomatous changes. However, the bladder is involved most frequently and will therefore be discussed most extensively.

- Collecting system and ureteral lesions have a high (~60%) likelihood of spreading to the bladder, as this disease is a field defect. Rate of contralateral spread is ~5%, so patients require lifelong surveillance.
- Nephroureterectomy is treatment of choice.
- As with bladder cancer (see below), advanced disease has poor prognosis.
- Presentation and risk factors are similar to bladder (see below).

- Second most common cancer of the GU tract.
- Men are affected three times more than women.
- Peak incidence occurs between the ages of 60 and 70.
- Ninety-eight percent of bladder cancers are epithelial; in the United States, most are transitional cell carcinomas.
- Nontransitional cell carcinomas, such as squamous cell and adenocarcinomas have a worse prognosis compared to transitional cell carcinoma.
- Squamous cell carcinoma (SCC) tends to arise secondary to chronic irritation and inflammation (indwelling catheter, recurrent UTI, schistosomiasis).
- Adenocarcinoma tends to be metastatic or direct spread from adjacent organ (large bowel, uterus, uracus).
- Transitional cell carcinoma (by far the most common!) may result from cigarette smoking (twofold increased risk), dye, or chemical exposures.

SIGNS AND SYMPTOMS

- Gross and microscopic hematuria are the most common presenting symptom (80–95%).
- Other symptoms include dysuria urinary frequency, urgency, and ureteral obstruction.

DIAGNOSIS AND STAGING

- Urine cytology for exfoliated malignant cells (poor sensitivity, high specificity).
- Intravenous pyelography (IVP)—ureteral obstruction with hydronephrosis or filling defect.
- Cystoscopy with tumor biopsy.
- Additional staging may be obtained via CT of abdomen and pelvis and endoscopic resection of a bladder neoplasm.

- **Superficial:**
  - Tis: Carcinoma in situ, mucosal involvement.
  - Ta: No invasion.
- **Invasive:**
  - T1: Submucosal involvement.
  - T2: Involvement of bladder muscularis.
  - T3: Involvement of perivesical fat.
  - T4: Involvement of adjacent viscera.
- **Metastatic:** Uses TNM system.

TREATMENT

- Transurethral resection of bladder tumor (TURBT): Endoscopic resection is necessary for initial evaluation of the lesion to assess for depth of invasion. Superficial localized tumors can be treated with TURBT and surveillance (Tis–T1).
- Intravesical chemotherapy using BCG (bacillus Calmette-Guérin) or mitomycin has been shown to have preventative effects after TURBT for lesions up to and including T1.
- Radical cystectomy is the treatment of choice in patients with T2 and greater disease who can tolerate a surgery of this magnitude. Resection of the iliac lymph nodes during this surgery has shown to be both diagnostic and therapeutic.
- The oncologic indications for partial cystectomy are the same as for radical cystectomy. However, the former is generally performed when the tumor(s) are in a location in the bladder, and of a sufficiently small size, amenable to a bladder-sparing procedure. Lymph node dissection is also performed with this surgery.
- Neoadjuvant chemotherapy before (partial) cystectomy improves survival.
- XRT is a reasonable option for muscle invasive (T2–T3) lesions for poor surgical candidates. There is not as much long-term data on this modality.
- The prognosis of metastatic urothelial cancer is poor. However, chemotherapeutic agents have been shown to prolong survival. Commonly used agents are cisplatin, methotrexate, gencitabine doxorubicin, cyclophosphamide, and vinblastine.

PROGNOSIS

The survival rate of patients with metastatic disease is generally < 2 years.

Orthopedics

- Categorized by anatomical location (proximal or middle third of shaft), direction of fracture line (transverse, oblique, spiral), and whether it's simple or comminuted.
- Patient presents with loss of function, pain, tenderness, swelling, abnormal motion, and often deformity.

Open Fracture

- Fracture communicates with the external environment due to a breach of the overlying soft tissue.
- **True orthopedic emergency:** Almost always results in bacterial contamination of soft tissues and bone.
- Prognosis dependent on extent of soft tissue injury and by type/level of bacterial contamination.
- **Treatment plan:** Prevent infection, restore soft tissues, achieve bone union, avoid malunion, and institute early joint motion and muscle rehabilitation.

Pathologic Fracture

- Occurs due to minimal trauma on a bone weakened by preexisting disease.
- **Predisposing conditions:** Primary or metastatic carcinoma, cysts, enchondroma, giant cell tumors, osteomalacia, osteogenesis imperfecta, scurvy, rickets, and Paget's disease.
- Orthopedic surgeon must not only treat the broken bone but should also diagnose and treat the underlying condition.

Stress or Fatigue Fracture

- A complete fracture resulting from repetitive application of minor trauma.
- Most stress fractures occur in the lower extremities and commonly affect individuals involved in sports and military recruits ("march fracture").
- Pathophysiology of stress fractures is unclear but possibly due to inability of the fatigued muscle to protect bone from strain.
- If the patient is seen within first 2 weeks of onset of symptoms, the plain radiograph is likely to be normal.
- Patients usually complain of pain only with activity.
- **Treatment:** Decrease physical activity.

Comminuted Fracture

Fracture in which the bone is divided into more than two fragments by fracture lines.

Osteoporosis is the most common pathologic condition associated with pathologic fractures.

Suspect violence or battering if fracture occurs on normal bone and history reveals trivial trauma.

Incidence of stress fractures by site:
Metatarsals: > 50% stress fractures
Calcaneus: 25%
Tibia: 20%
Tarsal navicular: Basketball players

- Fracture involving the physis. Occur irregularly through the weak zone of hypertrophic cartilage (Figure 27-1).
- **Types I and II**: Fracture is transverse and does not travel vertically across the germinal cell layer. Prognosis for normal healing is good.
- **Types III and IV**: Fracture traverses the growth plate in a vertical fashion often causing angular deformity from continued growth. Surgical intervention necessary.
- **Type V**: Crush injury to the physis such that metaphysis and epiphysis are impacted on one another. No visible fracture line. Poor prognosis with high risk of growth plate arrest.

Greenstick fracture: Think of a young, moist twig, which would break without snapping apart!

Greenstick Fracture

- An incomplete and angulated fracture of the long bones. A transverse crack that hangs on to its connection.
- Very common in children, rarely seen in adults.
- Since kids have "softer," less brittle bone and thicker (leathery) periosteal membrane, they get incomplete fractures with unique patterns.

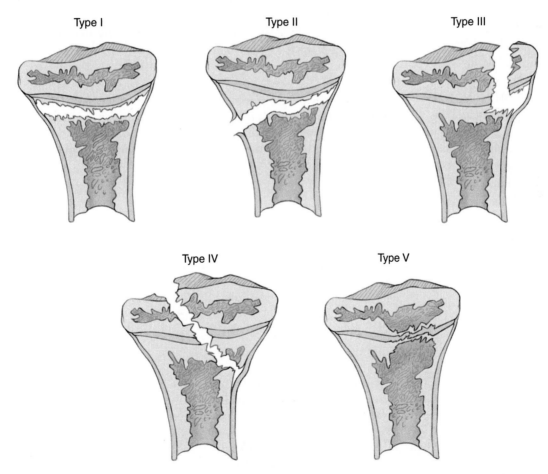

Type I   Type II   Type III

Type IV   Type V

FIGURE 27-1. **Salter-Harris classification of fractures.**

DEFINITION

An acute respiratory distress syndrome caused by release of fat droplets from the marrow as may occur following a long bone fracture.

COMMON CAUSES

- Long bone fracture.
- Burns.
- Severe infection.
- Inhalation anesthesia.
- Metabolic disorders.
- Cardiopulmonary bypass.
- Decompression sickness.
- Others: Hemoglobinopathy, collagen disease, diabetes, renal homo-transplantations.

PATHOPHYSIOLOGY

- Microdroplets of fat are released into the circulation at the site of fracture, occluding pulmonary circulation causing ischemic and hemorrhagic changes.
- Another theory: Release of free fatty acids from the marrow have toxic effects in all tissues, especially the lung.

SIGNS AND SYMPTOMS

- Symptoms may occur immediately or 2–3 days after trauma.
- Shortness of breath with respiratory rate above 30.
- Confusion, restlessness, disorientation, stupor, or coma.
- Fleeting petechial rash on chest, axilla, neck, and conjunctiva.
- Fever, tachycardia.

DIAGNOSIS

- **Hallmark finding:** Arterial hypoxemia. Arterial $PO_2 < 60$ mmHg is suggestive.
- Chest x-ray (CXR): Progressive snowstorm-like infiltration.
- Cryostat—frozen section of clotted blood reveals presence of fat.
- Absence of fat globules in urine makes diagnosis unlikely; however, their presence is not specific for fat embolism.

TREATMENT

- Administer oxygen to decrease hypoxemia and monitor PO_2 to maintain it over 90 mmHg.
- In severe hypoxemia: Mechanical ventilatory support.
- Use of ethanol, heparin, hypertonic glucose, or steroids has been suggested but their effectiveness is questionable.
- Prevent fat embolism syndrome by careful stabilization of fractures and effective treatment of shock.

Classic triad for fat embolism:
- Confusion
- Dyspnea
- Petechiae on chest

Typical scenario: A 25-year-old male complains of difficulty breathing. His family notes he is acting a little confused, and that he has a spotty purplish rash. Two days ago, he sustained a femur fracture after a high-speed motor vehicle collison. *Think:* Fat embolism syndrome.

PROGNOSIS

Mortality from fat embolism thought to be as high as 50% following multiple fractures.

> ▶ **SHOULDER DISLOCATIONS**

See Table 27-1.

COMPLICATIONS COMMON TO ALL DISLOCATIONS

Axillary artery injury (more common with luxatio erecta), venous injury, injury to nerves of brachial plexus (most common being axillary nerve):

- Palpate radial pulse to check axillary artery.
- Check motor component of axillary nerve by assessing strength of the deltoid muscle.
- Check sensory component of axillary nerve by assessing sensation over the lateral part of upper arm.
- Do a neurologic exam to evaluate all brachial nerve lesions.

TABLE 27-1. Shoulder Dislocations

	ANTERIOR DISLOCATION	POSTERIOR DISLOCATION	INFERIOR DISLOCATION (LUXATIO ERECTA)
Features	High risk of recurrence 70% occur in patients younger than 30 years of age	Diagnosis missed in 60% of cases Often precipitated by a convulsion, seizure, electrical shock, and falls	< 1% of all shoulder dislocations
Types	Subcoracoid (most common), subclavicular, subglenoid	Subacromial (most common), subglenoid, subspinous	
Mechanism of injury	Abduction and external rotation of the arm causes strain on anterior capsule and glenohumeral ligaments	Internal rotation and adduction (when one falls on an arm that is forwardly flexed and internally rotated)	Hyperabduction always results in detachment of rotator cuff
Signs and symptoms	■ Arms held to the side ■ Patient resists medial rotation and adduction ■ Prominent acromion ■ Loss of normal rounded shoulder contour	■ Patient holds arm medially rotated and to the side ■ Abduction limited ■ External rotation limited ■ Prominence of the coracoid process and posterior part of shoulder ■ Flattening of anterior aspect of shoulder	■ Patient in severe pain ■ Arm held in 180° elevation ■ Arm appears shorter compared to opposite side ■ Humeral head often felt along the lateral chest wall

HIGH-YIELD FACTS

Orthopedics

473

COMPLICATIONS SPECIFIC TO TYPE OF DISLOCATION

Anterior Dislocation
- Rotator cuff tear
- Glenoid labral lesions
- Coracoid fractures
- Greater tuberosity fractures (seems to decrease recurrence)
- Hill-Sachs deformity (compression fracture of the posterolateral humeral head)

Posterior Dislocation
- Fractures of the lesser tuberosity
- Fractures of posterior glenoid rim and proximal humerus humeral head)

Inferior Dislocation
- Rotator cuff tear
- Fractures of greater tuberosity

RADIOGRAPH

Anterior Dislocation
- Obtain anterior, posterior, and axillary views
- Look for Hill-Sachs deformity in the posterolateral portion of humeral head (occurs in 50%)

Posterior Dislocation
- Look for loss of the normal elliptical pattern produced by the overlap of humeral head and posterior glenoid rim
- Look for the greater tuberosity rotated internally

Inferior Dislocation
- Top of humerus is displaced downward

TREATMENT

Anterior Dislocation
- Reduction (Hennipen technique, Stimson technique, traction and countertraction and lateral traction)
- Immobilize shoulder
- Surgery if needed

Posterior Dislocation
- Apply longitudinal traction (Stimson technique)
- Surgery if needed, although neurovascular complications are rare

Inferior Dislocation
- Rotate arm inferiorly while applying traction longitudinally along the humerus with counter-traction in the supraclavicular region
- Surgical repair of rotator cuff

DEFINITION

A condition in which increased pressure within a limited space compromises the circulation and function of tissues within that closed space.

CAUSES

- Fractures.
- Soft tissue crush injuries.
- Vascular injuries.

- Drug overdose with prolonged limb compression.
- Burn injuries.
- Trauma.
- Muscle hypertrophy and nephrotic syndrome.

SIGNS AND SYMPTOMS

- Clinical presentation often indefinite and confusing.
- Hallmark finding: First sign in leg is paresthesia at the first web space (i.e., between great and second toes). Pain in a conscious and fully oriented person that is out of proportion to injury or findings.
- Pain: Deep, unremitting, and poorly localized. Pain increases with passive stretching of involved muscle.
- Pallor: Not necessary for diagnosis, may not be present.
- Paresthesias: Of cutaneous distribution supplied by the compressed nerve is an early sign.
- Paralysis: Occurs after ischemia is well established.
- Pulselessness: Shown to occur late at times. Pulse may be present.
- Compartment may get tense on palpation.

DIAGNOSIS

Measure pressure within compartment with commercially available monitors.

- Pressure < 30 mmHg usually will not produce a compartment syndrome.
- Pressure > 30 mmHg is an indication for fasciotomy.

TREATMENT

Complete fasciotomy: Goal is to decompress all tight compartments and salvage a viable extremity.

Do not delay treatment of compartment syndrome! Elevation of pressure to > 30 mmHg for > 8 hours leads to irreversible tissue death.

▶ OSTEOMYELITIS

Acute

PATHOPHYSIOLOGY

- Bacteria lodge in end artery of metaphysis and multiply.
- Local increase in serum and white blood cells (WBCs).
- Decrease in blood flow and pressure necrosis.
- Pus moves to haversian and medullary canals.
- Goes beneath the periosteum.

CAUSE

- Route of infection is mainly hematogenous, rarely trauma.
- Most cases of acute hematogenous osteomyelitis caused by *Staphylococcus aureus*.

SIGNS AND SYMPTOMS

- History of infection (e.g., skin or throat) or trauma.
- Significant pain in the affected area, anorexia, fever, irritability, nausea, malaise, rapid pulse.
- Limited joint motion, tenderness, swelling of soft tissue, and guarding apparent on physical exam.

Most common site for acute osteomyelitis is the metaphyseal end of a single long bone (especially around the knee).

DIAGNOSIS

- Elevated WBCs, erythrocyte sedimentation rate (ESR), and C-reactive protein; ± anemia.
- Deep circumferential soft-tissue swelling with obliteration of muscular planes.

DIFFERENTIAL DIAGNOSIS

- Septic arthritis: Swelling and tenderness directly on the joint with intense pain on joint movement, high WBC, and positive culture.
- Rheumatic fever: More insidious onset, less local and constitutional symptoms.
- Ewing's sarcoma: Early symptoms are more insidious and less intense and present with bone destruction.

TREATMENT

- **Medical:** Infection must be diagnosed early. Intravenous antibiotics (usually oxacillin or cloxacillin 8–16 g adult) started soon after obtaining specimen for culture. Monitor temperature, swelling, pain, WBC, and joint mobility.
- **Surgical:** Open drainage of abscess if antibiotics fail or signs of abscess appear. After surgical drainage, wound is left open to heal by secondary intention.

Chronic

EPIDEMIOLOGY

Often seen in lower extremities of a diabetic patient.

PATHOPHYSIOLOGY

- Untreated acute osteomyelitis results in a cavity walled off by an involucrum containing granulation tissue, sequestrum, and bacteria.
- Drainage of pus into surrounding soft tissue and skin via sinus tracts.
- Persistent drainage can lead to carcinoma.
- Bone fragments and exudates unreachable by antibiotics.
- Result is severely deformed bone and pathologic fracture.

CAUSE

- Usually an end result of untreated or treatment failed acute osteomyelitis. Occasionally due to trauma or surgery.
- Cause is usually polymicrobial—difficult to eradicate.

SIGNS AND SYMPTOMS

- Characterized by persistent drainage following an episode of acute osteomyelitis or onset of inflammation and cellulitis following an open fracture.
- Fever, pain, mild systemic symptoms, tenderness.
- Easy to diagnose when drainage is present and x-ray shows bone destruction and deformity. In cases with absence of drainage, radionuclide imaging studies are very helpful.

DIAGNOSIS

Radiographic findings:

- Areas of radiolucency within an irregular sclerotic bone.
- Irregular areas of destruction present. Often, periosteal thickening can be seen.

DIFFERENTIAL DIAGNOSIS

- Acute suppurative arthritis.
- Rheumatic fever: Examine synovial fluid.
- Cellulitis: Absence of soft tissue swelling on radiographs.

TREATMENT

- Varies from open drainage of abscess or sequestrectomy to amputation.
- Most effective: Extensive debridement of all necrotic and granulation tissue along with reconstruction of bone and soft tissue defects with concomitant antibiotics.
- Excellent adjunct: Temporary placement of polymethylmethacrylate beads in the wound for a depot administration of antibiotics.

COMPLICATIONS

- Soft tissue abscess.
- Septic arthritis due to extension to adjacent joint.
- Metastatic infections to other areas.
- Pathologic fractures.
- If significant spinal involvement, paraplegia.

▶ BRODIE'S ABSCESS

- Subacute pyogenic osteomyelitis in the metaphysis.
- Roentgenographic finding: Lucent lesions surrounded by sclerotic bone.
- Usually caused by *S. aureus* and *Staphylococcus albus*.

▶ SEPTIC BURSITIS

- Infection of the superficial bursa commonly affecting the bunion, olecranon, and prepatellar bursa.
- Most common offending organism is *S. aureus*.
- Clinically presents with painful bursal swelling, often along with intense cellulitis. Systemic signs of sepsis often present along with regional lymphadenopathy.
- Treatment: Aspirate bursa for culture and sensitivity. Give broad-spectrum antibiotic. Take care not to aspirate the joint since passing the needle through the area of cellulitis might spread it to the joint!

Low back pain is the leading cause of an orthopedic visit.

EPIDEMIOLOGY

- Four out of five people suffer from low back pain sometime in life.
- Incidence 15–20%, males > females.
- Most patients with low back pain have no systemic disorder.
- Often, back pain is a symptom of a systemic illness such as primary or metastatic neoplasm, infectious disease, or an inflammatory disorder.

HISTORY

- Very important, although often the only presenting complaint is pain that is poorly localized.
- Character of pain needs to be described: *What is the pain like? Does it radiate? When does it occur? How does it interfere with sitting, standing, walking? What factors make the pain better or worse? How many episodes have you had? Any other symptoms along with back pain?*
- Give patient a diagram and ask patient to mark areas of pain.
- History of pain development and how it affects everyday life.
- History of weight loss, malaise, fever, gastrointestinal (GI) or genitourinary (GU) illnesses.
- Psychological assessment in patients with chronic pain.

PHYSICAL EXAMINATION

- Straight leg-raising test: Positive in nerve root irritation.
- Check for reflexes and motor and sensory deficits.
- Check presence of nonorganic signs (Waddell's signs) when patient responds to axial loading, local touch, and simulated rotation.
- Check spine for range of motion.
- Bowel and bladder symptoms are suggestive of cauda equina syndrome.
- Leg and buttock pain are suggestive of herniated disk.

DIAGNOSIS

- X-rays of lumbar spine especially if patient is > 50 years of age and has history of other medical illnesses or trauma.
- Magnetic resonance imaging (MRI) of the lumbar spine if x-rays are negative: Great for assessing neural tissue.
- Computed tomography (CT) scan if MRI not helpful.
- Technetium bone scan and gallium scan can be done if an infection of the spine is suspected.

TREATMENT

- Rule out a serious pathologic condition.
- Goal is early return to normal activities.
- Patients with acute low back pain should avoid sitting or lifting and use mild analgesics and anti-inflammatory drugs.
- Physical and occupational therapy programs prove to be helpful.
- Antidepressants often help those with pain persistent for 3 months.
- Other questionable treatments: Transcutaneous electrical nerve stimulation (TENS), traction, manipulation with radicular signs, biofeedback, acupuncture, trigger point injections, and muscle relaxants.

HIGH-YIELD FACTS

Orthopedics

- Occur due to uncontrolled cellular proliferation of a single clone of cells whose regulatory mechanisms are defective.
- Benign tumors are 200 times more likely to occur than malignant ones.
- A careful history and physical is very crucial and will reveal the duration of the mass, onset of pain, other associated symptoms, and the chronological sequence of these symptoms.
- A thorough physical exam consists of evaluation of patient's general health status. The mass should be noted for size, location, consistency, mobility, tenderness, local temperature, and change with position. Note any muscular atrophy.

RADIOGRAPHY

- Never diagnose a bone tumor without an x-ray.
- Bone reacts to a benign or malignant tumor by bone production or destruction.
- An x-ray appearance shows a combination of bone production and bone destruction.
- Three patterns of x-ray appearance:
    - **Permeative:** Implies a rapidly spreading intramedullary tumor; tumor replaces marrow and fat.
    - **Moth eaten:** Implies a poorly circumscribed, slow-growing malignant tumor.
    - **Geographic:** Implies a well-circumscribed slow-growing tumor, therefore bone has time to react and results in sclerotic margins.

Benign Bone Tumors

Patient is usually asymptomatic, and the x-ray shows a well-defined lesion with sclerotic margins.

OSTEOID OSTEOMA

SIGNS AND SYMPTOMS

- Most common osteoid-forming benign tumor (10%).
- Male-to-female ratio is 2:1 to 3:1, three fourths of cases between ages 5 and 25.
- Most common sites: Diaphysis of long tubular bones, especially the proximal femur.
- Local tenderness and dull aching pain that is localizable, tends to be more severe at night and relieved by nonsteroidal anti-inflammatory drugs (NSAIDs).
- Pain can radiate and mimic other diseases (sciatica if present in vertebra).

RADIOGRAPHY

Localized area of bone sclerosis with a central radiolucent nidus. Little sclerosis seen if it is present in cancellous bone.

Emergency causes of low back pain: **FACTOID**
Fracture
Abdominal aortic aneurysm
Cauda equine syndrome
Tumor (cord compression)
Other (osteoarthriris [OA], severe musculoskeletal pain, other neurological syndromes)
Infection (e.g., epidural abscess)
Disk herniation/rupture

HIGH-YIELD FACTS

Orthopedics

HISTOLOGY

Usually measures < 1 cm. Circumscribed, highly vascular nidus made of fibroconnective tissue and woven bone.

TREATMENT AND PROGNOSIS

Mostly treated symptomatically with aspirin or NSAIDs. If this fails, surgical intervention to remove the nidus. Prognosis is excellent.

OSTEOBLASTOMA

EPIDEMIOLOGY

- One percent of benign bone tumors. Larger than osteoid osteomas.
- Male > female, most patients between ages 10 and 35 years.
- Most common sites: Mostly axial skeleton, less common in jaw, hands, and feet. One third to one half of cases are in the vertebral column.

SIGNS AND SYMPTOMS

Pain is the major complaint. Tenderness and swelling may be present over the lesion.

RADIOGRAPHY

Nonspecific x-ray findings, which may be interpreted as osteoid osteomas, aneurysmal bone cysts, or malignant tumors.

HISTOLOGY

Histologically similar to osteoid osteoma.

TREATMENT AND PROGNOSIS

- Vigorous curettement of the lesion. Prognosis is generally good except occasionally can become locally aggressive or recur locally if they are not adequately excised.
- Have potential to undergo malignant transformation and metastasize.

OSTEOCHONDROMA

- An outgrowth of bone capped by cartilage.
- Most common benign tumor of the bone (45%) with most patients in their first two decades of life.
- Usually solitary. Originates in childhood from growing epiphyseal cartilage plate. Mostly stage I lesions.
- Most common sites: Metaphysis of long bones of extremities; rarely in flat bones, vertebrae, or clavicle.

SIGNS AND SYMPTOMS

May be asymptomatic; patient may complain of pain, mass, or impingement syndromes.

RADIOGRAPHY

Shows a mushroom-like bony prominence.

HISTOLOGY

Trabecular, cancellous bone continuous with the marrow cavity and covered by hyaline cartilage cap.

Multiple hereditary osteochondroma is an autosomal dominant disorder in which multiple bones have osteochondromas (1% risk of malignant transformation).

TREATMENT AND PROGNOSIS

- Surgical excision if the patient complains of pain or if it enlarges after puberty.
- Rarely undergo malignant transformation to chondrosarcoma (< 1%).

ENCHONDROMA

- Neoplasm consisting of mature hyaline cartilage (chondroma).
- A centrally located chondroma. Can be single or multiple.
- Ten percent of benign tumors. Peak incidence in ages 20–50 years.
- Most common sites: Tubular bones of hands and feet.
- Chondromas can arise close to cortex or periosteum (ecchondroma) or in relation with synovium, tendons, or joints (synovial chondroma).
- Stage I or stage II lesions.

SIGNS AND SYMPTOMS

Asymptomatic until a pathologic fracture brings attention to it.

RADIOGRAPHY

Geographic lysis in a well-circumscribed area with spotty calcifications.

HISTOLOGY

Consists of hyaline cartilage often with active nuclei. Interpretation depends on size, location, and growth.

TREATMENT AND PROGNOSIS

No treatment if patient is asymptomatic. If pathologic fracture occurs, then allow fracture to heal. Perform a simple excision and bone grafting procedure.

GIANT CELL TUMOR

- Thought to arise from mesenchymal stromal cells supporting the bone marrow.
- Five to ten percent of benign bone tumors. Peak incidence in 30s.
- Female-to-male ratio is 3:2.
- Most common sites: Around the knee (distal femur, proximal tibia), distal radius, and sacrum.
- Mostly stage II or III lesions.

SIGNS AND SYMPTOMS

- Pain, swelling, and local tenderness; often presents with arthritis or joint effusions due to proximity to the joint.
- May also present with a pathologic fracture.

RADIOGRAPHY

- A radiolucent lesion occupying the epiphysis and extending into the metaphysis; asymmetrical with bone destruction.
- Occasional "soap bubble" appearance due to a thin subperiosteal bone shell.

HISTOLOGY

Abundant mononuclear stromal cells interspersed with a lot of giant cells with numerous nuclei.

Ollier's disease: Enchondromas in multiple bones. More likely for malignant transformation. Can result in bowing and shortening of long bones.

Factors that predispose to malignancy:
- Size (> 4.5 cm)
- Location (long and axial bones)
- Growth (active and painful)

TREATMENT AND PROGNOSIS

- Curettage and bone grafting (recurrence rate > 50%).
- Aggressive curettage with adjuvant phenol, hydrogen peroxide, or liquid nitrogen (recurrence rate 10–25%).
- Important to obtain chest x-ray every 6 months for 2–3 years for monitoring.
- Often recurs after incomplete removal.

Malignant Tumors

Metastatic tumors are much more common than primary tumors.

OSTEOSARCOMA

- Tumor made of a malignant spindle cell stroma producing osteoid.
- Many subtypes of osteoid forming sarcomas.
- Peak incidence in ages between 10 and 30 years, male > female.
- Most common sites: Around the knee (distal femur, proximal tibia), proximal humerus, rarely mandible.

Osteosarcoma can occur secondary to Paget's disease.

SIGNS AND SYMPTOMS

- Pain associated with a tender mass.
- Dilated veins may be visible on the skin over the mass.
- Constitutional symptoms may be present.

RADIOGRAPHY

- X-ray shows a poorly defined lesion in the metaphysis with areas of bone destruction and formation.
- Codman's triangle: Due to new bone formation under the corners of the raised periosteum.
- Sun-ray appearance: Occurs when the bone spicules are formed perpendicular to the surface of the bone.

HISTOLOGY

- Spindle-shaped tumors cells with odd, hyperchromatic nuclei showing a high mitotic rate. Giant cells may be present.
- High-dose methotrexate, doxorubicin, cisplatin, and ifosfamide along with surgical intervention.
- Tumors hematogenously metastasize to the lung.
- Surgery plus chemotherapy: Five-year survival is about 60%.
- Better prognosis if the tumor is in a small bone.

CHONDROSARCOMA

- Low-grade malignant tumor that derives from cartilage cells.
- Seven to twelve percent of primary bone tumors; male > female.
- Peak incidence between ages 30 and 60 years.
- Most common sites: Pelvis, femur, flat bones, proximal humerus, scapula, upper tibia, and fibula.

SIGNS AND SYMPTOMS

Pain and swelling over months or years.

RADIOGRAPHY

- Central chondrosarcomas show well-defined radiolucent areas with small, irregular calcifications to ill-defined areas breaking through the cortex.
- Peripheral chondrosarcomas look like large, lobulated masses hanging from the surface of a long bone with calcification.

HISTOLOGY

Varies from well-differentiated hyaline cartilage with little nuclear atypia to highly anaplastic spindle cell tumor with little cartilaginous differentiation.

TREATMENT AND PROGNOSIS

- Surgical resection of the tumor.
- Do not respond to radiation or chemotherapy.
- Prognosis better than osteosarcoma since chondrosarcoma grows slowly and metastasizes late.

EWING'S TUMOR

- Tumor of small round cells arising in the medullary cavity.
- Seven percent of primary bone tumors.
- Ninety percent of cases between ages 5 and 25 years; male > female.
- Most common sites: Diaphysis or metaphysis of long bones, pelvis, and scapula; potential to occur anywhere in the body.

SIGNS AND SYMPTOMS

- Pain that increases with time and is more severe at night.
- Local swelling and a tender mass.
- Malaise, fever, leukocytosis, mild anemia, increased ESR.
- Often mimic subacute osteomyelitis, syphlitic osteoperiostitis, or other tumors.

RADIOGRAPHY

- Shows lytic bone lesions with a permeative pattern.
- Elevations and permeations of the periosteum give rise to lamellated "onion skin" appearance.

HISTOLOGY

Area contains densely packed small round cells containing glycogen with little intercellular stroma arranged in sheets, cords, or nests.

TREATMENT AND PROGNOSIS

- Vincristine, cyclophosphamide, actinomycin D, and adriamycin along with surgery.
- Advanced metastatic disease: Five-year survival is 30%.
- Surgically resectable lesion treated with drugs and surgery has a 70% chance of 5-year survival.
- Males have worse prognosis.

MULTIPLE MYELOMA

- A malignant plasma cell tumor with multiple site involvement.
- Most common primary malignant tumor of the bone (45%).

Ewing's sarcoma is the most lethal of all bone tumors.

Ewing's sarcoma usually occurs after age 5. If patient < 5 years of age, think metastatic neuroblastoma instead.

- Ninety percent of cases in patients over the age of 40 years; male > female.
- Most common sites: Vertebral column, ribs, skull, pelvis, femur, clavicle and scapula; can occur anywhere in the body.

SIGNS AND SYMPTOMS

- Bone pain.
- Weight loss, weakness, neurologic impairment if pathologic fractures in the vertebrae present.
- Pathologic fractures or deformities.
- Susceptibility to infections.
- Amyloidosis.
- Kidney damage due to protein plugging of renal tubules.

LABS

- Increased serum calcium due to bone reabsorption.
- Elevated uric acid due to increased cell turnover.
- Monoclonal gammopathy, Bence Jones proteinuria, increased ESR, and rouleaux formation.
- Anemia due to marrow suppression.

RADIOGRAPHY

Classically shows sharply punched out lesions giving a soap-bubble appearance or often shows diffuse demineralization.

HISTOLOGY

Marrow aspirate shows larger-than-normal plasma cells with many nuclei, a nucleoli, and showing mitotic activity.

TREATMENT AND PROGNOSIS

- Chemotherapy with melphalan, often with prednisone.
- Bisphosphonates and other bone absorption–reducing agents help in reducing pathologic fractures.
- Untreated cases rarely survive more than 6–12 months.
- Chemotherapy induces remission in about 50–70% of cases.
- Poor prognosis with 90% of patients dying within 2–3 years.

Metastatic Tumors

- Metastatic tumors comprise 95% of all malignant bone tumors, primary bone tumors 5%.
- Spread via direct extension, lymphatics, vascular system, or intraspinal seeding.
- In children: Bone metastasis most likely from a neuroblastoma.
- Most common sites: Vertebral column, ribs, pelvis, upper ends of femur and humerus.

SIGNS AND SYMPTOMS

- Pain (most common symptom).
- Spine involvement: Neurologic symptoms due to pressure on nerve roots or spinal cord.
- Hypercalcemia and anemia.

Classic triad for multiple myeloma: **PAM**
"Punched out" lytic lesions
Atypical plasma cells
Monoclonal gammopathy

Two percent of myeloma cases will present with
POEMS:
Polyneuropathy
Organomegaly
Endocrinopathy
M-component spike
Skin changes/Sclerosis of bone

Most likely site of origin for metastatic tumors: **Breast, Lungs, Thyroid, Kidney, Prostate**

- Pathologic fractures are common.
- Increased acid phosphatase in prostatic metastasis.

DIAGNOSTIC WORKUP

- Order complete blood count (CBC), ESR, liver and renal panels, alkaline phosphatase, and serum protein electrophoresis.
- Plain CXR, x-ray of most commonly involved bones.
- Staging bone scan (more sensitive than x-ray).

RADIOGRAPHY

- Lesions may be multiple or solitary (kidney), well or poorly circumscribed, osteoblastic or osteolytic (majority).
- Osteoblastic: Breast and prostate.

HISTOLOGY

Generally, primary tumors produce matrix for the tumor stroma, whereas epithelial tumors form clusters in fibrous tissue.

TREATMENT AND PROGNOSIS

- Radiation as palliative treatment along with chemotherapy.
- Surgical intervention aims at relieving pain and prevents pathologic fractures.
- Radioactive iodine for thyroid carcinoma metastasis.
- Tamoxifen for metastatic carcinoma of the breast.
- Bilateral orchiectomy, estrogens, or antiandrogens for metastatic prostate tumors.
- Poor prognosis with average survival time being 19 months after suffering a pathologic fracture.

The Hand

Muscles

- Intrinsic muscles of the hand have their origin and insertion in the hand. See Table 28-1.
- Extrinsic muscles of the hand have their muscle bellies in the forearm and their tendon insertions in the hand. See Table 28-2.

Bones

- There are 27 bones in the hand: 5 metacarpals, 14 phalanges, and 8 carpals.
- Each finger has one metacarpal.
- Each finger or digit has three phalanges—proximal, middle, and distal.

TABLE 28-1. Intrinsic Muscles of the Hand

MUSCLE	INNERVATION	FUNCTION
Thenar Group		
Abductor pollicis brevis	Median	Abduction of thumb
Adductor pollicis brevis	Median	Adduction of thumb
Flexor pollicis brevis	Median	Flexes thumb MCP joint
Opponens pollicis	Ulnar (deep branch)	Opposes—pulls thumb medially and forward across palm
Remainder of Hand		
Palmar interossei	Ulnar	▪ Adduct finger toward center of third digit ▪ Flex MCP, extend PIP and DIP
Dorsal interossei	Ulnar	▪ Abduct finger from center of third digit ▪ Flex MCP, extend PIP and DIP
Lumbricals	First and second: Median Third and fourth: Ulnar (deep branch)	Flex MCP, extend PIP and DIP
Palmaris brevis	Ulnar (superficial branch)	Aids with hand grip
Hypothenar Group		
Abductor digiti minimi	Ulnar (deep branch)	Abducts little finger
Flexor digiti minimi	Ulnar (deep branch)	Flexes little finger
Opponens digiti minimi	Ulnar (deep branch)	Aids little finger with cupping motion of hand

TABLE 28-2. **Extrinsic Muscles of the Hand**

MUSCLE	COMPARTMENT	INNERVATION	FUNCTION
Flexor carpi radialis	Anterior	Median	Flexes and abducts hand at wrist
Palmaris longus	Anterior	Median	Flexes hand
Flexor carpi ulnaris (humeral and ulnar heads)	Anterior	Ulnar	Flexes and abducts hand at wrist
Flexor digitorum superficialis (humeroulnar and radial heads)	Anterior	Median	▪ Flexes middle phalanx ▪ Assists with flexion of proximal phalanx and hand
Flexor digitorum profundis	Anterior	Median and ulnar nerves	▪ Flexes distal phalanx ▪ Assists in flexion of middle and proximal phalanx and wrist
Extensor carpi radialis longus	Lateral	Radial	Extends and abducts hand at wrist
Extensor carpi radialis brevis	Posterior	Radial	Extends and abducts hand at wrist
Extensor digitorum	Posterior	Radial	Extends fingers and hand
Extensor digiti minimi	Posterior	Radial	Extends little finger MCP joint
Extensor carpi ulnaris	Posterior	Radial	Extends and adducts hand at wrist
Abductor pollicis longus	Posterior	Radial	Abducts and extends thumb
Extensor pollicis longus	Posterior	Radial	Extends distal phalanx of thumb
Extensor pollicis brevis	Posterior	Radial	Extends thumb MCP joint
Extensor indici	Posterior	Radial	Extends index finger MCP joint

- The thumb has only two phalanges—a proximal phalanx and a distal one.
- The joints between the phalanges are the metacarpophalangeal (MCP), proximal interphalangeal (PIP), and distal interphalangeal (DIP).
- The thumb has only MCP and DIP joints.
- Carpal bones (see Figure 28-1):
  - Scaphoid
  - Lunate
  - Triquetrum
  - Pisiform
  - Trapezium
  - Trapezoid
  - Capitate
  - Hamate

The wrist bones are easily remembered by the saying: **Some Lovers Try Positions That They Can't Handle.**

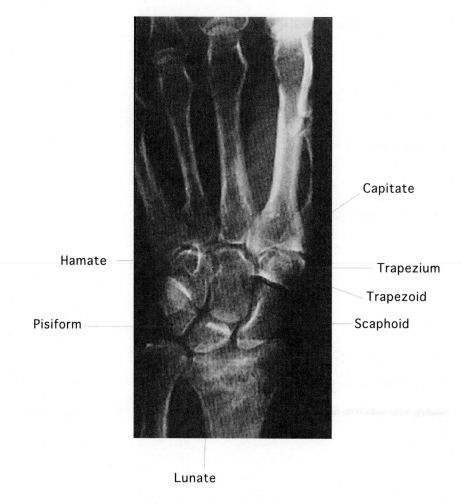

FIGURE 28-1. Bones of the wrist on AP radiograph.

The radial nerve does not innervate any of the intrinsic muscles of the hand. See Table 28-3 for clinical maneuvers to test function of the hand.

Nerves

- **Sensory:**
  - Radial: Sensory to lateral aspect of dorsum of hand and lateral 3.5 fingers.
  - Median: Sensory to skin on lateral half of palm.
  - Ulnar: Sensory to skin on medial aspect of dorsum of hand, hypothenar eminence, and medial 1.5 fingers.
- **Motor:** See Tables 28-1 and 28-2 for muscles innervated by the radial, median, and ulnar nerves.

Tendons

ZONES OF THE HAND

- Two main groups: Flexors and extensors.
- Extensor tendon lacerations can usually be repaired in the emergency department (ED).
- Flexor tendons are more difficult and usually require operative repair.

TABLE 28-3. Clinical Maneuvers for Testing Muscles of the Hand

PATIENT MANEUVER	MUSCLE TESTED
Making a fist	
Bending the tip of the thumb	Flexor pollicis longus
Bending each individual fingertip against resistance while PIPs are stabilized by examiner	Flexor digitorum profundus
Bending each individual fingertip against resistance while DIPs are stabilized by examiner	Flexor digitorum superficialis
Bring thumb out to side and back	Extensor pollicis brevis and abductor pollicis longus
Flexing and extending a fist at the wrist	Extensor carpi radialis longus and brevis
Raising thumb only while rest of hand is laid flat	Extensor pollicis longus
Making a fist with little finger extended alone	Extensor digiti minimi

- The flexor and extensor tendons are grouped into zones (see Figures 28-2 and 28-3).
- Flexor tendon injury repair timetable by zone:
  - Zones I and II: 1–3 weeks.
  - Zones III–V: Immediate.
  - Zone IV injuries are technically difficult because tendons lie within the carpal tunnel.
  - Zone V tendon injuries are relatively easy to fix, but functional outcome is often poor due to associated nerve injury.

▶ **HISTORY**

Focused hand history:
- Hand dominance.
- Time of injury.
- Status of tetanus immunization.
- Occupation.
- Cause and mechanism of injury.

A flexor tendon injury will present with a straight finger (unopposed extensors).

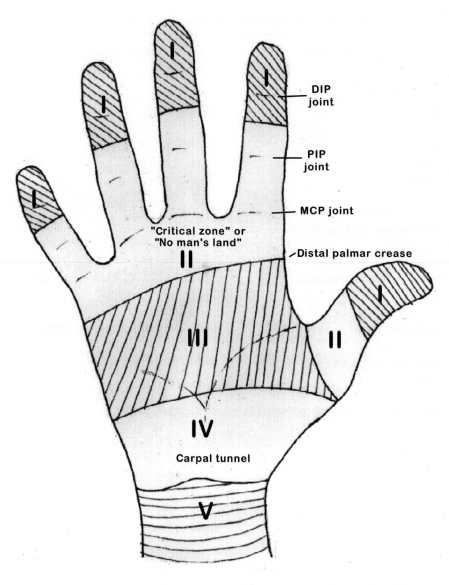

FIGURE 28-2. **Flexor tendon zones of the hand.**

(Artwork by Elizabeth N. Jacobson, Mayo Medical School.)

▶ **PHYSICAL EXAMINATION**

See Figure 28-4.

1. Sensibility:
   ■ Pinprick (two-point discrimination): Normal is < 6 mm when the points are static and < 3 mm when the points are moving. Abnormal values seen with underlying nerve injury.
   ■ Immersion test: Skin on palm of hand should wrinkle within 10 minutes when immersed in water. Failure to do so suggests underlying nerve injury.
2. Strength:
   ■ Test grip
   ■ Fromment's sign

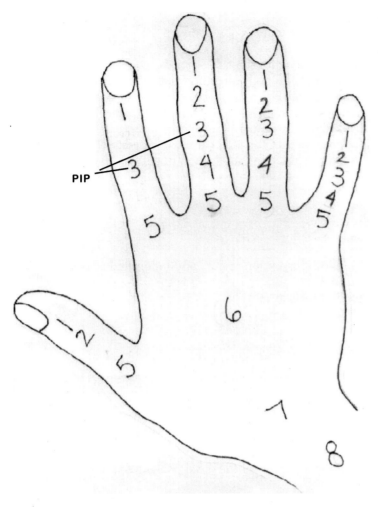

FIGURE 28-3. Extensor tendon zones of the hand.

(Artwork by Elizabeth N. Jacobson, Mayo Medical School.)

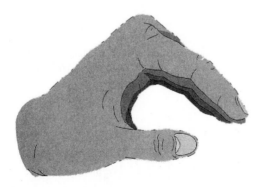

FIGURE 28-4. "Safe" position of hand.

Flexor zone II (also called "no man's land") is the worst place for a tendon laceration because the tendon must slide in a small tunnel, and much care at surgery, as well as a long rehabilitation period, is required to achieve a good functional outcome.

3. Vascular:
   - Capillary refill: Normal is < 2 seconds.
   - Allen test:
     - Patient makes a tight fist for 20 seconds.
     - Examiner occludes both ulnar and radial arteries by holding direct pressure.
     - Examiner releases ulnar artery—a normal (patent) ulnar artery will perfuse the hand within 5–7 seconds (color returns).
     - Test is repeated with the radial artery released to check ulnar flow.
4. Motor and sensory function: See section under Nerves for which nerves supply which muscles and sensory areas.

▶ NERVE BLOCKS

- Used to anesthesize a portion of the hand innervated by certain nerve(s) (see Figure 28-4).
- Advantages over local anesthesia:
  - Does not distort area you want to examine/suture.
  - Eliminates need for multiple injections.

▶ INFECTIONS OF THE HAND

Felon

DEFINITION

Infection of the pulp space of any of the distal phalanges (see Figure 28-5).

ETIOLOGY

Caused by minor trauma to the dermis over the finger pad.

COMPLICATIONS

Results in increased pressure within the septal compartments and may lead to cellulitis, flexor tendon sheath infection, or osteomyelitis if not effectively treated.

TREATMENT

- Using a digital block, perform incision and drainage (I&D) with longitudinal incision over the area of greatest induration but not over the flexor crease of the DIP.

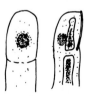

FIGURE 28-5. **Felon (infection of pulp space).**

(Reproduced, with permission, from LeBlond RF, DeGowin RL, Brown DD. *DeGowin's Diagnostic Examination*, 8th ed. New York: McGraw-Hill, 2004: 729.)

- Drain may be placed and wound checked in 2 days.
- Antibiotics: Usually first-generation cephalosporin or anti-*Staphylococcus* penicillin.

Paronychia

DEFINITION

Infection of the lateral nail fold (see Figure 28-6).

ETIOLOGY

Caused by minor trauma such as nail biting or manicures.

TREATMENT

- Without fluctuance, this may be treated with a 7-day course of antibiotics, warm soaks, and retraction of the skin edges from the nail margin.
- For more extensive infections, unroll the skin at the base of the nail and at the lateral nail or I&D at area of most fluctuance using a digital block. Pus below the nail bed may require partial or total removal of the nail. Warm soaks and wound check in 2 days. Antibiotics are usually not necessary unless area is cellulitic.

Tenosynovitis

ETIOLOGY

This is a surgical emergency requiring prompt identification. Infection of the flexor tendon and sheath is caused by penetrating trauma and dirty wounds (e.g., dog bite). Infection spreads along the tendon sheath, allowing involvement of other digits and even the entire hand, causing significant disability.

ORGANISMS

- Polymicrobial.
- *Staphylococcus* most common.
- *Neisseria gonorrhoeae* with history of sexually transmitted disease (STD).

TREATMENT

- Immobilize and elevate hand.
- Immediate consultation with hand surgeon.
- Parenteral antibiotics; first-generation cephalosporin and penicillin, or β-lactamase inhibitor.

Kanavel signs of tenosynovitis: STEP
Symmetrical swelling of finger.
Tenderness over flexor tendon sheath.
Extension (passive) of digit is painful.
Posture of digit at rest is flexed.

FIGURE 28-6. Paronychia.

(Reproduced, with permission, from LeBlond RF, DeGowin RL, Brown DD. *DeGowin's Diagnostic Examination*, 8th ed. New York: McGraw-Hill, 2004: 729.)

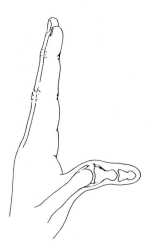

FIGURE 28-7. Gamekeeper's thumb.

(Reproduced, with permission, from Scaletta TA et al. *Emergent Management of Trauma.* New York: McGraw-Hill, 1996: 220.)

Gamekeeper's thumb is commonly associated with ski pole injury (see Figure 28-7).

► **GAMEKEEPER'S THUMB**

DEFINITION

Avulsion of ulnar collateral ligament of first MCP joint.

ETIOLOGY

- Forced abduction of the thumb.
- Can be associated with an avulsion fracture of the metacarpal base.

SIGNS AND SYMPTOMS

Inability to pinch.

DIAGNOSIS

Application of valgus stress to thumb while MCP joint is flexed will demonstrate laxity of ulnar collateral ligament.

TREATMENT

- Rest, ice, elevation, analgesia.
- Thumb spica cast for 3–6 weeks for partial tears.
- Surgical repair for complete tears.

Carpal tunnel syndrome is the most common entrapment neuropathy.

► **CARPAL TUNNEL SYNDROME**

DEFINITION

Compression of the median nerve resulting in pain along the distribution of the nerve (see Figure 28-8).

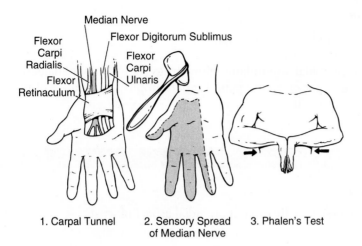

1. Carpal Tunnel   2. Sensory Spread   3. Phalen's Test
                      of Median Nerve

FIGURE 28-8. Carpal tunnel syndrome.

(Reproduced, with permission, from LeBlond RF, DeGowin RL, Brown DD. *DeGowin's Diagnostic Examination*, 8th ed. New York: McGraw-Hill, 2004: 736.)

ETIOLOGY

- Idiopathic/overuse (most common).
- Tumor (fibroma, lipoma).
- Ganglion cyst.
- Tenosynovitis of flexor tendons secondary to rheumatoid arthritis or trauma.
- Edema due to pregnancy, thyroid or amyloid disease.
- Trauma to carpal bones.
- Gout.

RISK FACTORS

Repetitive hand movements.

EPIDEMIOLOGY

More common in women 3:1.

SIGNS AND SYMPTOMS

- Pain and paresthesia of volar aspect of thumb, digits 2 and 3, and half of digit 4.
- Activity and palmar flexion aggravate symptoms.
- Thenar atrophy: Uncommon but irreversible and indicates severe long-standing compression.
- Sensory deficit (two-point discrimination > 5 mm).

DIAGNOSIS

- Tinel's test: Tapping over median nerve at wrist produces pain and paresthesia.
- One minute of maximal palmar flexion produces pain and paresthesia.
- Consider erythrocyte sedimentation rate (ESR), thyroid function tests (TFTs), serum glucose, and uric acid level to look for underlying cause.

Typical scenario: A 37-year-old female presents with pain in her right wrist and fingers, accompanied by a tingling sensation. The pain awakens her from sleep, and she is unable to perform her duties as a word processor. *Think:* Carpal tunnel syndrome.

TREATMENT

- Treat underlying condition.
- Rest and splint.
- Nonsteroidal anti-inflammatory drugs (NSAIDs) for analgesia.
- Surgery for crippling pain, thenar atrophy, and failure of nonoperative management.

▶ GANGLION CYST

DEFINITION

A synovial cyst, usually present on radial aspect of wrist.

ETIOLOGY

Idiopathic.

SIGNS AND SYMPTOMS

- Presence of mass that patient cannot account for.
- May or may not be painful.
- Pain aggravated by extreme flexion or extension.
- Size of ganglia increases with increased use of wrist.
- Compression of median or ulnar nerve may occur (not common).

DIAGNOSIS

Radiographs to ascertain diagnosis; since a ganglion cyst is a soft tissue problem only, no radiographic changes should be noted.

TREATMENT

- Reassurance for most cases.
- Wrist immobilization for moderate pain.
- Aspiration of cyst for severe pain.
- Surgical excision for cases involving median nerve compression and cosmetically unacceptable ganglia.

▶ MALLET FINGER

DEFINITION

Rupture of extensor tendon at its insertion into base of distal phalanx (see Figure 28-9).

ETIOLOGY

- Avulsion fracture of distal phalanx.
- Other trauma.

SIGNS AND SYMPTOMS

Inability to extend DIP joint.

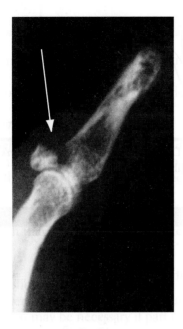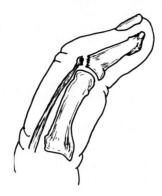

FIGURE 28-9. Mallet finger.

(Reproduced, with permission, from Schwartz DT, Reisdorf EJ. *Emergency Radiology*. New York: McGraw-Hill, 2000: 40.)

TREATMENT

- Splint finger in extension for 6–8 weeks.
- Surgery may be required for large avulsions of distal phalanx and for injuries that were not splinted early.

▶ TRIGGER FINGER

DEFINITION

Stenosis of flexor digitorum, tendon sheath leading to nodule formation within the sheath (see Figure 28-10).

RISK FACTORS

- Rheumatoid arthritis
- Middle-aged women
- Congenital

SIGNS AND SYMPTOMS

Snapping sensation or click when flexing and extending the digit.

TREATMENT

- Splinting of MP joint in extension.
- Injection of corticosteroid into tendon sheath.
- Surgical repair if above fail.

TABLE 28-4. Common Hand and Wrist Injuries (continued)

INJURY	DESCRIPTION	TREATMENT

Colles' fracture	▪ Distal radius fracture with dorsal angulation
	▪ Most commonly caused by fall on outstretched hand
	▪ "Dinner fork deformity" is classic
		▪ Short arm cast for 4–6 weeks with volar flexion and ulnar deviation
		▪ Surgical repair for:
		  ▪ Open fracture
		  ▪ Comminuted fracture
		  ▪ Intra-articular displacement > 2 mm

Smith fracture	▪ Distal radius fracture with volar angulation ▪ Most commonly caused by direct trauma to dorsal forearm	Surgical repair needed for most cases
Galeazzi fracture	▪ Distal one third radial fracture with dislocation of distal radioulnar joint ▪ Commonly caused by fall on outstretched hand with forearm in forced pronation or direct blow to back of wrist	Surgical repair needed for most cases
Monteggia fracture	▪ Proximal one third ulnar fracture with dislocation of the radial head ▪ Commonly caused by fall on outstretched hand with forearm in forced pronation or direct blow to posterior ulna ▪ May note injury of radial nerve	▪ Surgical repair for adults ▪ Closed reduction for children (children can tolerate a greater degree of displacement)

Nightstick fracture	▪ Isolated fracture of the ulnar shaft	▪ Long arm cast for 3–6 weeks
		▪ Surgical repair for:
		  ▪ Angulation > 10°
		  ▪ Displacement > 50%

Classified: Awards and Opportunities

American Association for the Surgery of Trauma

AAST provides medical student scholarships to attend the annual meeting. You may be sponsored by a member of the AAST to attend next year's annual meeting. You would be required to send a letter of recommendation by a member of the AAST for approval by the AAST Board of Managers. Once approved, your registration fee and banquet fee will be waived. The AAST will also cover the cost of your hotel room. In addition, you will be provided with an approximately $75 stipend for food/miscellaneous items. You/your institution are responsible for your travel arrangements. Contact the AAST for the deadline for medical student scholarship applications (CV and letter of recommendation from an AAST member), generally June of each year. For consideration, medical students should send their letters of recommendation and curriculum vitae (CV) to:

Robert C. Mackersie, MD
Trauma/Critical Care
UCSF-San Francisco General Hospital
1001 Potrero Avenue, Ward 3A
San Francisco, CA 94110
Phone: (415) 206-4622
Fax: (415) 206-5484
E-mail: rmackersie@sfghsurg.ucsf.edu

New York Academy of Medicine—Ferdinand C. Valentine Student Research Grants in Urology

Eligibility: Open to medical students who plan to conduct a New York–based research project in urology

Application Deadline/Start Date: Generally each February

Additional Information: www.nyam.org/

Oregon Health and Science University—Campagna Scholarship in Neurological Surgery

Eligibility: Open to students who have completed their M1 or M2 year who are interested in participating in a mentored neurosurgical research project in Portland, Oregon.

Application Deadline/Start Date: Generally each February

Additional Information: www.ohsu.edu/ohsuedu/academic/som/neurosurgery/news-and-events/campagna-scholarship.cfm

Society for Clinical and Vascular Surgery—Peter B. Samuels Essay Award Competition

Open to students, residents, and fellows in a university, affiliated hospital, or in a surgical or vascular surgical residency in the United States or Canada. Submissions must be original papers on a subject related to vascular surgery that have not been previously published or presented. Abstracts may be based on either experimental or clinical observations or it may be analytical, based on analysis and review of previous published data on the anatomy, physiology, pathology, biochemistry, or genetics of the vascular system and its disease.

Finalists for this award will be notified and must submit seven copies of the manuscript to the Society's office before the deadline specified for the annual symposium. The 2009 award was $1,000 cash prize, plus round-trip coach airfare reimbursement and 3 nights' hotel accommodations.

Society for Clinical and Vascular Surgery—Allastair Karmody Poster Competition

First-round winners will each receive a cash award ($500 in 2009). The Karmody Poster Competition winner will receive an additional cash award.

- The competition is limited to fellows, residents, and medical students.
- All abstracts accepted for poster presentation will be considered. No additional field needs to be marked during the abstract submission process.
- Submissions must be original papers on a subject related to vascular surgery that have not been previously publishd or presented.
- Abstracts may be based on either experimental or clinical observations, or they may be analytical, based on analysis and review of previously published data on the anatomy, physiology, pathology, biochemistry, or genetics of the vascular system and its disease.

Roswell Park Cancer Institute—Summer Oncology Research Program

Expand your horizons in the care and treatment of the cancer patient by participating in state-of-the-art clinical research. Explore the mysteries of the cancer cell by participating in a basic scientific research program. Or participate in both! Special emphasis is placed on cancer prevention through lectures and practical experiences. The Roswell Park program provides competitive stipend support (projected at $350 per week) for students in the health professions (medicine, dentistry, osteopathy) to engage in clinical and/or basic scientific research for an 8-week period. Some funding is available to defray costs of room. The program runs from early June through the end of July (contact Roswell Park directly for specifics); however, dates of participation may be changed to accommodate your academic schedule. **Applications:** Generally due in February of each year

Additional Information:
Arthur M. Michalek, PhD, FACE
Senior Vice President
Department of Educational Affairs
Roswell Park Cancer Institute
Carlton and Elm Streets
Buffalo, NY 14263
Phone: (716) 845-2339
E-mail: arthur.michalek@roswellpark.org

University of Texas M. D. Anderson Cancer Center—Medical Student Summer Research Program in Biomedical Sciences

Research educational appointments for college students at the University of Texas M. D. Anderson Cancer Center provide firsthand experience in the areas of cancer research and insight into the varied career opportunities available in the biomedical sciences. To qualify for a college student research appointment, the applicant must be classified as a college freshman, sophomore, junior, or nongraduate senior at the time of appointment. The applicant should be pursuing a career in sciences and have a transcript that demonstrates a record of academic achievement. The appointment policy limits an individual to a 1-year appointment, which may be renewed upon the recommendation of the faculty mentor. College students seeking individual appointments should contact the faculty members or department administrators in the departments of interest to obtain information about available positions and the eligibility requirements of each program.

SIGN AAN Neurology Medical Student Programs

The Student Interest Group in Neurology (SIGN) program is a network of more than 150 chapters in medical schools across the United States and Canada. SIGN fosters medical student interest in neurology by providing opportunities to participate in clinical, research, and service activities in neurology, increasing the student's neurologic knowledge, and creating an interest in the AAN.

Free SIGN membership will enable you to:
- Socialize with students, residents, and faculty who share your interest in neurology
- Shadow neurologists
- Attend patient presentations and seminars
- Develop experience, leadership, and valuable contacts
- Join the nationwide SIGN network
- Meet other SIGN members at the Annual Meeting

Apply for SIGN scholarships:
- $3,000 Summer Research Scholarship
- $1,000 AAN Annual Meeting Scholarship

www.aan.com/go/education/awards

Medical Student Summer Research Scholarship in Neurology

Application Deadline: Generally each February

Sponsored by the AAN's Undergraduate Education Subcommittee, the Medical Student Summer Research Scholarship program offers members of the AAN's Student Interest Group in Neurology (SIGN) program a summer stipend of approximately $3,000 to conduct a project in either an institutional, clinical or laboratory setting where there are ongoing programs of research, service or training, or a private practice. Only applicants from schools with established SIGN chapters are eligible to apply. The project is to be conducted through a U.S. or Canadian institution of the student's choice and jointly designed by the student and sponsoring institution. More than one student from an institution may apply, but only one student will be selected from an institution. The scholarship program was established to stimulate individuals to pursue careers in neurology in either research or practice settings.

The AAN will award up to twenty $3,000 scholarships to first or second-year AAN medical student members who have a supporting preceptor and a project with clearly defined goals. Third-year AAN medical student members who are on an official summer break will also be considered with accompanying documentation. One graduating medical student from each institution is eligible to receive the award.

The project is to be conducted through a U.S. or Canadian institution of the student's choice and jointly designed by the student and sponsoring institution. Only applicants from schools with established SIGN chapters are eligible to apply. More than one student from an institution may apply, but only one student will be selected from an institution.

Applicants must be AAN medical student members at the time of application submission.

AAN Medical Student Prize for Excellence in Neurology

Application Deadline: Generally each February

This award recognizes excellence in clinical neurology among graduating medical students. Only one medical student per institution should be nominated for the Medical Student Prize for Excellence. Awarded annually to a graduating medical student who exemplifies outstanding scientific achievement and clinical acumen in neurology or neuroscience, and outstanding personal qualities of integrity, compassion, and leadership. A Certificate of Recognition and a check for $200 will be presented on behalf of the AAN during the graduation or awards ceremony at each institution.

Application Procedure: Each department chair will designate a faculty committee that will select the award winner. The award winner will be selected based on outstanding performance in the neurology clerkship and outstanding personal and professional qualities, as noted in the award description.

Preference should be given to students choosing neurology as a career.

Submit material to calementi@aan.com, fax to (651) 361-4837 or mail to:

Medical Student Prize for Excellence in Neurology
Cheryl Alementi
American Academy of Neurology
1080 Montreal Avenue
St. Paul, MN 55116

Application Deadline: The deadline to nominate a medical student for the Medical Student Prize for Excellence is generally in February of each year.

Medical Student Essay Award—Roland P. Mackay Award

This award seeks to stimulate interest in the field of neurology as an exciting and challenging profession by offering highly competitive awards for the best essay. Essays are judged on the basis of the quality of the scholarship and on suitability for an audience of general neurologists.

This award is given for the best essay in historical aspects.

Presentation: Recipients are expected to give a poster presentation based on the selected manuscript at the AAN Annual Meeting.

Recipient will receive:
- Certificate of Recognition and $350 prize
- Complimentary registration for 61st Annual Meeting
- One-year complimentary subscription to *Neurology* journal
- Reimbursement for 61st Annual Meeting travel, lodging, and meal expenses (up to 2 days)
- Recognition at Awards Luncheon at Annual Meeting

Eligibility:
- Must be enrolled and in good standing in an accredited medical school in North America
- Must submit an original, lucid essay targeted to general neurologists (essay cannot be a previously published manuscript for Mackay)
- Must have spent less than 1 year on a project leading to the submitted essay

Applicants should submit one complete set of the following materials:
- Completed application form
- Essay using the following guidelines (essays will not be returned):
  - Must be typed, double-spaced using a standard font
  - Maximum length of 30 pages
  - Only deceased persons may be subjects of biographical papers
  - Letter attesting to eligibility criteria and identifying award category
  - Maximum 200-word abstract
  - Letter from a faculty sponsor detailing the extent of technical or financial support received, the student's individual contribution to the project, and verifying that the student is the sole author of the essay

For more information, please contact Kyle Krause at kkrause@aan.com or (651) 695-2733.

Michael S. Pessin Stroke Leadership Prize

Sponsored by the AAN and endowed by Dr. Pessin's family, friends, and colleagues, this award recognizes emerging neurologists who have a strong interest in and have demonstrated a passion for learning and expanding the field of stroke research. Applicants should have an active involvement in providing patients with the highest quality of compassionate care. This award is intended to stimulate and reward individuals in the developmental stages of their careers, who demonstrate a passion for stroke.

Presentation: Recipient is expected to give a 10-minute presentation on a topic of their choice during a scientific session at the AAN Annual Meeting.

Recipient will receive:
- Certificate of Recognition and $1,500 prize
- Complimentary registration for Annual Meeting
- Recognition at Awards Luncheon at Annual Meeting

Eligibility:
- Must be a medical student, resident, fellow, or junior faculty member involved in or considering a career in neurology, emphasizing the care of stroke patients
- Must be no more than 5 years from completion of most recent training program and no higher academic rank than assistant professor
- Additional consideration will be given to those involved in clinical research aimed at enhancing the understanding of stroke or improving acute treatment protocols

Application Procedure: Applicants should submit one complete set of the following materials:
- Completed application form
- Current curriculum vitae

For more information, please contact Franziska Schwarz at fschwarz@aan.com or (651) 695-2807.

Medical Student Essay Award–Extended Neuroscience Award

This award seeks to stimulate interest in the field of neurology as an exciting and challenging profession by offering highly competitive awards for the best essay. Essays are judged on the basis of the quality of the scholarship and on suitability for an audience of general neurologists.

This award is given for the best essay in Neuroscience.

Presentation: Recipients are expected to give a poster presentation based on the selected manuscript at the AAN Annual Meeting.

Recipient will receive:
- $1,000 prize
- Complimentary registration for Annual Meeting
- One-year complimentary subscription to *Neurology* journal
- Reimbursement for Annual Meeting travel, lodging, and meal expenses (up to 2 days)
- Recognition at Awards Luncheon at Annual Meeting

Eligibility:
- Must be enrolled and in good standing in an accredited medical school in North America
- Must submit an original, lucid essay targeted to general neurologists
- Must have spent more than one year on a project leading to the submitted essay

Applicants should submit one complete set of the following materials:
- Completed application form
- Essay using the following guidelines (essays will not be returned):
  - Must be typed, double-spaced using a standard font
  - Maximum length of 30 pages
  - Only deceased persons may be subjects of biographical papers
  - Letter attesting to eligibility criteria and identifying award category
  - Maximum 200-word abstract
  - Letter from a faculty sponsor detailing the extent of technical or financial support received, the student's individual contribution to the project, and verifying that the student is the sole author of the essay

For more information, please contact Kyle Krause at kkrause@aan.com or (651) 695-2733.

Medical Student Essay Award–G. Milton Shy Award

This award seeks to stimulate interest in the field of neurology as an exciting and challenging profession by offering highly competitive awards for the best essay. Essays are judged on the basis of the quality of the scholarship and on suitability for an audience of general neurologists.

This award is given for the best essay in clinical neurology.

Presentation: Recipients are expected to give a poster presentation based on the selected manuscript at the AAN Annual Meeting.

Recipient will receive:
- Certificate of Recognition and $350 prize
- Complimentary registration for Annual Meeting
- One-year complimentary subscription to *Neurology* journal

- Reimbursement for Annual Meeting travel, lodging, and meal expenses (up to 2 days)
- Recognition at Awards Luncheon at Annual Meeting

Eligibility:
- Must be enrolled and in good standing in an accredited medical school in North America
- Must submit an original, lucid essay targeted to general neurologists (essay cannot be a previously published manuscript for Shy)
- Must have spent less than 1 year on a project leading to the submitted essay

Applicants should submit one complete set of the following materials:
- Completed application form
- Essay using the following guidelines (essays will not be returned):
  - Must be typed, double-spaced using a standard font
  - Maximum length of 30 pages
  - Only deceased persons may be subjects of biographical papers
  - Letter attesting to eligibility criteria and identifying award category
  - Maximum 200-word abstract
  - Letter from a faculty sponsor detailing the extent of technical or financial support received, the student's individual contribution to the project, and verifying that the student is the sole author of the essay

For more information, please contact Kyle Krause at kkrause@aan.com or (651) 695-2733.

Medical Student Essay Award—Saul R. Korey Award

This award seeks to stimulate interest in the field of neurology as an exciting and challenging profession by offering highly competitive awards for the best essay. Essays are judged on the basis of the quality of the scholarship and on suitability for an audience of general neurologists.

This award is given for the best essay in experimental neurology.

Presentation: Recipients are expected to give a poster presentation based on the selected manuscript at the AAN Annual Meeting.

Recipient will receive:
- Certificate of Recognition and $350 prize
- Complimentary registration for Annual Meeting
- One-year complimentary subscription to *Neurology* journal
- Reimbursement for Annual Meeting travel, lodging, and meal expenses (up to 2 days)
- Recognition at Awards Luncheon at Annual Meeting

Eligibility:
- Must be enrolled and in good standing in an accredited medical school in North America
- Must submit an original, lucid essay targeted to general neurologists (essay cannot be a previously published manuscript for Korey)
- Must have spent less than 1 year on a project leading to the submitted essay

Application Procedure: Applicants should submit one complete set of the following materials:
- Completed application form
- Essay using the following guidelines (essays will not be returned):

510

- Must be typed, double-spaced using a standard font
- Maximum length of 30 pages
- Only deceased persons may be subjects of biographical papers
- Letter attesting to eligibility criteria and identifying award category
- Maximum 200-word abstract
- Letter from a faculty sponsor detailing the extent of technical or financial support received, the student's individual contribution to the project, and verifying that the student is the sole author of the essay

For more information, please contact Kyle Krause at kkrause@aan.com or (651) 695-2733.

University of California at Davis Ophthalmology Summer Fellowship

Department will offer summer fellowship stipend of $2,000 for expenses and supplies for a medical student to pursue a research project. Students first must find a project and a mentor for the summer project. Then the student will need to write up the project proposal with a budget and submit it to the Department of Ophthalmology Research Committee. The committee will award the stipends based on the quality of the submitted proposal.

Additional funding besides a summer stipend for medical student research is available. Students first must find a project and a mentor for the project. Then the student will need to write up the project proposal with a budget and submit it to the Department of Ophthalmology Research Committee. The committee will award the stipends based on the quality of the submitted proposal.

The projects are of two types:

1. (Short Projects) These projects should be completed in a relatively short time frame (e.g., 2 to 3 months). A student could start it on a 4- to 8-week rotation and then write the project up at a later time. The type of projects that would be appropriate might be:
   a. Case reports
   b. Chart reviews on particular projects asking a limited and specific question

2. (Long Projects) These projects would be more long-range projects that would take 6 to 12 months. The student would be taking off from medical school to do the project.
   a. The projects may be prospective clinical projects with a well-defined question, mentor, research plan, and budget with funding defined.
   b. The project may be a laboratory project with a well-defined question, mentor, research plan, and budget with funding defined.

Web site: www.ucdmc.ucdavis.edu

Harvard-Longwood Research training in Vascular Surgery Summer Research Fellowships in Vascular Surgery:

- This experience is supported by the William J. von Liebig Summer Research Fellowship program.
- Four student research fellowships available starting (generally) on June 1.

- Program runs 10–12 weeks over the summer, with research training in molecular and cell biology, coagulation and thrombosis, atherogenesis, intimal hyperplasia, prosthetic/host interactions, and thrombosis.
- Trainees will pursue a program of intense research activity, which will be carried out under the guidance of a selected faculty advisor based at one of four Harvard Medical School hospitals.
- Applicants should have a minimum of 1 year of medical school at an LCME accredited school.
- Student will receive a $5,000 stipend for the summer.
- Application deadline is generally January.

For more information, contact:

Leena Pradhan, PhD
William J. von Liebig Summer Research Fellowship
Harvard Institutes of Medicine
4 Blackfan Circle, Room 130
Boston, MA 02115
Phone: (617) 667-0096
Fax: (617) 975-5300
E-mail: lpradhan@bidmc.harvard.edu

NYU Hospital for Joint Diseases Department of Orthopaedics (Year-Long Fellowship)

- One-year fellowship for medical students interested in pursuing a career in orthopaedics.
- The program is centrally located at the Hospital for Joint Diseases and Bellvue Medical Center with some travel to Jamaica Hospital in Queens, New York.
- Responsibilities will include participation in ongoing studies, maintenance of the Orthopaedic Trauma Service database, and submission of IRB protocols.
- Applicants should be in medical school or a recent graduate.
- A monthly stipend is given to help offset the cost of New York City housing, which is not provided.
- For more information, go to: www.med.nyu.edu/orthosurgery/research/opp.html

For more information, please contact:
Kenneth Egol
E-mail: kenneth-egol@nyumc.org

American Otological Society Medical Student Research Training Fellowships

Purpose: To further the study otosclerosis, Méniére's disease, and related ear disorders.

The American Otologic Society, Inc., through its Research Fund, is offering Research Grant Awards and full time Research Training Fellowships to study otosclerosis, Méniére's disease, and related ear disorders in United States or Canadian institutions only. Proposals may include investigation of the management and pathogenesis of these disorders, and underlying processes.

Research Training Fellowship: For physicians only (residents and medical students), fellowship will support 1–2 years' full-time research conducted outside of residency training; $35,000 for stipend, $5,000 for supplies (and up to 10% indirect costs).

Applications must be accompanied by sponsoring institution documentation stating that facilities and faculty are appropriate for requested research. Research conducted during the Research Training Fellowship can be on any topic related to ear disorders.

Deadline: Grant and fellowship applications must be postmarked by January 31.

Information and materials may be obtained from www.americanotologicalso ciety.org/forms.html or by contacting:

Lloyd B. Minor, MD, Executive Secretary
Research Fund of the American Otological Society, Inc.
Johns Hopkins University, School of Medicine
Department of Otolaryngology–Head & Neck Surgery
601 N. Caroline Street, JHOC 6210
Baltimore, MD 21287-0910
Phone: (410) 955-1080
Fax: (410) 955-6526
E-mail: lminor2@jhmi.edu

The NYU Urology Summer Fellowship

This is an 8-week opportunity for two students between their first and second years of medical school to learn more about this exciting and diverse surgical subspecialty. This summer experience will allow students to spend time in the operating room observing procedures in urologic oncology, female and male incontinence, infertility, erectile dysfunction, stone disease, and pediatric urology. Students will also spend time in the clinic observing urological outpatient procedures and office visits with patients before and after surgery. Summer fellows will attend teaching conferences and journal clubs run by faculty and residents.

To round out this exciting summer experience, students will be assigned to work with one of the Urology attending physicians on a clinical research project. For highly motivated students, this is a great opportunity to take a project from the start and create abstracts and manuscripts eligible for submission to national conferences and peer-reviewed journals for publication. Students will have the opportunity and are strongly encouraged to continue this research following completion of the summer fellowship. Finally, at the end of the fellowship, students will give a short oral presentation to the Department of Urology on a topic to be decided. This summer program will provide students with great exposure to this surgical subspecialty and research opportunities that can lead to medical conference presentations and publications.

Eligibility and Salary: Students must be between their first and second years of medical school to apply.

A stipend of $800 is provided. In addition to the stipend, students may receive additional funds in the amount of $2,100 through the NYU School of Medicine Office of Financial Aid if they qualify for work study. However, work-study eligibility is not required to apply.

How to Apply: Please forward a one-page cover letter addressed to Dr. William Huang, Director of the Urology Summer Fellowship, describing your interest in the fellowship, along with your resume, to Sabine Gay, program coordinator, at Sabine.Gay@nyumc.org. For further information, call (646) 825-6310.

Application Deadline and Important Dates: Students must submit applications by February 15 for the upcoming summer.

Notification of acceptance into this program will be in mid-March. The fellowship program runs from mid-June to early August.

The William J. von Leibig Summer Research Fellowship in Vascular Surgery at Harvard Medical School

Available June 1. Four medical student research fellowships are available for 10–12 weeks of summer research training in molecular and cell biology, biomechanics, coagulation and thrombosis, and angiogenesis, with a focus on clinically relevant problems such as atherogenesis, intimal hyperplasia, prosthetic/host interactions, and thrombosis. Trainees will pursue a program of intense research activity. This training program is designed to provide medical students an initial exposure to vascular surgery research.

Students will carry out their research projects under the guidance of a faculty advisor, selected form renowned vascular researchers based at four Harvard Medical School hospitals: Beth Israel Deaconess Medical Center, Brigham and Women's Hospital, Children's Hospital (Boston), and the Joslin Diabetes Institute, as well as the Massachusetts Institute of Technology.

Selection of trainees is based on candidates' demonstrated ability. Applicants should be medical students who have completed at least 1 year of study at an LCME accredited school. Students must be U.S. citizens or permanent residents (green card holders).

Interested applicants are encouraged to submit a personal statement, together with a curriculum vitae, dean/advisor or program director's letter, and two letters of recommendation. Selection is based on merit only, without bias to gender, race, color, or ethnic origin.

Support: A $5,000 stipend for the summer and appointment at Harvard Medical School as a Research Fellow in Surgery.

Student Program Director:
Frank W. LoGerfo, MD
Chief, Division of Vascular Surgery
Beth Israel Deaconess Medical Center
William V. McDermott Professor of Surgery
Harvard Medical School

Contact:
Leena Pradhan, PhD
William J. von Liebig Summer Research Fellowship
Harvard Institutes of Medicine
4 Blackfan Circle, Room 130
Boston, MA 02115
Tel: 617-667-0096
Fax: 617-975-5300
E-mail: lpradhan@bidmc.harvard.edu

The American Association of Neurological Surgeons (AANS) through the Neurosurgery Research and Education Foundation (NREF)

The new AANS Medical Student Summer Research Fellowship (MSSRF) program. The fellowship is open to medical students in the United States or Canada who have completed 1 or 2 years of medical school and wish to spend a summer working in a neurosurgical laboratory, mentored by a neurosurgical investigator who is a member of the AANS and will sponsor the student.

This year, 15 Medical Student Summer Research Fellowships will be awarded in the amount of $2,500 per award.

To be considered for this award, applications need to be received by February 1. Awardees will be notified and posted on the AANS web site by March 31.

Submit completed applications to:

AANS Medical Student Summer Research Fellowship
c/o American Association of Neurological Surgeons
5550 Meadowbrook Drive
Rolling Meadows, IL 60008-3852

or e-mail application and all supporting documents to nref@aans.org.

For more information about this medical student summer research fellowship program, contact the Development Department, toll free at (888) 566-2267 or info@aans.org.

The Orthopedic Research and Education Foundation

The Orthopaedic Research and Education Foundation sponsors a Medical Student Summer Orthopaedic Research Fellowship. Our goal is to encourage medical students considering a career in orthopaedics to gain experience in basic, clinical, or translational research.

The Orthopaedic Research and Education Foundation (OREF) is an independent organization that raises funds to support research and education on diseases and injuries of bones, joints, nerves, and muscles. OREF-funded research enhances clinical care, leading to improved health, increased activity, and a better quality of life for patients.

Fellowship Description:
- Medical students with an interest in orthopaedics are eligible to apply.
- The medical student needs to identify an investigator at a U.S. institution with an ongoing orthopaedic research project who is willing to provide research training to the student and act as his/her mentor.
- OREF will provide $2,500 as salary support for the student, payable directly to the sponsoring institution. OREF will reimburse the institution for FICA taxes of up to $200 and up to $200 for supplies, if requested. No other fringe benefits are authorized.
- This program is intended to be a summer research fellowship. A minimum of 8 weeks' full-time work on a specific project is required. The research project should be one that the student is not already involved in.
- At the completion of the program, the medical student is required to complete an evaluation form provided by OREF. The mentor will also complete an evaluation form.

Orthopaedic Research and Education Foundation (OREF)
6300 North River Road, Suite 700
Rosemont, IL 60018-4261
847-698-9980/847-698-9981
Web site: http://www.oref.org

University of Wisconsin–Madison–Surgery Summer Research Experience for Medical Students

The decrease in the number of physicians interested in pursuing a career as a clinician-scientist is well documented in lower numbers of NIH applications and in AAMC questionnaires. The Department of Surgery at the University of Wisconsin is uniquely qualified to direct a short-term summer research experience for medical students who are interested in research related to diabetes, obesity, endocrine disorders, nutritional disorders, digestive diseases, liver disease, kidney disease, and urologic disease. The overall program goal of this Department of Surgery training program is to provide six medical students with a focused, mentored 12-week research and training experience that will help students discern their career path, preferably toward a career that involves biomedical research. During this experience, all students will plan and complete a research project, complete a learning contract, attend an established curriculum in effective research and academic conduct, and write an abstract for submission and presentation at a medical meeting. The training program will foster the development of knowledge, competence, skills, professional attitudes, and experience required to understand what is involved in successful academic careers in laboratory or clinically based research related to the goals of the NIDDK. The four specific objectives of this program are to:

1. Expose medical students, early in their training, to the excitement and challenges of a research career through participation in an individual, mentored training experience.
2. Encourage students to pursue a research career through participation in a focused 12-week research experience in a research program of relevance to the mission of NIDDK.
3. Provide a didactic curriculum emphasizing research issues.
4. Increase the pool of medical students who pursue further research activities by partnering medical students with physicians and scientists who will serve as role models for a career combining patient care and scientific research. The training program includes plans to follow up with trainees later in their career to evaluate whether their summer surgical research experience in the Department of Surgery led to additional research training and a career as a clinician-scientist.

Contact: Herbert Chen, MD, University of Wisconsin–Madison

The CNS/CSNS Medical Student Summer Fellowship in Socioeconomic Research

Award Amount: $2,500

Number of Awards: 2

Purpose: The CNS/CSNS Medical Student Socioeconomic Fellowship supports a medical student conducting research on a socioeconomic issue impacting neurosurgical practice.

516

Eligibility: The fellowship is open to all medical students in the United States and Canada. The fellow will spend 8–10 weeks conducting supervised research on a socioeconomic topic of importance to neurosurgery.

Requirements: The fellow must submit a final report to the CNS Fellowships Committee by December 1 following completion of the summer fellowship. Any publications resulting from supported research must acknowledge the support.

Eligible Expenses: Financial support is exclusively for stipend support to the student.

Application Requirements:
- Complete the online CNS/CSNS Medical Student Fellowship Application.
- Two reference letters.
- Curriculum vitae of applicant.
- Curriculum vitae of proposed mentor.
- Attach a headshot photograph.

Congress of Neurological Surgeons
Elad I. Levy, MD
Chairman, CNS Fellowships Committee
10 North Martingale Road, Suite 190
Schaumburg, IL 60173
Phone: (847) 240-2500
Fax: (847) 240-0804
Toll Free: (877) 517-1CNS
E-mail: info@1CNS.org

Fight for Sight—Summer Student Fellowships

Awards of $2,100 are offered to currently enrolled undergraduates, medical students, or graduate students who wish to explore ophthalmology or eye research as a career. Students are expected to complete a short, independent project during the summer months under the guidance of a senior scientist or clinician. The goal of this award is to advance the skills needed to initiate and carry out research in a scientific environment. Lab employees are not eligible for this fellowship.

Go to www.fightforsight.com/grant_IGP.php for more information.

The Hospital for Special Surgery—Medical Student Summer Research Fellowship

This is an 8-week program of mentored research designed to introduce students who have completed their first year of medical school to research opportunities in orthopaedic basic science, translational science, and clinical research in orthopaedics.

The fellowship program is built around a summer research project that is directed by an orthopaedic surgeon or scientist at the Hospital for Special Surgery (HSS). Both clinical and basic science projects are offered, and these are detailed below.

The fellowship program includes the opportunity for weekly observation of orthopaedic surgical procedures with a variety of clinical faculty. In addition, a

CLASSIFIED: AWARDS AND OPPORTUNITIES

weekly seminar series and discussion group provides the opportunity for students to expand their understanding of the fundamentals of medical research and clinical orthopaedics.

The 8-week program runs from late June through mid-August (in 2009: June 22 to August 14) and includes a $2,400 stipend. Up to 15 fellowship awards will be granted.

To apply for the program, eligible students should first contact an orthopaedic surgeon or scientist who is offering a research project that is of interest (see list below). Once the student has been accepted by the surgeon or scientist, the student and mentor may apply for the fellowship together. Alternatively, if a student has an established working relationship with a faculty member, projects not listed can be submitted for consideration.

Students who have completed their first year in an accredited U.S. medical school are eligible to apply. Preference will be given to those students attending Weill Cornell Medical College.

Download the Fellowship Application Form.

The applications must be sent to Lizandra Portalatin (portalatinl@hss.edu) by April 3. Students and mentors will be notified of the award by May 1.

For questions, contact Chisa Hidaka, MD, Assistant Scientist, Hospital for Special Surgery, at hidakac@hss.edu or (212) 774-2384.

Fellowship Coordinators: Chisa Hidaka, MD, and Jo A. Hannafin, MD, PhD

The American Association of Thoracic Surgery—Medical Student Internship

The Summer Intern Scholarship Program was established in 2007 to introduce the field of cardiothoracic surgery to first- and second-year medical students from North American medical schools. In the 2 years since its inception, the Summer Intern Scholarship has offered 100 medical students the opportunity to broaden their educational experience by providing scholarships to spend 8 weeks during the summer working in an AATS member's cardiothoracic surgery department.

Web site: www.aats.org/MSSR/medicalStudents.html

INDEX